Diabetes: Current and Future Developments

(Volume 2)

(Diabetes and the Eye: Latest Concepts and Practices)

Edited by

Douglas R. Lazzaro
Department of Ophthalmology,
NYU Langone Health,
NYU Grossman School of Medicine,
USA

&

Samy I. McFarlane
Department of Medicine,
Division of Endocrinology,
State University of New York-Downstate Medical Center,
Brooklyn, New York,
USA

Diabetes: Current and Future Developments

Volume # 2

Diabetes and the Eye: Latest Concepts and Practices

Editors: Douglas R. Lazzaro and Samy I. McFarlane

ISSN (Online): 2717-5855

ISSN (Print): 2717-5847

ISBN (Online): 978-981-14-6646-5

ISBN (Print): 978-981-14-6644-1

ISBN (Paperback): 978-981-14-6645-8

need for a court order if at any point you breach any terms of this License Agreement. In no event will any delay or failure by Bentham Science Publishers in enforcing your compliance with this License Agreement constitute a waiver of any of its rights.

3. You acknowledge that you have read this License Agreement, and agree to be bound by its terms and conditions. To the extent that any other terms and conditions presented on any website of Bentham Science Publishers conflict with, or are inconsistent with, the terms and conditions set out in this License Agreement, you acknowledge that the terms and conditions set out in this License Agreement shall prevail.

Bentham Science Publishers Pte. Ltd.
80 Robinson Road #02-00
Singapore 068898
Singapore
Email: subscriptions@benthamscience.net

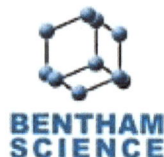

**BENTHAM
SCIENCE**

CONTENTS

FOREWORD

Diabetes mellitus is certainly one of the most important public health problems of the 21st century. Its protean impacts on the eye are well known to all ophthalmologists, who deal with diabetic ocular complications virtually every day. Diabetic eye disease still accounts for much preventable blindness in working age adults, despite the many advances in understanding of pathophysiology and treatment over the last three decades. It is therefore a great pleasure for me to write a foreword to this comprehensive textbook on diabetes and the eye, edited by my colleagues, Douglas R. Lazzaro, and Samy I. McFarlane. Of interest to a wide audience, this book will enhance education of trainees in ophthalmology, and will serve as a definitive resource for practicing ophthalmologists and other physicians who manage diabetes for years to come. This text not only sheds light on the current state of our understanding of ocular manifestations of diabetes, but also looks towards the future when a better understand of the risk factors for diabetic eye disease and improved treatments will reduce the burden of this disease on our society, truly a noble goal. Happy reading!

Kathryn Colby
Elisabeth J Cohen Professor and Chairman
Department of Ophthalmology
NYU Grossman School of Medicine
NYU Langone Health System
New York
USA

PREFACE

Diabetic eye disease is a heterogeneous group of disorders that affect the diabetic population and include diabetic retinopathy, cataract, macular edema, glaucoma, as well as other manifestations of the anterior and posterior segments of the eye. Among these manifestations, diabetic retinopathy and cataract are the most common cause of visual impairment and blindness. In fact people with diabetes are 25 times more likely to develop blindness compared to the general population, and diabetes is the most common cause of blindness among adults 20-74 years of age.

While diabetic retinopathy affects nearly 60% of patients with type 2 diabetes, in type 1 diabetes it is almost universal to develop diabetic retinopathy 15- 20 years after the diagnosis of diabetes is made.

With the rapid rise of obesity, diabetes has become the modern-day epidemic with its attendant complications including diabetic eye disease that leaves millions of people visually disabled, significantly decreasing the quality of life and markedly increasing the risk of injury.

In this volume on Diabetes and the Eye: Latest Concepts and Practices, we have assembled a group of renowned scholars with special expertise in diabetic eye disease, addressing a wide range of topics in a highly scientific, yet easy to read format that will benefit the generalist as well as the specialist and will appeal to the student, the graduate and the practicing physician who commonly encounter diabetic eye disorders, putting practical, yet cutting edge information at their fingertips.

Topics covered in this volume include the epidemiology and trends of the diabetes epidemic and diabetic eye disorders, the pathophysiologic mechanisms of diabetic eye disease and the various manifestations of diabetic complications in the eye. We highlight the latest research findings, the cutting edge diagnostic methods and the most recent developments in the management of retinopathy and other complications. We also discuss future directions and the latest developments in this exciting and rapidly developing field.

Douglas R. Lazzaro
Department of Ophthalmology
NYU Langone Health
NYU Grossman School of Medicine
USA

&

Samy I. McFarlane
Department of Medicine
State University of New York-Downstate Medical Center
Brooklyn, New York
USA

List of Contributors

Agemy, Steven   New York Eye and Ear Infirmary of Mount Sinai, NY, USA

Albano, Alessandro   SUNY Downstate College of Medicine, Brooklyn, NY, USA

Ali, Ferhina S.   The Retina Service of Wills Eye Hospital, Professor of Ophthalmology Thomas Jefferson University 840 Walnut Street, Suite 1020 Philadelphia, PA 19107, USA

Arepalli, Sruthi   The Cole Eye Institute, Cleveland Clinic, Cleveland, OH, USA

Azam, Zaki   SUNY-Downstate College of Medicine, Brooklyn, NY, USA

Cao, Frank   SUNY Downstate College of Medicine, SUNY Downstate Medical Center, Brooklyn, NY, USA

Danias, John   SUNY Downstate College of Medicine, SUNY Downstate Medical Center, Brooklyn, NY, USA

DeBacker, Julie   NYU School of Medicine, NYU Langone Health, NY, USA

Ehlers, Justis P.   The Cole Eye Institute, Cleveland Clinic, Cleveland, OH, USA

Garg, Sunir J.   The Retina Service of Wills Eye Hospital, Professor of Ophthalmology Thomas Jefferson University 840 Walnut Street, Suite 1020 Philadelphia, PA 19107, USA

Gelman, Rony   Department of Ophthalmology, State University of New York, Downstate Medical Center, NY, USA

Groysman, Anna Y.   Department of Medicine, Division of Endocrinology, State University of New York, Downstate-Medical Center, Brooklyn, NY, USA

Hendrick, Andrew M.   Department of Ophthalmology, Emory University, Atlanta, GA, USA

Joseph, Bogaard   Department of Ophthalmology and Visual Sciences, Medical College of Wisconsin, Milwaukee, USA

Kaiser, Peter K.   The Cole Eye Institute, Cleveland Clinic, Cleveland, OH, USA

Kim, Judy E.   Department of Ophthalmology and Visual Sciences, Medical College of Wisconsin, Milwaukee, USA

Lazzaro, Douglas R.   Department of Ophthalmology, NYU Langone Health, NY, USA

Lopez, Jennifer   Medical Center, NYU Langone, NY, USA

McFarlane, Samy I.   Department of Medicine, Division of Endocrinology, State University of New York, Downstate-Medical Center, Brooklyn, NY, USA

Rizzuti, Allison E.   Medical Center, NYU Langone, NY, USA

Shah, Gaurav K.   The Retina Institute, Saint Louis, Missouri, USA

Shrier, Eric   SUNY- Downstate College of Medicine, Brooklyn, NY, USA

Skwiersky, Samara   Department of Medicine, Division of Endocrinology, State University of New York, Downstate-Medical Center, Brooklyn, NY, USA

Soni, Lina   Department of Medicine, Division of Endocrinology, State University of New York, Downstate-Medical Center, Brooklyn, NY, USA

Sun, Lucy   SUNY Downstate Medical Center, NY, USA

Vangipuram, Gautam   The Retina Institute, Saint Louis, Missouri, USA

CHAPTER 1

Diabetes Epidemic, Epidemiology, Statistics and Trends

Andrew M. Hendrick[*]

Department of Ophthalmology, Emory University, Atlanta, GA, USA

Abstract: The incidence of diabetes mellitus is increasing worldwide. Over time, diabetes is associated with the development of diabetic retinopathy, a major cause of vision loss globally. Research has demonstrated factors associated with the onset and progression of the disease. Despite advancements in understanding the importance of optimizing care, the cases of vision loss due to diabetic retinopathy are also increasing. The epidemic of this systemic disease and the retinal manifestations will be discussed in detail in this chapter.

Keywords: Diabetes mellitus, Diabetic retinopathy, Epidemic, Epidemiology, Population, Type 1 Diabetes mellitus, Type 2 Diabetes mellitus.

INTRODUCTION

Diabetes mellitus (DM) is a chronic health condition defined by the presence of impaired glucose regulation leading to hyperglycemia. Normal blood sugar levels depend on the effective use of insulin, a peptide hormone responsible for triggering glucose uptake into cellular spaces (among many other critical metabolic effects). In people with diabetes mellitus, insulin is not used effectively; this is either due to underproduction as seen in type 1 diabetes mellitus (T1DM), or end-tissue resistance to the effects of insulin as seen in type 2 diabetes mellitus (T2DM). Longstanding and/or poorly controlled elevated blood sugar levels are major determinants of complications from DM such as cardiovascular disease, nerve damage, renal disease, and eye disease including retinopathy [1].

The two major subdivisions of diabetes mellitus have several distinguishing characteristics. T1DM results from an auto-immune attack of the insulin-producing pancreatic islet cells, typically during childhood. The onset of T1DM can be dramatic with diabetic ketoacidosis but can be more insidious, characterized by poor growth. T1DM requires insulin injections as the fulcrum of

---

[*] **Corresponding Author Andrew M. Hendrick:** Department of Ophthalmology, Emory University, Atlanta GA, USA; E-mail: ahendrick@emory.edu

therapy to normalize blood sugar levels and are required for survival. In contrast, T2DM results from dysfunction of insulin response, such that circulating glucose levels remain elevated [2]. It is often unclear when T2DM onset begins and symptoms can be poorly recognized for years in some cases. Although previous nomenclature described T2DM as adult-onset, children are increasingly affected [3]. Therapies are directed at lifestyle improvement, weight and dietary management, along with medicines taken both orally and injectable insulin [2].

Our world is in the midst of a diabetes mellitus epidemic with rising rates of people affected across the globe. Factors driving the increase include population aging, economic development, increased urbanization, sedentary lifestyle, and increased consumption of unhealthy foods [2]. Diabetes is a major driver of healthcare costs, morbidity and mortality worldwide [2]. The risk of developing complications is tied directly to the adequacy of medical management. Managing the disease and associated health-related consequences, such as blinding complications of retinopathy, is becoming increasingly important as all societies struggle with this burden. This chapter will discuss the epidemiology of diabetes mellitus, with a focus on diabetic retinopathy (DR) and the implications for vision loss.

Epidemiology of Diabetes Mellitus

T1DM accounts for nearly 10% of DM cases and the incidence has slightly increased over time, with considerable variation by region and sampling technique [3]. Data from US based studies indicate the incidence of T1DM increased from 14.8/100,000 (95% CI 14.0 – 15.6) from 1978-1988 to 23.9/100,000 (95% CI 22.2-25.6) from 2002-2004 and was noted to increase in both Hispanic and non-Hispanic youth [4]. The prevalence of T1DM for adults in the US is estimated to be 0.55% (95% CI 0.46-0.66) [5].

90% of all people with DM have T2DM, also known as adult-onset diabetes. As a result, global estimates of diabetes are predominantly reflective of change due to T2DM. T2DM is increasingly more common - likely due to the strong association with obesity, population aging, inactive lifestyle and poor dietary habits [6]. Fig. **(1)** demonstrates a graphical estimate of worldwide numbers of people with diabetes over since 2000. These estimates represent a compilation of best-available data sources, but high-quality data are not universally available. In 2015, the International Diabetes Federation estimated that the worldwide burden of diabetes mellitus (DM) affected 415 million people and would increase to 642 million globally by the year 2040 [2]. Current estimates demonstrate a global prevalence of ~9% of all adults with only half of individuals being formally diagnosed with DM [2]. The International Diabetes Federation predicts that low-

and middle-income countries will be disproportionately affected by this epidemic and are expected to have the greatest increase in prevalence [2]. This is critical because of the magnitude of impact: Approximately 75% of all individuals with T2DM live in low- and middle-income countries [2].

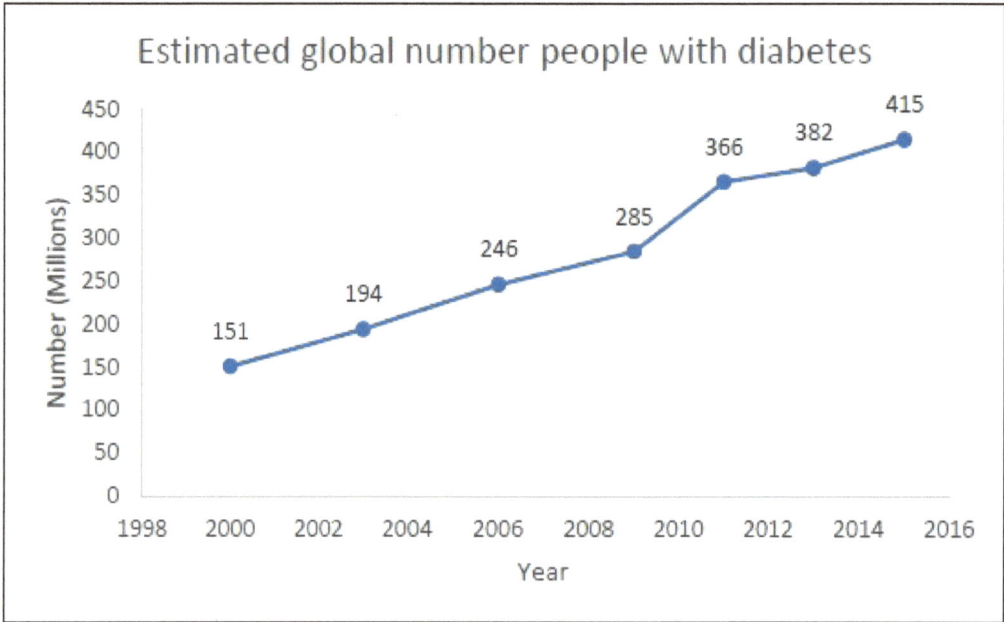

Fig. (1). Estimated number of people with diabetes over time worldwide (in millions) [2].

The fallout from chronic hyperglycemia on the human body is accumulative over time. Morbidity and disability that arises from serious complications of diabetes include cardiovascular disease, kidney disease, neuropathy, limb amputation, and retinopathy. These complications, in turn, lead to an increased demand for medical care, reduce the quality of life, and place stress on families including financial burden. Altogether, diabetes-related care incurs an estimated $673 billion (12%) of global healthcare expenditure and 8% of all-cause mortality [7]. The presence of T2DM increases the risk of heart attack comparable to the risk attributable to having had a prior heart attack [8]. Actual risk varies by study, but the prevalence of coronary heart disease in T2DM is around 21% (ranges between 12-32%) [8]. Similarly, stroke risk is also increased nearly three-fold in people with diabetes compared to those without [8]. Interestingly, the presence of diabetic retinopathy serves as an independent risk factor predicting a higher likelihood of systemic comorbidities such as both stroke and heart disease [9 - 11]. Furthermore, T2DM is a leading cause of renal failure and lower limb amputation [12, 13]. It is estimated that T2DM accounts for estimated up to 21-

54% of all cases of end-stage renal disease [12, 14], and the prevalence of end-stage renal disease is 10-fold greater in people with diabetes compared to those without [7]. Similarly, lower limb amputations are estimated 10 to 20 times more likely in people with diabetes compared to those without [13].

Epidemiology of Diabetic Retinopathy

Ocular complications of diabetes include a spectrum of pathologies that range from refractive error and increased risk of cataract formation to cranial nerve palsies and blindness from diabetic retinopathy (DR) [15]. DR results from damage to the retinal neurons and microvasculature that occurs more commonly in individuals with longstanding DM [16]. Retinopathy is the most serious ocular complication of diabetes and is a leading cause of significant vision loss globally [17]. Importantly, most DR is largely preventable [18] and affects working age adults [19]. As a result, screening and treatment of DR contributes to taking otherwise productive individuals from the workplace, creating economic burden and impacting quality of life. Both the onset and progression of DR is mitigated with blood glucose control [20] and blood pressure management [1]. Other factors commonly associated with DR progression include the socioeconomic status of the individual, degree of dietary compliance, level of physical activity, and geographic location [10].

Earliest estimates on the epidemiology of DR came from the Wisconsin Epidemiologic Study of Diabetic Retinopathy (WESDR). The WESDR was a population-based study conducted on a predominantly Caucasian cohort with both T1DM and T2DM in the 1980's. In this study, which has now accrued decades of follow up, it became possible to understand the increased risk of diabetic retinopathy progression over time [16, 21]. At 4 years, 10 year, and 14 years, the cumulative incidence of DR in people with T1DM was 59%, 89%, and 96%, respectively. After 25 years, 97% of people with type 1 DM had DR, 43% of them PDR, and 29% had DME [22, 23]. People with T2DM have an estimated cumulative incidence of DR that is lower than people with T1DM, but due to the greater prevalence, the impact in the overall population is greater. Studies in the UK report the 4-year cumulative incidence of DR at 26% [24], 6 years at 38-41% [1, 25], and 66% at 10 years [26]. Similar results are seen in US based studies with reports of the 4-year cumulative incidence of DR at 22-34% [27, 28] and 72% at 14 years [29]. In contrast, a study based in urban China demonstrated a higher 5 year cumulative incidence of DR at 46.9%, which was attributed to a longer disease duration in their cohort [30].

At the time of WESDR, it was not yet established that euglycemia was critical for risk factor modification in preventing retinopathy progression [1, 31]. Despite advances in pharmacotherapy and knowledge regarding the importance of lifestyle, glycemic control and comorbidity management, data from the WESDR remains pertinent, as it demonstrates the natural history of diabetic retinopathy is to progress through advancing severity stages. More recent studies indicate declining rates of DR, PDR, and DME in patients with T1DM, which is likely significantly improved by advancements in systemic management [25, 32].

The prevalence of DR is widely varied due to variations in timing and characteristics of the snapshot of the defined population [19]. A multitude of studies examining diverse populations report wide variations in prevalence of diabetic retinopathy and are summarized in (Fig. **2**). Global estimates indicate over one third of people with DM have DR, and that one third of those have visually threatening diabetic retinopathy (VTDR) [33]. VTDR represents a higher risk category of 'severe NPDR' or worse and includes all eyes with DME. This study further concluded that the global prevalence of PDR is 7.5%, and DME is 6.8% [33]. Prevalence of any DR and PDR was higher in people with T1DM, compared to individuals with type 2 diabetes (77.3 *vs.* 25.2% for any DR, 32.4 *vs.* 3.0% for PDR) [33].

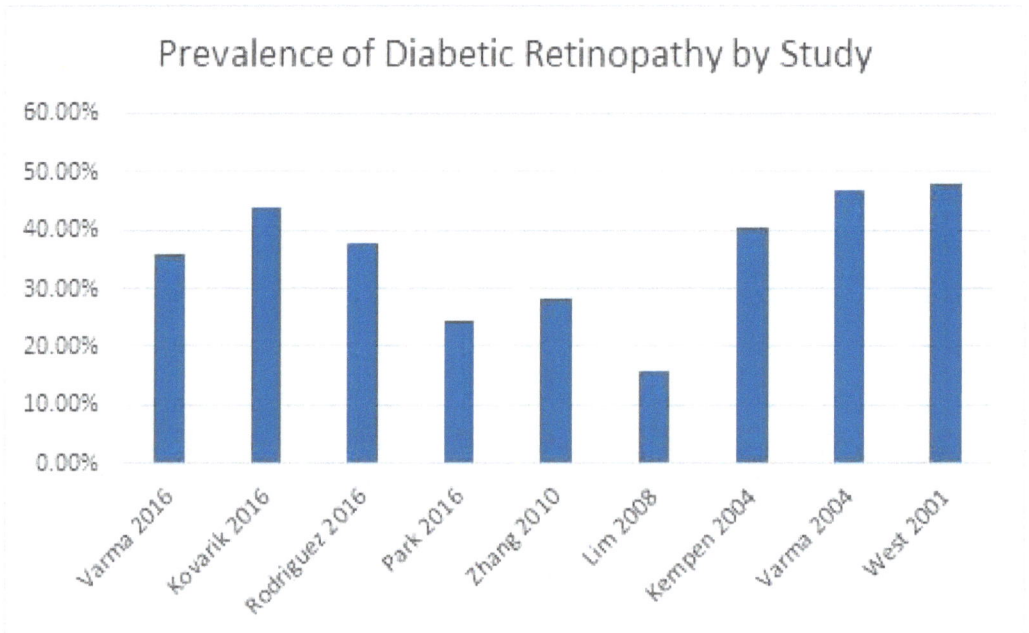

Fig. (2). The prevalence of diabetic retinopathy varies depending on the population characteristics and sampling techniques employed [34 - 42].

The epidemiology of DME is of great interest due to its impact on quality of vision, but difficult to compare due to variations in definition of the disease.

Studies vary with use of clinical examination, fundus photography and optical coherence tomography based definitions [43]; in addition, variations in subject selection and population characteristics make cross study comparisons less robust in their validity. WESDR reported the 14 year cumulative incidence of DME in people with T1DM was 26.1%, which increased to 29% by 25 years of follow up [22, 44]. Among population-based studies of DME, the prevalence of DME in people with T1DM ranges between 4.2 and 7.9% [33]. In people with T2DM, prevalence of DME is reported between 1.4 and 12.8% [33].

Racial and ethnic impact on the epidemiology of DR is of great interest because of the wide differences in the reported rates of DR prevalence and the implications for environmental *versus* genetic influence. From the US, the third National Health and Nutrition Examination Survey (NHANES III) was a cross sectional study from the Center for Disease Control and Prevention from 1988-1994 to determine if racial and or ethnic differences modulated the risk of developing DR. This study demonstrated that Mexican-American participants had higher rates of DR compared to non-Hispanic white participants (33.4% *vs* 18.2%) [45]. In general, trends are seen in most studies such that Western societies have higher prevalence of DR than Eastern societies [19]. Of great concern is the impact that Westernization has on development of DM and DR. As evidenced in the Singapore Indian Eye Study, increased industrialization and urbanization in an Asian country was associated with rates of DR in Asian eyes that are similar to rates reported in Western populations [46]. Interestingly, in the same study, three major ethnic groups in Singapore had differing prevalence of DR. The Malays and Indians have a higher prevalence of DR (33.4% in Malays, 33.0% in Indians) compared to the Chinese (25.4%). Urban and rural differences in DR prevalence also indicate an important impact of the environment on health outcomes [47, 48].

Genetics also contribute to susceptibility of DR onset and severity. Analysis of the Diabetes Control and Complications Trial (DCCT) indicates that glycemic control, as was reflected by hemoglobin A1c levels, was beneficial in reducing the incidence of DR [31]. It also showed a significant association for an inheritable tendency to developing advanced severity of DR in families with both type 1 and T2DM, independent of shared risk factors [49]. Similar findings were demonstrated in a study that included Mexican Americans with both T1DM and T2DM and severe DR [50 - 53]. A meta-analysis confirming the presence of variations in a gene that affects the aldose reductase pathway (*AKR1B1*) was found to be significantly associated with DR onset in T1DM, regardless of ethnicity [54]. Other genes of interest include the adipose most abundant gene transcript-1 (apM-1) which encodes for adiponectin [55], vascular endothelial growth factor (VEGF) gene polymorphisms [56 - 59], The overall importance of genetics in determinants of diabetes related complications is an ongoing area of investigation.

Screening of Diabetic Retinopathy

Due to the asymptomatic nature of DR, individuals with diabetes should be properly screened for signs of DR and the progressive stages of DR. At a minimum, screening guidelines suggest a dilated fundus examination on an annual basis for T2DM and T1DM, beginning 5 years after diagnosis [18]. People with evident DR need more frequent follow up to determine if treatment may become indicated, thereby requiring more exams as disease severity worsens. Screening for and timely treatment of DR reduces the likelihood of developing severe vision loss by up to 94% and are also highly cost-effective [60].

Studies suggest that there is poor adherence to recommended guidelines such that an estimated nearly half of people with diabetes do not routinely receive an eye exam [61]. Screening can alternatively be considered remotely using telemedicine in some systems. Telemedicine involves the use of remote interpretation of point of care fundus photography. While remote screening does not fully replace a comprehensive eye exam, it improves access to individuals who have limited access to ophthalmic care, such as in resource poor or geographically remote locations. Research has consistently validated telemedicine-based screening efforts as both effective and cost-effective tools with substantial cost savings to healthcare systems [62].

CONCLUSION

Overall, type 1 diabetes represents a minority of cases of diabetes mellitus with indications that the disease is becoming slightly more common over time. Although people with T1DM have higher rates of ocular complications than people with T2DM, incident retinopathy has reduced with improved control of systemic management. In contrast, type 2 diabetes is much more prevalent, and the prevalence is increasing over time worldwide with substantial regional variation. Similar increasing trends are noted when examining the epidemiology of diabetic retinopathy.

Detecting, diagnosing, and managing diabetes mellitus and the associated retinopathy is an increasingly important societal burden of great public health importance that current projections indicate will only worsen without change. The increased potential for death and disability, due to associations of DR with stroke, heart attack, amputation and kidney failure, supports a multifaceted approach to management and treatment. Glycemic control is fundamental to optimizing the health-related morbidity in the diabetic patient, but the duration disease over time remains an important driver of complications. Racial, ethnic, genetic and environmental influences are increasingly understood as contributors of disease status. Screening programs are critical to detect disease and provide framework to connect the patient to treatment when indicated.

CONSENT FOR PUBLICATION

Not applicable.

CONFLICT OF INTEREST

The author declares no conflict of interest, financial or otherwise.

ACKNOWLEDGEMENTS

Declared none.

REFERENCES

[1]   Stratton IM, Kohner EM, Aldington SJ, *et al.* UKPDS 50: risk factors for incidence and progression of retinopathy in Type II diabetes over 6 years from diagnosis. Diabetologia 2001; 44(2): 156-63.
        [http://dx.doi.org/10.1007/s001250051594] [PMID: 11270671]

[2]   International Diabetes Federation. IDF Diabetes Atlas, eB. Belgium: International Diabetes Federation 2015.

[3]   Maahs DM, West NA, Lawrence JM, Mayer-Davis EJ. Epidemiology of type 1 diabetes. Endocrinol Metab Clin North Am 2010; 39(3): 481-97.
        [http://dx.doi.org/10.1016/j.ecl.2010.05.011] [PMID: 20723815]

[4]   Vehik K, Hamman RF, Lezotte D, *et al.* Increasing incidence of type 1 diabetes in 0- to 17-year-old Colorado youth. Diabetes Care 2007; 30(3): 503-9.
        [http://dx.doi.org/10.2337/dc06-1837] [PMID: 17327312]

[5]   Bullard KM, Cowie CC, Lessem SE, *et al.* Prevalence of Diagnosed Diabetes in Adults by Diabetes Type - United States, 2016. MMWR Morb Mortal Wkly Rep 2018; 67(12): 359-61.
        [http://dx.doi.org/10.15585/mmwr.mm6712a2] [PMID: 29596402]

[6]   van Dieren S, Beulens JW, van der Schouw YT, Grobbee DE, Neal B. The global burden of diabetes and its complications: an emerging pandemic. Eur J Cardiovasc Prev Rehabil 2010; 17 (Suppl. 1): S3-8.
        [http://dx.doi.org/10.1097/01.hjr.0000368191.86614.5a] [PMID: 20489418]

[7]   Group IDFDA. IDF Diabetes Atlas Group. Update of mortality attributable to diabetes for the IDF Diabetes Atlas: Estimates for the year 2013. Diabetes Res Clin Pract 2015; 109(3): 461-5.
        [http://dx.doi.org/10.1016/j.diabres.2015.05.037] [PMID: 26119773]

[8]   Einarson TR, Acs A, Ludwig C, Panton UH. Prevalence of cardiovascular disease in type 2 diabetes: a systematic literature review of scientific evidence from across the world in 2007-2017. Cardiovasc Diabetol 2018; 17(1): 83.
        [http://dx.doi.org/10.1186/s12933-018-0728-6] [PMID: 29884191]

[9]   Cheung N, Wang JJ, Rogers SL, *et al.* ARIC (Atherosclerosis Risk In Communities) Study Investigators. Diabetic retinopathy and risk of heart failure. J Am Coll Cardiol 2008; 51(16): 1573-8.
        [http://dx.doi.org/10.1016/j.jacc.2007.11.076] [PMID: 18420100]

[10]   Cheung N, Wang JJ, Klein R, Couper DJ, Sharrett AR, Wong TY. Diabetic retinopathy and the risk of coronary heart disease: the Atherosclerosis Risk in Communities Study. Diabetes Care 2007; 30(7): 1742-6.
[http://dx.doi.org/10.2337/dc07-0264] [PMID: 17389333]

[11]   Cheung N, Rogers S, Couper DJ, Klein R, Sharrett AR, Wong TY. Is diabetic retinopathy an independent risk factor for ischemic stroke? Stroke 2007; 38(2): 398-401.
[http://dx.doi.org/10.1161/01.STR.0000254547.91276.50] [PMID: 17194880]

[12]   Bell S, Fletcher EH, Brady I, *et al.* Scottish diabetes research network and scottish renal registry. End-stage renal disease and survival in people with diabetes: a national database linkage study. QJM 2015; 108(2): 127-34.
[http://dx.doi.org/10.1093/qjmed/hcu170] [PMID: 25140030]

[13]   Moxey PW, Gogalniceanu P, Hinchliffe RJ, *et al.* Lower extremity amputations--a review of global variability in incidence. Diabet Med 2011; 28(10): 1144-53.
[http://dx.doi.org/10.1111/j.1464-5491.2011.03279.x] [PMID: 21388445]

[14]   Lok CE, Oliver MJ, Rothwell DM, Hux JE. The growing volume of diabetes-related dialysis: a population based study. Nephrol Dial Transplant 2004; 19(12): 3098-103.
[http://dx.doi.org/10.1093/ndt/gfh540] [PMID: 15507475]

[15]   Jeganathan VS, Wang JJ, Wong TY. Ocular associations of diabetes other than diabetic retinopathy. Diabetes Care 2008; 31(9): 1905-12.
[http://dx.doi.org/10.2337/dc08-0342] [PMID: 18753669]

[16]   Klein R, Klein BE, Moss SE, Davis MD, DeMets DL. The Wisconsin epidemiologic study of diabetic retinopathy. III. Prevalence and risk of diabetic retinopathy when age at diagnosis is 30 or more years. Arch Ophthalmol 1984; 102(4): 527-32.
[http://dx.doi.org/10.1001/archopht.1984.01040030405011] [PMID: 6367725]

[17]   Leasher JL, Bourne RR, Flaxman SR, *et al.* Vision loss expert group of the global burden of disease study. Global estimates on the number of people blind or visually impaired by diabetic retinopathy: a meta-analysis from 1990 to 2010. Diabetes Care 2016; 39(9): 1643-9.
[http://dx.doi.org/10.2337/dc15-2171] [PMID: 27555623]

[18]   American Academy of Ophthalmology Retina/Vitreous Panel.. Preferred Practice Pattern®Guidelines. Diabetic Retinopathy. C.A.A.o.O.A.a.w.a.o.p

[19]   Lee R, Wong TY, Sabanayagam C. Epidemiology of diabetic retinopathy, diabetic macular edema and related vision loss. Eye Vis (Lond) 2015; 2: 17.
[http://dx.doi.org/10.1186/s40662-015-0026-2] [PMID: 26605370]

[20]   Nathan DM, Genuth S, Lachin J, *et al.* Diabetes Control and Complications Trial Research Group. The effect of intensive treatment of diabetes on the development and progression of long-term complications in insulin-dependent diabetes mellitus. N Engl J Med 1993; 329(14): 977-86.
[http://dx.doi.org/10.1056/NEJM199309303291401] [PMID: 8366922]

[21]   Klein R, Klein BE, Moss SE, Davis MD, DeMets DL. The Wisconsin epidemiologic study of diabetic retinopathy. IV. Diabetic macular edema. Ophthalmology 1984; 91(12): 1464-74.
[http://dx.doi.org/10.1016/S0161-6420(84)34102-1] [PMID: 6521986]

[22]   Klein R, Knudtson MD, Lee KE, Gangnon R, Klein BE. The Wisconsin Epidemiologic Study of Diabetic Retinopathy XXIII: the twenty-five-year incidence of macular edema in persons with type 1 diabetes. Ophthalmology 2009; 116(3): 497-503.
[http://dx.doi.org/10.1016/j.ophtha.2008.10.016] [PMID: 19167079]

[23]   Klein R, Knudtson MD, Lee KE, Gangnon R, Klein BE. The Wisconsin Epidemiologic Study of Diabetic Retinopathy: XXII the twenty-five-year progression of retinopathy in persons with type 1 diabetes. Ophthalmology 2008; 115(11): 1859-68.
[http://dx.doi.org/10.1016/j.ophtha.2008.08.023] [PMID: 19068374]

[24]   Thomas RL, Dunstan F, Luzio SD, *et al.* Incidence of diabetic retinopathy in people with type 2 diabetes mellitus attending the Diabetic Retinopathy Screening Service for Wales: retrospective analysis. BMJ 2012; 344e874
       [http://dx.doi.org/10.1136/bmj.e874] [PMID: 22362115]

[25]   Younis N, Broadbent DM, Harding SP, Vora JP. Incidence of sight-threatening retinopathy in Type 1 diabetes in a systematic screening programme. Diabet Med 2003; 20(9): 758-65.
       [http://dx.doi.org/10.1046/j.1464-5491.2003.01035.x] [PMID: 12925058]

[26]   Jones CD, Greenwood RH, Misra A, Bachmann MO. Incidence and progression of diabetic retinopathy during 17 years of a population-based screening program in England. Diabetes Care 2012; 35(3): 592-6.
       [http://dx.doi.org/10.2337/dc11-0943] [PMID: 22279031]

[27]   Varma R, *et al.* Four-year incidence and progression of diabetic retinopathy and macular edema: the Los Angeles Latino Eye Study. Am J Ophthalmol 2010; 149(5): 752-61.e1-3.
       [http://dx.doi.org/10.1016/j.ajo.2009.11.014]

[28]   Tudor SM, Hamman RF, Baron A, Johnson DW, Shetterly SM. Incidence and progression of diabetic retinopathy in Hispanics and non-Hispanic whites with type 2 diabetes. San Luis Valley Diabetes Study, Colorado. Diabetes Care 1998; 21(1): 53-61.
       [http://dx.doi.org/10.2337/diacare.21.1.53] [PMID: 9538971]

[29]   Lee ET, Lee VS, Kingsley RM, *et al.* Diabetic retinopathy in Oklahoma Indians with NIDDM. Incidence and risk factors. Diabetes Care 1992; 15(11): 1620-7.
       [http://dx.doi.org/10.2337/diacare.15.11.1620] [PMID: 1468294]

[30]   Tam VH, Lam EP, Chu BC, Tse KK, Fung LM. Incidence and progression of diabetic retinopathy in Hong Kong Chinese with type 2 diabetes mellitus. J Diabetes Complications 2009; 23(3): 185-93.
       [http://dx.doi.org/10.1016/j.jdiacomp.2008.03.001] [PMID: 18479945]

[31]   Group, DR. The effect of intensive treatment of diabetes on the development and progression of long-term complications in insulindependent diabetes mellitus. N Engl Med 1993; 329: 977-86.
       [http://dx.doi.org/10.1056/NEJM199309303291401]

[32]   Kytö JP, Harjutsalo V, Forsblom C, Hietala K, Summanen PA, Groop PH. FinnDiane Study Group. Decline in the cumulative incidence of severe diabetic retinopathy in patients with type 1 diabetes. Diabetes Care 2011; 34(9): 2005-7.
       [http://dx.doi.org/10.2337/dc10-2391] [PMID: 21868777]

[33]   Yau JW, Rogers SL, Kawasaki R, *et al.* Meta-analysis for eye disease (META-EYE) study group. Global prevalence and major risk factors of diabetic retinopathy. Diabetes Care 2012; 35(3): 556-64.
       [http://dx.doi.org/10.2337/dc11-1909] [PMID: 22301125]

[34]   Varma R, Wen G, Jiang X, *et al.* Chinese American Eye Study Group. Prevalence of diabetic retinopathy in adult chinese american individuals: the Chinese American eye study. JAMA Ophthalmol 2016; 134(5): 563-9.
       [http://dx.doi.org/10.1001/jamaophthalmol.2016.0445] [PMID: 27055063]

[35]   Kovarik JJ, Eller AW, Willard LA, Ding J, Johnston JM, Waxman EL. Prevalence of undiagnosed diabetic retinopathy among inpatients with diabetes: the diabetic retinopathy inpatient study (DRIPS). BMJ Open Diabetes Res Care 2016; 4(1)e000164
       [http://dx.doi.org/10.1136/bmjdrc-2015-000164] [PMID: 26925238]

[36]   Rodriguez NM, Aguilar S. Prevalence of diabetic retinopathy in a clinic population from puerto rico. Optom Vis Sci 2016; 93(7): 750-3.
       [http://dx.doi.org/10.1097/OPX.0000000000000854] [PMID: 27046091]

[37]   Park DW, Mansberger SL. Eye disease in patients with diabetes screened with telemedicine. Telemed J E Health 2017; 23(2): 113-8.
       [http://dx.doi.org/10.1089/tmj.2016.0034] [PMID: 27328169]

[38] Zhang X, Saaddine JB, Chou CF, *et al.* Prevalence of diabetic retinopathy in the United States, 2005-2008. JAMA 2010; 304(6): 649-56.
[http://dx.doi.org/10.1001/jama.2010.1111] [PMID: 20699456]

[39] Lim A, Stewart J, Chui TY, *et al.* Prevalence and risk factors of diabetic retinopathy in a multi-racial underserved population. Ophthalmic Epidemiol 2008; 15(6): 402-9.
[http://dx.doi.org/10.1080/09286580802435179] [PMID: 19065433]

[40] Kempen JH, O'Colmain BJ, Leske MC, *et al.* Eye Diseases Prevalence Research Group. The prevalence of diabetic retinopathy among adults in the United States. Arch Ophthalmol 2004; 122(4): 552-63.
[http://dx.doi.org/10.1001/archopht.122.4.552] [PMID: 15078674]

[41] Varma R, Torres M, Peña F, Klein R, Azen SP. Los Angeles Latino Eye Study Group. Prevalence of diabetic retinopathy in adult Latinos: the Los Angeles Latino eye study. Ophthalmology 2004; 111(7): 1298-306.
[http://dx.doi.org/10.1016/j.ophtha.2004.03.002] [PMID: 15234129]

[42] West SK, Klein R, Rodriguez J, *et al.* Proyecto VER. Diabetes and diabetic retinopathy in a Mexican-American population: Proyecto VER. Diabetes Care 2001; 24(7): 1204-9.
[http://dx.doi.org/10.2337/diacare.24.7.1204] [PMID: 11423503]

[43] Virgili G, Menchini F, Murro V, Peluso E, Rosa F, Casazza G. Optical coherence tomography (OCT) for detection of macular oedema in patients with diabetic retinopathy. Cochrane Database Syst Rev 2011; (7): CD008081
[http://dx.doi.org/10.1002/14651858.CD008081.pub2] [PMID: 21735421]

[44] Klein R, Klein BE, Moss SE, Cruickshanks KJ. The Wisconsin Epidemiologic Study of Diabetic Retinopathy. XV. The long-term incidence of macular edema. Ophthalmology 1995; 102(1): 7-16.
[http://dx.doi.org/10.1016/S0161-6420(95)31052-4] [PMID: 7831044]

[45] Harris MI, Klein R, Cowie CC, Rowland M, Byrd-Holt DD. Is the risk of diabetic retinopathy greater in non-Hispanic blacks and Mexican Americans than in non-Hispanic whites with type 2 diabetes? A U.S. population study. Diabetes Care 1998; 21(8): 1230-5.
[http://dx.doi.org/10.2337/diacare.21.8.1230] [PMID: 9702425]

[46] Zheng Y, Lamoureux EL, Lavanya R, *et al.* Prevalence and risk factors of diabetic retinopathy in migrant Indians in an urbanized society in Asia: the Singapore Indian eye study. Ophthalmology 2012; 119(10): 2119-24.
[http://dx.doi.org/10.1016/j.ophtha.2012.04.027] [PMID: 22709419]

[47] Liu L, Wu X, Liu L, *et al.* Prevalence of diabetic retinopathy in mainland China: a meta-analysis. PLoS One 2012; 7(9)e45264
[http://dx.doi.org/10.1371/journal.pone.0045264] [PMID: 23028893]

[48] Rema M, Premkumar S, Anitha B, Deepa R, Pradeepa R, Mohan V. Prevalence of diabetic retinopathy in urban India: the Chennai Urban Rural Epidemiology Study (CURES) eye study, I. Invest Ophthalmol Vis Sci 2005; 46(7): 2328-33.
[http://dx.doi.org/10.1167/iovs.05-0019] [PMID: 15980218]

[49] The Diabetes Control and Complications Trial Research Group. Clustering of long-term complications in families with diabetes in the diabetes control and complications trial. Diabetes 1997; 46(11): 1829-39.
[http://dx.doi.org/10.2337/diab.46.11.1829] [PMID: 9356033]

[50] Hallman DM, Huber JC Jr, Gonzalez VH, Klein BE, Klein R, Hanis CL. Familial aggregation of severity of diabetic retinopathy in Mexican Americans from Starr County, Texas. Diabetes Care 2005; 28(5): 1163-8.
[http://dx.doi.org/10.2337/diacare.28.5.1163] [PMID: 15855583]

[51] Arar NH, Freedman BI, Adler SG, *et al.* Family investigation of nephropathy and diabetes research

group. Heritability of the severity of diabetic retinopathy: the FIND-Eye study. Invest Ophthalmol Vis Sci 2008; 49(9): 3839-45.
[http://dx.doi.org/10.1167/iovs.07-1633] [PMID: 18765632]

[52]   Hietala K, Forsblom C, Summanen P, Groop PH. FinnDiane Study Group. Heritability of proliferative diabetic retinopathy. Diabetes 2008; 57(8): 2176-80.
[http://dx.doi.org/10.2337/db07-1495] [PMID: 18443200]

[53]   Monti MC, Lonsdale JT, Montomoli C, Montross R, Schlag E, Greenberg DA. Familial risk factors for microvascular complications and differential male-female risk in a large cohort of American families with type 1 diabetes. J Clin Endocrinol Metab 2007; 92(12): 4650-5.
[http://dx.doi.org/10.1210/jc.2007-1185] [PMID: 17878250]

[54]   Abhary S, Hewitt AW, Burdon KP, Craig JE. A systematic meta-analysis of genetic association studies for diabetic retinopathy. Diabetes 2009; 58(9): 2137-47.
[http://dx.doi.org/10.2337/db09-0059] [PMID: 19587357]

[55]   Zietz B, Buechler C, Kobuch K, Neumeier M, Schölmerich J, Schäffler A. Serum levels of adiponectin are associated with diabetic retinopathy and with adiponectin gene mutations in Caucasian patients with diabetes mellitus type 2. Exp Clin Endocrinol Diabetes 2008; 116(9): 532-6.
[http://dx.doi.org/10.1055/s-2008-1058086] [PMID: 18680072]

[56]   Wang H, Cheng JW, Zhu LS, *et al.* Meta-analysis of association between the -2578C/A polymorphism of the vascular endothelial growth factor and retinopathy in type 2 diabetes in Asians and Caucasians. Ophthalmic Res 2014; 52(1): 1-8.
[http://dx.doi.org/10.1159/000357110] [PMID: 24751925]

[57]   Han L, Zhang L, Xing W, *et al.* The associations between VEGF gene polymorphisms and diabetic retinopathy susceptibility: a meta-analysis of 11 case-control studies. J Diabetes Res 2014; 2014805801
[http://dx.doi.org/10.1155/2014/805801] [PMID: 24868559]

[58]   El-Shazly SF, El-Bradey MH, Tameesh MK. Vascular endothelial growth factor gene polymorphism prevalence in patients with diabetic macular oedema and its correlation with anti-vascular endothelial growth factor treatment outcomes. Clin Exp Ophthalmol 2014; 42(4): 369-78.
[http://dx.doi.org/10.1111/ceo.12182] [PMID: 23927080]

[59]   Kaidonis G, Burdon KP, Gillies MC, *et al.* Common Sequence Variation in the VEGFC Gene Is Associated with Diabetic Retinopathy and Diabetic Macular Edema. Ophthalmology 2015; 122(9): 1828-36.
[http://dx.doi.org/10.1016/j.ophtha.2015.05.004] [PMID: 26072347]

[60]   Schoenfeld ER, Greene JM, Wu SY, Leske MC. Patterns of adherence to diabetes vision care guidelines: baseline findings from the Diabetic Retinopathy Awareness Program. Ophthalmology 2001; 108(3): 563-71.
[http://dx.doi.org/10.1016/S0161-6420(00)00600-X] [PMID: 11237912]

[61]   Javitt JC, Aiello LP. Cost-effectiveness of detecting and treating diabetic retinopathy. Ann Intern Med 1996; 124(1 Pt 2): 164-9.
[http://dx.doi.org/10.7326/0003-4819-124-1_Part_2-199601011-00017] [PMID: 8554212]

[62]   Avidor D, Loewenstein A, Waisbourd M, Nutman A. Cost-effectiveness of diabetic retinopathy screening programs using telemedicine: a systematic review. Cost Eff Resour Alloc 2020; 18: 16.
[http://dx.doi.org/10.1186/s12962-020-00211-1] [PMID: 32280309]

CHAPTER 2

Recent Developments in Diabetes Evaluation and Management: Implications for the Practicing Clinicians

Anna Y. Groysman, Lina Soni, Samara Skwiersky and **Samy I. McFarlane**[*]

Department of Medicine, Division of Endocrinology, State University of New York, Downstate-Medical Center, Brooklyn, NY, USA

Abstract: Diabetes is a major public health problem affecting millions of people around the globe. In the United States alone, over 7.5 million have type 2 diabetes and an alarming 78 million adults have prediabetes and remain largely undiagnosed. This epidemic was ushered in by the ongoing epidemic of obesity and is caused in-part by sedentary life style and aging population. In this chapter we discuss the diabetes epidemic highlighting the major risk factor of diabetes, particularly type 2. We also discuss the complications of diabetes including microvascular complications as well as macrovascular disease including coronary heart disease and stroke, the major cause of morbidity and mortality in the diabetic population. Finally, we present the major therapeutic advances in diabetes including modern pharmacologic agents and their potential effects on cardiovascular risk. We also outline the recent technological advances in diabetes management including closed loop systems, artificial pancreas, stem cell therapy among other ongoing research bound to prevent and/or alleviate the effects of this ongoing epidemic.

Keywords: Complications, Diabetes, Glucose monitoring technology, Modern therapy, Risk factors.

INTRODUCTION

Diabetes mellitus is a progressively debilitating condition resulting in vascular complications, including cardiovascular, cerebrovascular, and peripheral vascular disease. This disease, together with microvascular diseases, including retinopathy, nephropathy, and peripheral neuropathy, lead to devastating complications and increased mortality. Although adults are generally afflicted with this condition, rising numbers of children, teenagers, and adolescents are also affected [1].

---

[*] **Corresponding Author Samy I. McFarlane:** Department of Medicine, Division of Endocrinology, State University of New York, Downstate-Medical Center, Brooklyn, NY, USA; Tel: 718-270- 3711; Fax: 718-270- 6358; E-mail: smcfarlane@downstate.edu

Driven mainly by a continuous rise in type 2 diabetes, the global epidemic of diabetes, according to data from the World Health Organization, reached over 422 million adults worldwide in 2014, exceeding the previous forecast of 439 million worldwide by 2030 [2].

Diabetes does not affect the population homogeneously and significant disparities exist that are worth noting. Diabetes disproportionally affects racial and ethnic minority groups. African Americans (13.2%), American Indians/Alaska Natives (15.9%), Asian Americans and Pacific Islanders (9.0%), and Latinos (12.8%) are about twice as likely to have been diagnosed with diabetes as non-Hispanic, white (7.6%) adults [6]. Diabetes has also been shown to disproportionally affect people living in rural *versus* urban areas. Individual factors, such as health literacy, communication barriers, and cultural differences, have been associated with diabetes disparities [7]

The observed disparities have been explained by numerous analyses. A fully adjusted study found that both the prevalence of diabetes and the likelihood of forgoing medical care among people diagnosed with diabetes were higher for those with lower incomes, racial/ethnic minority groups, lower incomes, and living in the South of the U.S [8]. Additionally, "food insecurity" is the inability to regularly obtain nutritious food without resorting to socially unusual practices. Unfortunately, one in seven people in America is "food insecure". This rate is higher among racial/ethnic minorities and in low-income households. The reason being that people are faced with the difficult choice of buying nutritious but more expensive food *versus* less expensive, high calorie, and low nutrient containing foods [9].

Many resources have been focused on developing modalities to achieve euglycemia in patients and to reduce the prevalence of macro-and microvascular complications. Unfortunately, the primary cause of mortality in patients with diabetes is cardiovascular disease. Within the next thirty years, the number of people living with diabetes is predicted to double and with it, the prevalence of incapacitating complications [3]. The incidence of diabetes increases with age and as the number of older adults in the United States is growing, so is the prevalence of the disease. The advent of insulin therapy has prolonged the lives of patients with type 1 diabetes (T1D), but every year of life comes with an increased risk of complications. As the prevalence of obesity rises in the United States, T2D occurs at an earlier age. This is because overweight and obese people tend to have an earlier onset of insulin resistance. Such factors are increasing the number of people who need medical care and require interventions to prevent the complications or progression of diabetes complications [4].

The risk of diabetes is increased with non-modifiable factors, such as age, a positive family history, and genetics. However, the list of modifiable risk factors is much longer. Overweight and obesity is rampant in the United States and is the leading cause of diabetes onset. Lack of physical exercise and poor dietary choices or options are significant contributors [2]. Less well-known risk factors include vitamin deficiencies and compositions of gut bacteria [5], which are now being identified and will be further discussed in this chapter.

This chapter aims to elucidate what is known about diabetes, as well as where we are headed. The novel risk factors of diabetes will be explained as well as the pervasive complications. The focus of the chapter will be a discussion of the many medical and technological treatment approaches that have been developed to improve glycemic control or hold a promise to finding a cure. Finally, evidence of diabetes prevention will be discussed as it is as vital as disease treatment in managing this pandemic.

RISK FACTORS OF DIABETES MELLITUS

Non-modifiable Risk Factors (Table 1)

Genetics

The pathophysiology of T2DM has not yet been fully delineated; however, studies find that there is a significant genetic component. This is supported by a high concordance rate in monozygotic twins (96%) to develop T2D. Even 40% of first degree relatives of T2D patients develop diabetes as compared to only 6% observed in the general population [10].

Susceptibility Loci

Since 2007, Genome-Wide Association Studies have identified linkage signals at the same or different chromosomes with T2DM. Seventy-five susceptibility loci that are related to T2DM have been identified. For example, IGF2BP2 is involved in pancreas development and stimulation of insulin action. Unsorted loci for T2DM pathogenesis still remain but may serve to be useful in understanding the condition to eventually find a cure [11, 12].

Modifiable Risk Factors (Table 1)

Lifestyle

Numerous environmental and lifestyle factors have been found to contribute to the development of T2DM. Obesity, which may contribute to the development of insulin resistance, has been found to be the greatest risk factor for T2D. A sedentary lifestyle, physical inactivity, alcohol consumption, and smoking are also major contributors to disease development. Additionally, a low fiber diet with a high glycemic index is associated with an increased risk of developing diabetes [13]. When controlled for BMI, high intake of total and saturated fat was associated with an increased risk of T2D. However, intake of linoleic acid, a polyunsaturated fat, decreased this risk [14]. Greater consumption of water high in sugar was associated with greater weight gain and an increased risk of developing T2D in women [15]. Obstructive sleep apnea (OSA) is a modifiable risk factor in the development of insulin resistance. Numerous studies have shown that the prevalence of prediabetes (20 to 67%) is significantly higher in patients with OSA than subjects who did not suffer from OSA [16].

Vitamins

Vitamin K

Vitamin K is well known for its active role in maintaining bone quality. Recent studies found that vitamin K1 or phylloquinone to benefit euglycemia. Higher intake of vitamin K1 was found to be correlated with increased insulin sensitivity and glycemic control [17]. Further studies are needed to understand the role of vitamin K in protection from diabetes.

Vitamin D

There is a growing evidence that decreased vitamin D may contribute to the development of T2D. One study showed that patients with T2D had lower 25-OHD3 concentrations than patients without diabetes [18]. When non-obese diabetic mice were rendered vitamin D deficient in early life, impaired glucose tolerance was observed by the age of 100 days. Diabetes incidence doubled at 200 days of life [19]. Vitamin D has also been found to have an immunomodulatory role. In the presence of 1a,25(OH)2D3, dendritic cells mature to become tolerogenic cells as seen by their lower expression of major histocompatibility complex class II molecules and adhesions that are necessary to fully stimulate T-cells. Furthermore, 1a,25(OH)2D3 suppresses the recruitment and activation of T cells [20]. Even more interesting is the findings of a study that showed chronic administration of 1a, 25(OH) reduced the incidence of insulitis and diabetes in non-obese diabetic mice [21]. What can be deduced from these findings is that vitamin D is essential for β-cell function and might protect against diabetes later in life [18].

Gut Bacteria

Recent studies have shown that gut microbes may influence the host's metabolic and immune activity and eventually influence the development of diabetes or obesity. Some mechanisms that explain this phenomenon is increased nutrient absorption from diet, increased cellular uptake of triglycerides, enhanced lipogenesis, reduced free fatty acid oxidation, and chronic low-grade inflammation, as well as altered intestinal barrier function. Furthermore, gut microflora in obese individuals has been found to have an increased capacity to extract energy from their diet [22].

Table 1. Modifiable and Non Modifiable Risk Factors of T2D [23].

Modifiable Risk Factors	Non-Modifiable Risk Factors

• Body Mass Index $\geq$ 25 kg/m^2
• Hypertension
• Dyslipidemia (low HDL cholesterol, high triglycerides)
• Cardiovascular Disease
• Impaired fasting glucose ($\geq$100mg/dL)
• Impaired glucose tolerance 2 hr plasma glucose $\geq$140 mg/dL)
• HbA1c > 5.7%
• Lifestyle
   o Sedentary lifestyle
   o Physical inactivity
   o Alcohol consumption
   o Smoking
   o Low fiber diet
   o Food with a high glycemic index
   o Consumption of saturated fats
   o Sweet drinks
   o Obstructive Sleep Apnea
• Vitamin Deficiencies
   o Vitamin K
   o Vitamin D
• Gut bacteria that cause increased:
   o Nutrient absorption
   o Cellular uptake of triglycerides
   o Lipogenesis
   o Chronic low-grade inflammation
   o Capacity to extract energy from the diet
	• Age > 45 years old
	• Family History of T2D (first degree relative)
	• Ethnicity (*i.e.* African American, Hispanic-American, Asian American, Pacific Islander)
	• Genetics
	   o Susceptibility Loci
	• History of gestational diabetes or of a baby weighing more than nine pounds

COMPLICATIONS OF DIABETES MELLITUS

The increased prevalence of diabetes has also resulted in a greater number of people experiencing micro-and macrovascular complications of diabetes. These will be discussed in this section and include cardiomyopathy, cerebrovascular accidents, cancer, neuropathy, nephropathy, and retinopathy (Fig. **1**).

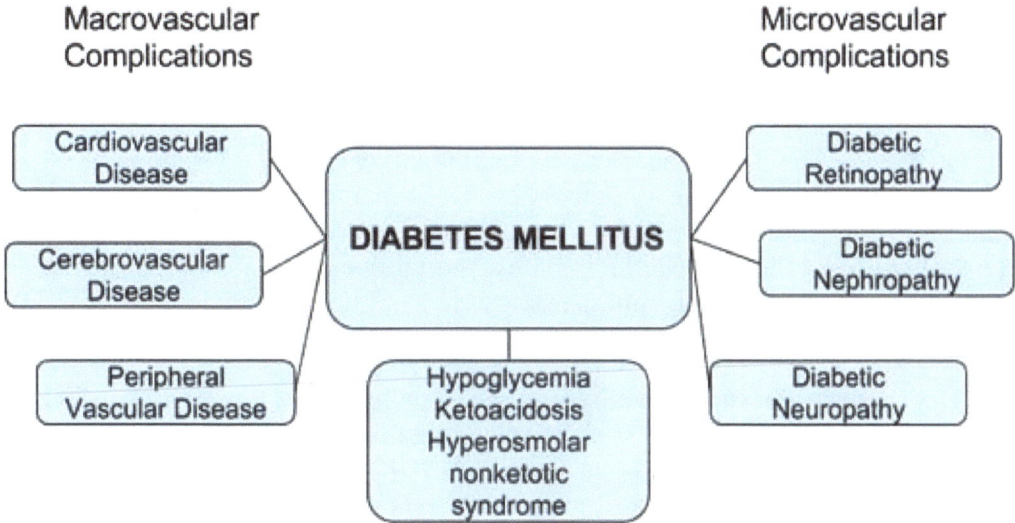

Fig. (1). Complications of Diabetes Mellitus: The complications of diabetes are numerous. Macrovascular complications include peripheral vascular disease and cardiovascular diseases, such as diabetic cardiomyopathy, cardiac autonomic neuropathy, and coronary artery disease. Cerebrovascular disease is suspected to be a result of macro-and microvascular complications. Microvascular complications include diabetic nephropathy, neuropathy, and retinopathy. Some of the metabolic complications of diabetes and its treatment include hypoglycemia, ketoacidosis, and hyperosmolar nonketotic syndrome.

Macrovascular Complications

Cardiovascular Diseases

There is overwhelming evidence that both T1D and T2D significantly increase the risk of cardiovascular diseases, including coronary heart disease, peripheral vascular disease, stroke, cardiomyopathy, and congestive heart failure. Alarmingly, complications of the aforementioned cardiovascular disease are now the primary cause of morbidity and mortality related to diabetes [4]. Cardiovascular disease-associated mortality with diabetes is about 65%. Thus, diabetes is now considered an equivalent risk of mortality as heart diseases [24]. The well known Framingham Heart Study has demonstrated that diabetic women have a five times greater frequency of heart failure; diabetic men have a two times greater risk as compared to their gender and age-matched control subjects [25].

Coronary artery disease is caused by accelerated atherosclerosis. Accumulation of lipids in cardiomyocytes and left ventricular hypertrophy contribute to contractile dysfunction and result in diabetic cardiomyopathy (DCM) [24]. The mechanism by which DCM occurs has not been fully elucidated. It is known that hyperglycemia, hyperlipidemia, and inflammation collectively induce the production of reactive oxygen species (ROS) that cause diabetic complications [26].

Persistent hyperglycemia causes increased glucose metabolism, which increases ROS production by mitochondria [27]. Oxidative stress thereafter can lead to reduced myocardial contractility and eventually cause myocardial fibrosis. Oxidative stress can also accelerate the rate of cardiomyocyte apoptosis and contribute to DNA damage in cells. This DNA damage can activate enzymes, such as poly ADP ribose polymerase (PARP). PARP can redirect glucose metabolism to another biochemical pathway that eventually results in increased production of advanced glycation end products. These products can crosslink protein, such as elastin and collagen, resulting in myocardial stiffness [4, 28].

Diabetes also causes cardiac autonomic neuropathy (CAN), which manifests as abnormalities in heart rhythm. It is suspected that the prevalence of CAN may be greater than 60% in people with chronic DM [24]. Patients with CAN have abnormal sympathetic tones resulting in increased peripheral vascular resistance and reduced vascular elasticity. This results in decreased myocardial perfusion, possibly contributing to ventricular dysfunction associated with diabetic CAN [24]. Prevention of diabetic cardiovascular events involve a combination of treatments that prevent hypertension, maintain normal lipid profiles, and routine administration of low-dose aspirin [29].

Cancer

Studies have shown that diabetes may increase the risk of cancers, such as breast, kidney, liver, and colorectal cancer [5]. The first mechanism that can explain this is hyperinsulinemia, which characterizes T2D. One study found that insulin-like growth factor-1 (IGF-1) and insulin are associated with adenomas and even more with advanced adenomas. Thus, IGF-1 and insulin may contribute to the development of adenomatous polyps that can eventually develop into colorectal cancer [30]. Furthermore, IGF-1 has an anti-apoptotic effect on cancer cells [31]. The more obvious explanation is that both T2D and cancers share many risk factors, including obesity, sedentary lifestyle, smoking, age, and a higher intake of saturated fats [32].

Cerebrovascular Accident

Diabetes is the fastest growing risk factor for stroke worldwide [33]. Diabetic patients are two to six times more susceptible to experiencing a stroke and are more likely to die or be disabled after the event. They are also less likely to benefit from intravenous tissue plasminogen activator therapy. These observations can be explained by deficits in cerebrovascular structure [34].

Stroke is considered a macrovascular complication since it is a result of accelerated atherosclerosis and carotid artery disease. However, there is new evidence that cerebral microcirculation is affected by diabetes and the brain is one of the organs that is a target [35]. Studies have noted that there is a thickening of the cerebral microvascular basement membrane due to collagen deposition and amorphous nodules. The basement membrane widens and, thus, compromises the integrity of vascular smooth muscle cells, pericytes, and astrocytic endfeet. Additionally, there is swelling of vascular smooth muscle mitochondria and endoplasmic reticulum [36]. While the association of diabetes and increased risk of stroke is well known, the underlying mechanism of this is not fully understood. Nevertheless, a step forward is the recognition that diabetes contributes to macro and microvascular complications in the brain. Perhaps understanding this mechanism will help identify novel therapeutic interventions to reduce the consequences of cerebrovascular complications in diabetic patients.

Peripheral Vascular Disease

Peripheral vascular disease, also known as peripheral arterial disease (PAD), results from accelerated atherosclerosis in the lower extremities that eventually can cause occlusion. PAD affects about 12 million people in the United States. Twenty percent of symptomatic patients with PAD have diabetes [37]. Due to shared pathophysiology, PAD is a marker for systemic vascular disease in cardiac, cerebral, and renal vessels. Systemic vascular disease contributes to an increased risk of myocardial infarction, stroke, and death [38]. Unfortunately, about 27% of people with PAD have a progression of symptoms over a 5 year period and about 4% experience limb loss. While this is not a high percentage, over the same course of time, 20% of patients sustain nonfatal events, such as myocardial infarction and stroke, and there is 30% mortality rate as well [39]. 30% of the patients who experience gangrene, tissue loss, or rest pain, have amputations, and about 20% die within 6 months [40].

Microvascular Complications

Neuropathy

Hyperglycemia induced oxidative stress can cause neural degeneration and rapid changes in glial cells [41]. It is by this process that diabetic neuropathy can occur. Diabetic neuropathy manifests as foot ulcers and nonhealing skin wounds since patients lose sensation in their feet. If not treated, these wounds can result in ulceration and cellulitis or osteomyelitis and gangrene. Unfortunately, some patients end up with amputations to prevent infection spread to other parts of the body. Diabetic neuropathy also manifests as sexual dysfunction in younger diabetic patients because of the oxidative stress in cavernous tissue [29].

Retinopathy

Diabetic retinopathy is the most common cause of new-onset blindness among patients between 20-74 years old. Within the first two decades of having diabetes, almost every patient with T1D and more than 60% of patients with T2D develop retinopathy [42]. Chronic hyperglycemia causes microvascular damage to retinal vessels resulting in increased vascular permeability. This permeability allows for the propagation of edema and hemorrhage into the retina or vitreous humor. Another mechanism by which diabetic retinopathy occurs is with redox-sensitiv--nuclear-transcriptional factor (NF-kB). It is a regulator of antioxidant enzymes in the retina. High glucose levels cause premature activation of NF-kB, which causes endothelial cell apoptosis [41].

Diabetic Kidney Disease

Diabetes is the most common reason for end-stage renal disease in the United States. The number of people initiating treatment for ESRD in 2008 is 18 fold of what it was in 1980. The term diabetic kidney disease encompasses the various complications of diabetes, including diabetic nephropathy, atheroembolic disease, ischemic nephropathy, and interstitial fibrosis [43]. Diabetes damages the microcirculation throughout the body, which contributes to microvascular complications, including nephropathy. This is caused by a decreased level of nitric oxide. In conditions of decreased insulin sensitivity, there is increased nitric oxide degradation and reduced production. A low serum level of nitric oxide causes reduced blood supply to kidneys and microcirculatory dysfunction [44]. Glycemic control and inhibition of the renin-angiotensin-aldosterone system (RAAS) have been the basis of therapy in patients with diabetic kidney disease. Furthermore, numerous trials have shown that improved glycemic control in patients with diabetes reduces the progression of diabetic kidney disease to end-stage renal disease [43, 45].

NEW THERAPEUTIC MODALITIES FOR TREATING DIABETES MELLITUS

The American Diabetes Association (ADA) recommends that metformin be used as the first-line pharmacological therapy if lifestyle changes alone are not successful in improving glycemic control [46]. The benefits of metformin are well established. Along with accomplishing glucose control, metformin lowers serum LDL cholesterol concentrations [47] and promotes modest weight reduction [48]. Observational studies even suggest that metformin may decrease the incidence of cancer by working through the Peutz-Jeghers protein, LKB1. This protein is a tumor suppressor that activates AMP-activated protein kinase, thereby inhibiting cell growth [49].

Despite its numerous benefits, after extended time on metformin, most patients require polytherapy due to the progressive nature of the disease and loss of insulin secretory function [50]. At this point, the ADA does recommend initiation of insulin for patients who are newly diagnosed and markedly symptomatic and/or have elevated glucose levels. Although this approach would improve glycemic control rapidly and effectively, it is important to take into account the burden on the patient with its use. Insulin burdens patients with the complexity of injection regimens, the need to frequently adjust doses, the risk of weight gain, and hypoglycemic episodes [51, 52]. Additionally, there has been suspicion of insulin increased risk of CVD and mortality in patients with T2D [52].

As an alternative to insulin therapy, the ADA recommends the use of a second oral agent or a GLP-1 receptor agonist. Unfortunately, there is no consensus on which drug to select, although algorithms provide some guidelines [46]. This is where patient-centered care depends on the good judgment of the clinician to select the appropriate glucose-lowering drug (GLD) for the patient. The clinician must take into account the medication cost, efficacy, potential side effects, hypoglycemic risks, the effect on weight, and patient preference [53]. The choices are many and include sodium-glucose co-transporter-2 (SGLT2) inhibitors, sulfonylureas, acarbose, dipeptidyl peptidase-4 (DPP-4) inhibitors, thiazolidinediones, or glucagon-like peptide-1 (GLP-1) receptor agonists [54, 55].

Previously, the most common next step in treatment for patients who required a second oral agent was sulphonylureas. Although the combination of metformin and sulphonylurea offers improved glycemic control, the latter is associated with hypoglycemia and weight gain. The danger of this is potential cardiovascular side effects, quality of life, as well as patients' adherence to treatment [56].

The ambiguity of selecting a second oral agent is now alleviated with evidence behind novel glucose-lowering agents for the treatment of T2D. These agents are sodium-glucose co-transporter-2 (SGLT2) inhibitors and dipeptidyl peptidase-4 (DPP-4) inhibitors. SGLT2 inhibitors lower blood glucose by preventing the kidney's re-uptake of glucose from the glomerular filtrate and promoting excretion of glucose in the urine [57]. DPP-4 inhibitors achieve glycemic control by preventing the degradation of incretin hormones. This results in a glucose-dependent increase in the stimulation of insulin secretion and inhibition of glucagon secretion. Both medications have the advantage of oral administration, low risk of hypoglycemia and weight gain, and, more importantly according to recent findings, cardiovascular safety [58].

DPP-4 and SGLT2 Inhibitors: The Next Second Line Oral Agents

An observational registry study used data from Swedish national registries to identify all patients with T2D as new users of oral glucose-lowering drugs (GLD), either DPP-4 inhibitors or SGLT2 inhibitors. The population studied had a 33% prevalence of CVD and a relatively short history of GLD treatment. The study has shown that compared with new initiation of insulin, dapagliflozin, an SGLT2 inhibitor, and DPP-4 inhibitors are to be associated with a decreased risk of fatal and non-fatal CVD (15%), all-cause mortality (44%), and severe hypoglycemia (74%). These findings make a significant argument for the use of these agents as a second-line oral agent when monotherapy fails [59, 60].

The study also assessed the separate contributions of dapagliflozin and DPP-4 inhibitors. When compared with insulin, dapagliflozin was associated with a 49% lower risk of fatal and non-fatal CVD and a 56% lower risk of all-cause mortality. The use of DPP-4 inhibitors was associated with a 41% lower risk of all-cause mortality. However, it was not superior to insulin in decreasing fatal and non-fatal CVD risk, with a hazard ratio of 1. Furthermore, the risk of hypoglycemia in DPP-4 inhibitors was 69% lower than that of insulin; there was no statistically significant difference in hypoglycemia risk when observing the effect of dapagliflozin. Conclusively, this study finds that the use of GLDs was associated with a lower risk of all-cause mortality, CVD, and severe hypoglycemia compared with the use of insulin [59, 60].

Although insulin has clear advantages for glycemic control and preventing complications of diabetes, evidence of its complications limits its benefits. These newer GLDs have been shown to have a lower risk of hypoglycemia and CVD. They may be therapeutic alternatives that beneficially lack risks of adverse effects [61].

The benefits of DPP-4 and SGLT2 are evident when compared with the use of insulin. Fortunately, two other observations studies from the U.S. and Sweden compared the use of sulfonylurea with insulin treatment after metformin monotherapy [60, 62]. The studies showed that patients treated with sulfonylurea had a lower all-cause mortality risk reduction as compared with insulin treated patients with T2D, 17% and 29%, respectively. The previously mentioned study demonstrated that patients treated with DPP-4 and SGLT2 inhibitors have a higher all-cause mortality risk reduction (44%) in patients with T2D as compared to those treated with insulin [60, 62]. This may be explained by the recent finding of novel GLDs to be safe and even cardioprotective [61]. Sulfonylureas, on the other hand, have been associated with higher risks of CVD in comparison to DPP-4 inhibitors, despite limited data [60]. These studies suggest that it is appropriate to use new GLDs as a second-line treatment of T2D because of their increased clinical utility. Furthermore, new guidelines are stating that sulfonylureas should be used with caution [63].

DPP-4 Inhibitors Compared to Sulfonylurea

A long-term study compared DPP-4 inhibitor, linagliptin, against a commonly used sulfonylurea, glimepiride. This study showed that for patients with T2D, whose blood glucose levels are not adequately controlled with metformin, linagliptin was non-inferior to glimepiride in lowering HbA1c, with a non-inferiority margin of 0.35%. This is important since HbA1c is a strong predictor of diabetes-associated morbidity and mortality as well as patient outcomes [59].

The study found that linagliptin was associated with significantly less hypoglycemia than glimepiride. Hypoglycemia should be avoided since it can negatively affect cognitive function, increase mortality and morbidity, decrease adherence to treatment, and worsen the quality of life [64]. The feared side effect of sulfonylureas is hypoglycemia since it improves insulin secretion independently of blood glucose concentrations. This results in intermittent episodes of hyperinsulinemic hypoglycemia and occurs in nearly 1 in 10 people who are treated with sulfonylurea [65, 66]. 10% of such episodes can be fatal [67].

DPP-4 inhibitors are much less likely to cause hypoglycemia since their mechanism of action depends on insulin secretion in response to raised blood glucose and tempers when glucose concentrations return to normal. This study found that patients taking sulfonylureas gained an average weight of 1.3kg, *versus* patients who were treated with linagliptin, who lost an average weight of 1.4 kg after 2 years. Despite their popularity in use, sulfonylureas are renowned for causing weight gain in patients with T2D, many of whom are already overweight or obese. The medical benefits of DPP-4 are many, but the cardiovascular benefits or risks are not yet known. A large trial, (CAROLINA, NCT01243424), is ongoing and was designed to evaluate the effect of linagliptin in comparison to glimepiride on cardiovascular outcomes [59].

The side effect profiles of oral agents are increasingly important to consider as we have more information on their effect on the cardiovascular system, glycemic control, incidence of hypoglycemic episodes, and ease of use. The study discussed supports the use of novel oral antiglycemic agents, including DPP-4 and SGLT2 inhibitors as a second-line therapy after metformin.

The Search for Superior Insulin as Demand for Higher Doses Rises

More than 90% of patients with T2D in the U.S. are overweight. Diabetic patients are less sensitive to exogenous insulin and require higher doses of insulin as the disease progresses. The challenge with administering higher doses of insulin is that they cannot be delivered with currently marketed insulin pen devices that only allow administration of a maximum of 80 units per injection. One unsatisfying solution is delivering large doses of insulin with a single injection using a syringe, which may be painful and can be physically challenging to deliver a large volume smoothly. A second, not much desirable solution is the addition of a second injection [68].

When considering optimal diabetes therapy for patients, the aim should be to select one that is simpler and requires less frequent dosing regimens. Less burden on the patient can result in better adherence and treatment outcomes [69]. Globally, about 30% of patients with T2D require the use of >60 units of basal insulin daily [70]. In response to the demand, Humulin R U-500 insulin was developed to deliver highly concentrated insulin. Between the years 2007-2008, its use increased by a staggering >70% in the U.S., reflecting the increased number of people requiring highly concentrated insulin for glycemic control [71].

Insulin Degludec

New insulin, Degludec (IDeg), has been developed in response to the growing need for higher insulin doses in patients who use prefilled pen devices. It is ultra-long-acting basal insulin that forms soluble multihexamers that slowly dissociate into monomers to produce a flat and consistent insulin effect lasting more than 42 hours [72]. Insulin Degludec has been found to offer a treatment advantage over basal insulin. A study demonstrated that when IDeg is used at 200 units/mL, it is associated with a lower frequency of injections, equivalent glycemic control, reduced rate of hypoglycemia, and improved patient-reported outcomes as compared to basal insulin [73].

Many patients who have T2D and are treated with insulin do not titrate their insulin dose adequately. Patients may fear the risk of hypoglycemia. Administration of large insulin volumes may be painful, which may also contribute to poor patient adherence [74]. A study showed that IDeg is superior to insulin glargine. The former can deliver as much as 160 units of insulin in a single injection rather than two injections needed by patients treated with the latter to maintain the same glycemic control.

IDeg uses a low-volume preparation at a high concentration. Treating patients with IDeg 200 units/ml resulted in similar HbA1c reductions as with the use of Insulin Glargine. IDeg had significantly better fasting plasma glucose reduction and a low rate of hypoglycemic episodes. An additional benefit is that there is no need for dose correction or calculation [75]. For a patient population that requires higher insulin doses, IDeg 200 units/ml may help overcome some of the barriers that patients experience when treating their diabetes.

Despite the exciting advantages of IDeg, it comes in prefilled insulin pen devices. Such devices are used by approximately 15% of the U.S. population. Perhaps, this is because they are more expensive than vial and syringes. The second reason is that insulin pen device use has been limited by the need to inject larger doses than what was previously available. IDeg 200 units/ml addresses the growing need for high insulin requirements of the growing population [75].

GPR40 Agonist

GPR40 is a G protein-coupled free fatty acid receptor that is highly expressed in pancreatic β-cells. Activation of GPR40 has been shown to improve glycemic control by promoting glucose-dependent insulin secretion. Fasiglifam (TAK-875) is one of the GPR40 agonists that has been shown to reduce fasting plasma glucose and HbA1c levels. Three novel GPR40 agonists have also been identified, AS2031477, AS1975063, and AS2034178, which may improve both acute glucose-dependent insulin secretion and chronic whole body glucose metabolism. The AS2034178 agonist has shown to decrease microvascular complications. GPR40 agonists are a new promising class of medications [76, 77].

Lixisenatide

Lixisenatide is a glucagon-like peptide (GLP)-1 receptor agonist. It was approved by the European Medicines Agency in 2013. This medication activates the GLP-1 receptors, thereby causing increased insulin secretion, decreased gastric motility to promote satiety, and inhibition of glucagon secretion. Lixisenatide was shown to reduce body weight, HbA1c, and fasting plasma glucose, as well as postprandial plasma glucose levels [78].

Lixisenatide is in the same family as exenatide of short-acting agents that promote delay in gastric emptying and blunt postprandial glucose excursions. Long term GLP-1 agonists, however, cause a desensitization of the gastric emptying effect, therefore the primary effect is mainly based on stimulation of insulin secretion and glucagon suppression. When comparing the two short term agents, lixisenatide and exenatide, a study found that lixisenatide taken once daily was noninferior to exenatide that was taken twice daily. Similar numbers of patients achieved the target HbA1c of 53mmol/mol. This was achieved with threefold fewer hypoglycemic events and with better gastrointestinal tolerability than that with exenatide [78].

Anti-Inflammatory Treatment

Hyperglycemia causes increased production of interleukin-1β in pancreatic cells. It is a pro-inflammatory cytokine that has been implicated in causing inflammatory β-cell destruction and leading to T1D. Increased levels of interleukin-1β lead to impaired insulin secretion and cell apoptosis. The expression of interleukin-1-receptor antagonist is decreased in β-cells of patients who have T2D. One study blocked interleukin-1with anakinra, a recombinant human interleukin-1-receptor antagonist. This improved hyperglycemia and β-cell secretory function. It also reduced markers of systemic inflammation. Further studies are still needed on long term use of anakinra and to test other interleukin-1 antagonists to prevent β-cell destruction [79].

Nitrates and Nitrites

Studies have shown that nitrates and nitrite may contribute to decreasing blood pressure and reducing oxidative stress [5]. One study demonstrated that inorganic nitrates could reduce visceral fat accumulation, normalize glucose tolerance, and lower serum triglycerides in endothelial nitric oxide deficient mice [80]. Thus, nitrates and nitrites may have roles in preventing and treating T2D. However, some harmful effects of this therapy are that high levels of nitrate can increase arterial pressure, may cause early-onset hypertension, cause kidney dysfunction, and hypothyroidism [81]. Nevertheless, this therapy holds promise for treating diabetes and is being investigated.

Antioxidant Therapy

It has been suggested that hyperglycemia causes four biochemical changes that are all activated by a common denominator, overproduction of superoxide radicals. First, there is glycation of proteins that interferes with their normal function contributing to the pathogenesis of diabetic complications, such as retinopathy, nephropathy, and neuropathy [82]. Second, there is an activation of protein kinase C, which contributes to vascular occlusion and the expression of pro-inflammatory genes. Third, there is increased shunting of glucose through the hexosamine pathway, which mediates increased transcription of genes for inflammatory cytokines. Fourth, there is an increased flux through the polyol pathway in which glucose is reduced to sorbitol, thereby reducing levels of NADPH and glutathione [83].

Production of ROS has been reported in diabetes as free radicals and oxidative stress contribute to the development of diabetic complications. Evidence confirms that oxidative stress is associated with endothelial dysfunction and predicts coronary vascular disease [84]. One study showed that vitamin C could decrease HbA1c levels and improve insulin action. It also showed that β-carotene might reduce oxidative LDL [85]. Vitamin E has been shown to reduce oxidative stress indicators, protein glycosylation, and insulin resistance. It also normalizes creatinine clearance [41].

Another study found that plants that contain antioxidant properties include cinnamic acids, coumarins, flavonoids, and monoterpenes. These plants can have a therapeutic effect on treating T2D [5]. The use of antioxidants offers an opportunity for controlling free radical production and increasing intracellular antioxidant defenses. This theory is still being investigated as it holds promise for diabetes treatment.

NEW TECHNOLOGIES FOR TREATMENT OF DIABETES MELLITUS

Glucose Monitoring

Prior to the advent of the continuous glucose monitoring system (CGMS), self-monitoring of blood glucose was the mainstay of guiding therapy for diabetes treatment. Blood glucose monitoring is key to informing patients' glycemic control, guiding treatment regimens, and outcomes. Since blood glucose fluctuates throughout the day and self-monitoring of blood glucose only reflects the glucose concentration at a specific point in time, it fails to be a reliable source.

CGMS has been a dream come true for patients with diabetes and for diabetologists [86]. CGMS gave a greater insight into the direction, magnitude, frequency, and duration of glucose fluctuations in response to exercise, meals, and insulin injections throughout the day. Additionally, smart pumps with bolus calculators and features for data upload have been used to guide clinical treatment [87]. With both of the advancements, diabetic management has become linked to technological innovations.

Although we can continuously track blood glucose levels and set an automatic basal level of insulin to be slowly delivered to the body, the challenge is that insulin requirements vary significantly. For individuals with T1D, insulin requirements may vary from one third to three times that of planned insulin delivery, even without acute illness [88]. Variable caloric intake, changes in physical activity, and aberrations in glucose turnover are among the factors that contribute to such changes in insulin requirements.

The use of CGMS and smart pumps has allowed us to elucidate treatment to progress to improved insulin dosing, but it still requires frequent re-adjustment of insulin requirements on behalf of the user [89]. The sensor augmented insulin pump (SAP), for example, uses the technology of CGMS and an insulin pump that sends glucose readings to the person wearing the device. The user then inputs the number of calories he/she intends to consume and the pump calculates the units of insulin that should be administered. This demands considerable participation on the part of the patient. Even the most diligent person may have trouble achieving optimal glycemic control. It is feasible to fine tune daytime insulin regimens while awake but is not easily done at night.

The Artificial Pancreas (Closed-loop Monitoring System)

The aim of achieving improved glycemic control with fewer burdens on the user has brought a joint effort to develop the "artificial pancreas," also known as the closed-loop stem. This system would emulate the functionality of β-cells, which release insulin in response to changes in glucose levels. Theoretically, the closed-loop system is intended to respond to blood glucose variability throughout the day and on a day to day basis. Its key advantage over the CGMS is that it autonomously and continuously modulates insulin delivery in response to the changes in glucose, irrespective of the time of food intake or the number of calories consumed and without the need for input from the user [89, 90].

The closed-loop system can individualize treatment based on patients' rate of metabolic glucose processing and daily level of physical activity. It relieves the user from performing a precise calculation of their carbohydrate intake. The adaptive features of the system also aim to minimize hyper-and hypoglycemic states by its capability to adapt to unforeseen changes in blood glucose levels and respond autonomously to improve glycemic equilibrium and reduce risks of hypo and hyperglycemic states (Fig. **2**) [89, 90].

Components of the Closed-loop Monitoring System

The closed-loop monitoring system is similar to the SAP in that it utilizes a continuous glucose monitor and an insulin pump. Its uniqueness is the presence of a third component: the control algorithm. Two forms of control algorithms have been employed, the proportional-integral-derivative (PID) controller and the model predictive controller (MPC). The PID controller assesses glucose changes from three viewpoints: **(1)** Proportional component: departure from target glucose; **(2)** Integral component: area under the curve between ambient and target glucose; **(3)** Derivative component: rate of change in ambient glucose. The MPC controller utilizes a mathematical model that links insulin delivery and meal ingestion to glucose changes. It compares the predicted glucose levels to actual glucose levels, updating the model, and calculating future insulin infusion rates to minimize the difference between the model's predicted glucose levels and the target glucose level [89].

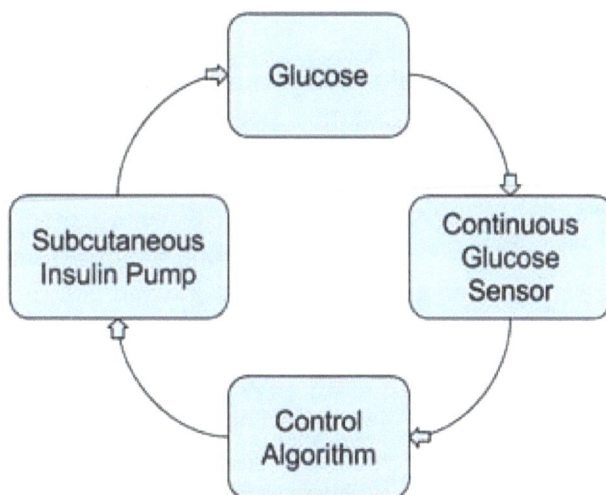

Fig. (2). The closed-loop system: Glucose measurements are detected by the continuous glucose sensor on the patient's stomach and are sent to a handheld device called the control algorithm. This algorithm computes and transmits the amount of insulin to be delivered *via* the subcutaneous insulin pump.

The Three-body Access Routes

Three-body access routes for the closed-loop system exist, but only two of them are practical. The subcutaneous-subcutaneous (S.C.-S.C.) approach utilizes the S.C. route for both glucose monitoring and insulin delivery. The intravenous-intraperitoneal (I.V.-I.P.) approach relies on intravenous glucose monitoring and intraperitoneal insulin delivery. The third approach is the I.V.-I.V. access, employing intravenous glucose sampling and intravenous insulin delivery. Its main use is in critically ill patients [91].

The minimally invasive S.C.-S.C. approach has the best potential to achieve application, as evidenced by the experience of more than 200, 000 external insulin pump users. However, this approach is limited by more than a 100 minutes time lag between times of insulin delivery to a peak of its detectable glucose-lowering effect. It is likely that users of this approach would have to enter information regarding their calorie intake and level of exercise to assist in the delivery of prandial insulin dose. This approach would not result in a fully closed loop system [92].

The I.V.-I.P. approach has a better potential of attaining a fully closed-loop system. The delays in the system are shorter than the S.C.-S.C. approach totaling about 70 minutes from the time of insulin delivery to the peak of its detectable glucose-lowering effect. However, with an implantable pump that would allow insulin to be infused intraperitoneally, a more physiological insulin delivery may be attained.

The disadvantage is that there is very limited experience with the use of implantable pumps. Only 1000 pumps have been used worldwide to date. Furthermore, this approach requires surgical intervention with a risk of infection and device failures requiring premature removal of the pump. The closed-loop system is limited by the speed of insulin absorption and glucose sensing inaccuracies. Several hurdles need to be overcome before an implantable closed-loop system can be made available for long-term glucose control [90, 92].

The Efficacy of the Closed-loop System

Numerous studies have been performed to evaluate the efficacy of the closed-loop system in outpatient transitional facilities but have not reached consensus on its effect on glycemic control. A study using 56 participants in a multicentre diabetes camp setting over a single night evaluated overnight closed-loop insulin delivery in comparison to the SAP. Compared with SAP therapy, the number of episodes of hypoglycemia with overnight closed-loop insulin therapy was significantly reduced ($p=0.003$). The study did not show improvement in the time spent in the target glucose range compared with SAP therapy [93]. However, another study showed that overnight closed-loop use for five consecutive nights in an outpatient translational facility actually resulted in significantly improved time spent within the target glucose range ($p<0.001$) as well as improved glucose levels overnight ($p<0.001$) when compared with SAP therapy [94].

To provide an objective assessment of closed-loop system performance, studies have also been done in unsupervised free-living home settings. The longest randomized home study lasted 3 months. Participants wore a closed-loop device or a SAP. Closed-loop therapy was found to improve the time in target glucose range by 11 percent ($p<0.001$) and reduce HbA1c levels ($p=0.002$). During 24 hours, the relative risk of time spent in hypoglycemia was reduced by closed-loop therapy by 19% $p=0.02$ [95]. Another study confirmed these findings and demonstrated a reduced average glucose level ($p<0.03$) when participants used the closed-loop system [96]. Despite the contradictory results when studied in the transitional outpatient settings, studies set in free-living home settings demonstrated that the closed-loop system is uniquely able to reduce mean glucose and the risk of hypoglycemia.

Bi-hormonal Therapy and the Closed-loop System

The closed-loop system is still being developed and refined. The use of bi-hormonal therapy (insulin and glucagon) is currently being explored to decrease the risk of hypoglycemia. A bi-hormonal system can deliver insulin but add glucagon to mitigate potential hypoglycemia due to insulin over delivery. Studies have compared the use of bi-hormonal and insulin-alone closed-loop systems. One study found that in a pediatric diabetes camp over the course of three consecutive nights, the time spent in hypoglycemia during the night was significantly reduced with the bi-hormonal system as compared to the insulin-alone system ($p=0.032$). The average glucose level was comparable in the two systems.

Bi-hormonal systems are limited due to their complexity and need for a second pump device to deliver glucagon. The user would be required to replace glucagon and the infusion setting every 24 hours A dual-chamber pump is currently being developed [97].

Adjunctive Therapies and the Closed-loop System

There has been a recent interest in the use of adjunctive therapies to improve glycemic control. Pramlintide and glucagon-like peptide-1 (GLP-1) are two adjunctive therapies that have been evaluated in combination with the closed-loop insulin delivery system. Pramlintide is an injectable analogue of amylin, a peptide hormone that is released by β-cells along with insulin. It slows gastric emptying, thereby improving cellular absorption of glucose, promoting satiety, and inhibiting inappropriate secretion of glucagon [98]. Exenatide is a GLP-1 agonist that augments pancreatic response to food intake, suppresses the pancreatic release of glucagon, promotes satiety, and slows down gastric emptying.

A study examined the use of either pramlintide or exenatide during closed-loop insulin delivery. They were compared with closed-loop insulin delivery alone during the course of 27 hours. The study demonstrated that co-administration of exenatide ($p<0.03$), but not pramlintide ($p>0.05$), resulted in a significantly greater decrease in glucose levels after lunch and dinner. Glucagon suppression was also greater with exenatide co-administration ($p<0.03$) but not with pramlintide ($p>0.05$) when compared with closed-loop insulin delivery alone. There was no increase in hypoglycemic episodes with either of the adjunctive therapies [99].

The Outlook of the Closed-loop Monitoring System

Significant resources have been allocated to the development and modification of the closed-loop monitoring system. Over $200 million in grants has been funded for this system. It is expected that the technology will be in clinical use by the end of the decade [100]. Nevertheless, with its ability to adjust insulin delivery in response to glucose levels without the user's constant manual adjustment, the system may help to achieve more stable glucose levels in patients.

Research on participants using closed-loop monitoring systems in transitional outpatient facilities and at home is promising. Bi-hormonal and adjunctive therapies are paving the road to expand diabetes care to a multimodal fashion combining the use of technology and novel hormonal analogues. Despite the exciting potential of utilizing technology to improve care, the use of wireless technology places closed-loop devices at cyber-security threats. The challenge faced is not only to develop a reliable therapy for glycemic control but also to secure patients' safety by preventing hacking of closed-loop monitoring systems [101].

Pancreas Allotransplantation

Conventional exogenous insulin therapy can improve glycemic control, but it cannot prevent the development of complications from T1D. This has spurred a search for alternative therapies. Pancreatic transplantation is one such solution. It is the key to restoring independence from insulin therapy, predominantly for patients with T1D. A well functioning pancreatic graft allows for a state of euglycemia that has shown to prevent and improve the complications of DM, such as nephropathy, neuropathy, macrovascular disease, and retinopathy. Transplantation can prolong and improve the quality of life of a diabetic patient [102].

Thus, so far, 23,000 pancreatic transplantations have been reported to the International Transplant Registry (IPTR) [102]. There are three types of a pancreas transplants. Pancreas-kidney (SPK) transplantation is commonly performed with a kidney transplant for patients with insulin-dependent DM and imminent or end-stage renal disease requiring dialysis. This procedure should be considered as an acceptable alternative to continued insulin therapy, especially for patients who plan to have a kidney transplant. As per the ADA recommendations, the addition of pancreas to the transplantation procedure does not jeopardize patient survival, and may improve kidney survival, and restore euglycemia [103]. Patients who undergo SPK transplantation have a significantly improved 10 year survival when compared to patients receiving kidney transplants alone, 23.4 years *versus* 12.9 years, respectively [104]. The pancreas after kidney transplants (PAK) involves transplantation of pancreas in patients who have already had a kidney transplant. However, pancreas survival is improved when done simultaneously with a kidney transplant [104].

Pancreas transplantation alone (PTA) is the least common form of transplantation since 30% of patients given a PTA eventually need a renal transplant due to the cumulative adverse effects of immunosuppression with calcineurin inhibitors [105]. However, this transplant is performed for patients with poorly controlled insulin-dependent T1D with adequate renal function [105]. The ADA requires patients to meet three criteria to undergo this procedure: (1) experience frequent and severe metabolic complications, such as hypoglycemia, hyperglycemia, or ketoacidosis that require medical attention; (2) clinical and emotional problems with the use of insulin therapy that are incapacitating; (3) consistent failure to prevent acute complications using exogenous insulin-based therapy [103].

SPK: Pancreas-kidney Transplantation

PAK: Pancreas after kidney transplantation

PTA: Pancreas transplantation alone

Like any transplantation, pancreatic transplantation has the disadvantage of requiring life-long immunosuppression as well as the surgical risks associated with undergoing a transplant procedure. Challenges that are faced with pancreatic transplantation also include scarcity of appropriate donor and graft loss. This limits the number of patients who can benefit from this treatment. Some of the factors that influence the long-term function of transplant (Fig. **3**) are the quality of the deceased donor. Thus, careful donor selection and type of transplantation influences short-term and long-term pancreatic graft function, thereby ensuring metabolic control and improved quality of life in diabetic patients [106].

Islet Cell Allotransplantation

A search for the ultimate cure for T1DM has not only set the fuel for research and attempts in pancreatic transplantation but also for identifying the optimal method for allogeneic islet transplantation. Islet cell transplantation is another means by which endogenous insulin production can occur. Unfortunately, this form of transplantation is far from perfect and faces similar challenges as those of pancreatic transplantation: a shortage of transplantable organs, need to select appropriate candidates for whom the procedure would be of greater benefit, a requirement of lifelong immunosuppression [107]. Islet transplantation is significantly less invasive than pancreatic transplantation. It has shown to slow down or halt the progression of complications secondary to DM. More importantly, it can significantly reduce the need for exogenous insulin use.

PERCENT OF GRAFT FUNCTION WITH APPROPRIATE FOLLOW UP TIME AFTER (X) YEARS BY TRANSPLANTATION TYPE

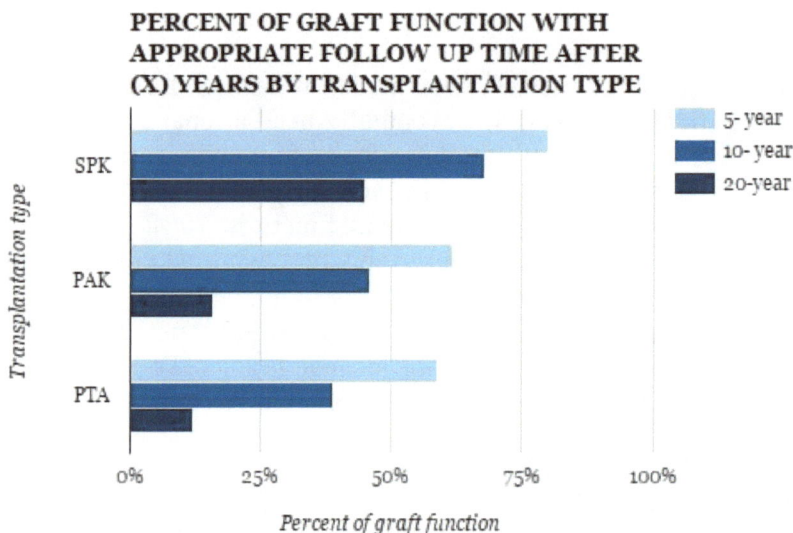

Fig. (3). For SPK transplantation with appropriate follow-up time, most recent 5-year, 10-year, and 20-year adequate graft function was 80%, 68%, and 45%, respectively, while for PAK transplantation, adequate graft function was 59%, 39%, and 12%, respectively. For PTA transplantation, the most recent 5-year, 10-year, and 20-year adequate graft function was 59%, 39%, and 12%, respectively.

Various anatomical sites have been attempted for islet transplantation. The liver has been the most common organ used for clinical transplantation. Unfortunately, about 50% to 75% of islet engraftments are lost after transplantation into the liver [108]. A study on Edmonton transplant patients showed that less than 10% of recipients remained insulin-independent five years after the transplant [109].

Islet graft loss can be explained by the occurrence of an instant inflammatory reaction as part of the body's innate immunity [110]. Other factors that contribute to this are hyperglycemia, high concentrations of drugs in the liver, and insufficient oxygen levels. Another issue is the infusion of islet cells into the portal system, which increases the regional pressure and substantially reduces the viability of transplanted islets. Recently, the bone marrow cavity has been suggested as an alternative site for islet cell transplantation. This transplantation is feasible and is similar to that of cord blood cell infusion into the bone marrow cavity for patients with acute leukemia. Additionally, it is a well-vascularized region allowing for adequate oxygen availability. The locally secreted factors in the bone marrow, such as epidermal growth factor receptor and vascular endothelial growth factor, may prevent apoptosis of islet graft cells. One group conducted a study in which they transplanted islet cells into the bone marrow cavity of diabetic Rhesus monkeys and were the first to show that this method can reverse diabetes [111].

Although islet transplantation is aggressively studied, the treatment often fails to produce durable and lifelong insulin independence. Specifically, one study aimed to assess short and long term results from pancreatic islet transplantation using the Edmonton protocol at the University of Chicago. Nine patients underwent the transplantation and were followed for up to 10 years, during which they received maintenance immunosuppression. Five of nine patients dropped out in the early phase of the study due to poor islet function and side effects of immunosuppression. However, the remaining four patients achieved a euglycemic state without the use of exogenous insulin. The study showed that this procedure offered durable, long term insulin-free glycemic control in only highly selected patients with brittle diabetes. For this group, the transplantation provided stable control of diabetic neuropathy and retinopathy without impaired renal function. These results were achieved, however, with close supervision throughout the study [112].

Rejection remains one of the greatest challenges in long term graft survival. More information is going to be available in regard to recipients' auto- and alloimmune responses to grafts. As knowledge grows regarding the immune processes in islet transplantation, eventually, superior patient-donor matching will be feasible [107].

Becoming Insulin Free with Stem Cells (Table 2)

While Islet cell and pancreatic transplantation are promising solutions to treating T1D, they require the use of immunosuppressants that cause diabetogenic and nephrotoxic side effects. They also increase the risk of infections. The numerous challenges associated with transplantation have led researchers to study stem cells as a potential therapeutic option. Stem cells pose a significant potential for a cure since they have the capacity to self-renew and to differentiate into specialized cells that can be directed to self-replenish glucose responsive and insulin producing cells for transplantation. Furthermore, stem cells are able to establish peripheral tolerance of β-cells by remodeling the immune response as well as by inhibiting autoreactive T cell function. Such immunomodulatory properties of stem cells can be used to halt β-cell destruction, facilitate endogenous β-cell regeneration, decrease islet graft rejection, and preserve residual β-cell mass [113].

In a search for a cell therapy that facilitates a renewable supply of β-cells, Kroon *et al.* showed that human embryonic stem cells (hESC) derived from pancreatic endoderm could generate glucose responsive cells after engraftment into mice. To test their therapeutic potential, streptozotocin was used to induce hyperglycemia in mice. The hESC successfully responded to attain a euglycemic state in mice. One of the limitations of this approach has been allo- and autoimmune destruction. A remaining theme of stem cell use is the potential for these cells to become teratogenic or tumorigenic *in-vivo* [114].

Induced pluripotent stem cells (iPSC) have also been demonstrated to be a reliable source for the generation of large quantities of β-cells. One study used non-obese diabetic (NOD) mice as a model for T1D that is very similar to that of humans. They induced the iPSCs of NOD mice to differentiate into functional pancreatic β-cells. After engraftment into diabetic mice, the cells produced insulin in response to glucose and normalized blood glucose levels in mice. Although these are exciting findings, there are still several limitations. While the aforementioned study did not detect tumorigenesis or teratoma formation in mice, long-term data is needed to show that this will not occur [115].

Among other stem cells, hematopoietic stem cells (HSC) have been the subject of much research. Couri *et al.* showed that after transplantation of autologous non-myeloablative HSCs, the majority of patients achieved "insulin independence with good glycemic control" [116]. Interestingly, HSCs do not differentiate into insulin producing cells, but instead, may aid in the preservation of existing β-cells. The HSCs likely improve β-cell mass *via* neovascularization, decreasing apoptosis, and/or stimulating proliferation. The mechanism of action for these effects has not been established yet [113].

Immune reconstitution studies suggest that HSCs accomplish this by resetting the immune system towards a "tolerant phenotype by increasing regulatory T cell numbers and by regeneration of a different and more diverse TCR (T – cell receptor) repertoire" [117]. Voltarelli *et al.* have provided proof of principle that high-dose immunosuppression combined with autologous HSC transplantation act synergistically to down regulate the autoreactive cells and to reset the immune system to a phenotype that is more tolerable [117]. The concern with this approach is that it is an expensive and complex process that must be performed in specialized bone marrow transplantation centers. It has short and long term life-threatening complication risks. Despite their successful findings, Voltarelli *et al.* argued that simpler approaches may accomplish the same therapeutic goal for millions of people [117].

The role of HSCs in immunomodulation has sparked interest in testing combinational therapeutic approaches that would aim to "reset" destructive immunity to one that is more tolerant without the need to use chronic immunosuppressive agents. For example, Leventhal *et al.* developed an approach that combined HSCs and tolerogenic graft facilitating cells with non-myeloablative conditioning to result in successful engraftment. The approach resulted in "durable chimerism, and tolerance induction in recipients with highly mismatched related and unrelated donors." The study found that none of the recipients had engraftment syndrome or developed anti-donor antibodies. No participant experienced graft-*versus*-host disease. This study, among others, demonstrates a new method of attaining durable chimerism that can be applied to solid organ transplantation [118].

Lastly, a highly appealing approach is the use of hypo immunogenic-human adipose tissue-derived mesenchymal stromal cells (hADSCs) and umbilical cord blood-derived mesenchymal stromal cells (hUCB-MSCs) [113]. These cells have proven preclinical ability to differentiate into glucose-responsive and insulin-producing cells and can be derived from an abundantly available human donor tissue [119, 120]. This approach has a high cell proliferation capacity. Furthermore, these cells have the ability to secrete angiogenic and antiapoptotic, anti-inflammatory, and anti-fibrotic factors that improve wound healing and tissue repair [121]. Human adipose tissue-derived adult stem cells have been success-fully shown to restore near normoglycemia in diabetic mice within a month after transplantation. There are a number of such trials investigating the feasibility of using these cells to treat T1D [122].

The field of stem cell therapy is being directed to a combinatorial approach to cure T1D. This approach aims to combine the use of the latest immuno-suppressive and immunomodulatory drug regimens as well as bioengineering techniques [113]. The use of exogenous insulin is a temporary solution as the scientific community aims to "fix" the innate function of the body. Transplantation, while it offers a means for patients to produce their own insulin, requires immunosuppression that is accompanied by numerous side effects. Stem cells, however, resolve this problem. The combination of their regenerative ability and immunomodulatory effects give a promising hope to eventually find a cure.

Table 2. Use of stem cells to cure T1D.

Stem cells' capacities	Application
• Regenerative capacity to make insulin-producing cells	• Stem cells can be induced to differentiate into glucose-responsive insulin-producing cells. • Autologous or allogeneic insulin-producing cells can be transplanted into the recipient.

(Table 2) cont.....

Stem cells' capacities	Application
• Immunomodulatory properties especially in BM-HSCs and iPSCs	• Inhibit β-cell destruction • Preserve remaining β-cell mass • Facilitate β-cell regeneration • Decrease innate/alloimmune graft rejection • Prevent recurrence of autoimmunity

PREVENTION OF DIABETES MELLITUS

Screening

The ADA recommends glucose testing of adults aged 45 years or above. Testing should also be performed in adults of any age who are overweight or obese and have one more additional risk factor for diabetes. Children and adolescents who are overweight or obese with two or more additional risk factors should also be tested. It is suggested that if tests are normal, they should be performed every three years in a high-risk population [9].

Lifestyle Modification

The alarming increased prevalence of T2D parallels that of obesity and lack of physical activity in the general population. Numerous studies have shown that improving lifestyle habits, such as weight loss, exercise, and diet, are effective in causing a sustained reduction in the incidence of T2D among high-risk patients [2, 123]. The Diabetes Prevention Program trial is an NIH-sponsored multicenter randomized controlled trial aimed at diabetes prevention through lifestyle changes. Over three thousand participants with pre-diabetes were randomly assigned to a lifestyle modification program, a metformin 850 mg twice daily therapy, or a matching placebo group. The study was discontinued early, at three years due to the significant superiority of lifestyle changes compared to pharmacological treatment or placebo. Data demonstrated that lifestyle changes resulted in a 58% reduction in diabetes incidence, whereas metformin therapy resulted in a 31% reduction in diabetes incidence compared to placebo. Thus lifestyle changes were much more effective than metformin therapy across gender, age, BMI, and ethnic groups [124].

Recently, more emphasis has been placed on quality rather than the quantity of fats consumed in order to prevent diabetes. This is evidenced by one study that showed that consumption of a non-calorie-restricted traditional Mediterranean diet enriched with high-fat foods of vegetable origin decreased the incidence of diabetes by 52% in individuals who had a high cardiovascular disease risk [125].

Weight loss is a significant contributor to decreasing the risk of diabetes onset. One study showed that a weight loss of about 5.6 kg was associated with a 58% decrease in the incidence of diabetes [126]. Exercise has also been shown to improve sensitivity to insulin and promote peripheral glucose uptake. Exercise causes an increased translocation of insulin-responsive glucose transporter (GLUT-4) from intracellular reserves to the cell surface, thereby improving glucose uptake [127]. A systemic review has also shown that moderate-intensity exercise is associated with a significantly decreased incidence of diabetes [128]. Interestingly, one study showed that four hours of exercise per week resulted in an 80% decrease in the incidence of diabetes, even in the group that did not lose weight. One study showed a decrease in diabetes incidence as high as 80% after exercise [2].

From this discussion of numerous studies, it is evident that lifestyle modification including a healthy diet, moderate intensity exercise, and moderate weight loss are in combination and separately very effective methods of preventing diabetes in patients who are at risk. More importantly, the effect of lifestyle change is sustained over time [2]. As per the recommendations of the ADA, patients with pre-diabetes should be referred to a behavioral counseling program focused on diet change and physical activity. Patients should aim at losing 7% of body weight and perform at least 150 minutes of moderate physical activity every week [129].

Pharmacological Agents

Pharmacological agents have been associated with preventing diabetes in patients at risk. However, except for metformin, side-effects and lack of durable efficacy outweigh their benefits of preventing diabetes. Such medication includes thiazolidinediones, alpha-glucosidase inhibitors, liraglutide, insulin, and xenical [124].

Motivational Interviewing

Despite the evidence supporting the positive effects of lifestyle change in preventing diabetes, it is well known how difficult it is to make such change. This is where theory clashes with the reality of daily life that is complicated by lack of access to healthy food, cost of food, little time for self-care in the midst of other responsibilities. Motivational interviewing (MI) is a counseling strategy that has been designed to elicit patient's' motivation for changing their behavior.

MI focuses on patient-centered communication by asking open-ended questions. It follows four core principles: (1) resisting the reflex to be right; (2) understanding what would motivate the patient to make a change; (3) listening to the patient and summarizing and reflecting on what they say; (4) empowering the patient. MI also follows a "spirit" of interviewing that encourages collaboration with the patient and avoiding the urge to "dictate" solutions and stating what one thinks is the right solution. Instead, the physician or health counselor should elicit what it is that motivates the patient to change. They must find reasons that are meaningful to them. It is important to remember to respect the patient's desires and this means that the patient may not be ready to make a change when it might be desired by someone else. Finally, the spirit of MI involves actively promoting the patient's emotional welfare through compassion and understanding [130].

A systemic review analyzed 1,882 studies to evaluate the effectiveness of motivational interviewing by general practitioners for T2D patients. Only eight studies met the criteria. The results of this review showed that "two-thirds of the studies found a significant improvement in at least one of the following outcomes: total cholesterol, low-density lipoproteins, fasting blood glucose, HbA1c, body mass index, blood pressure, waist circumference, and physical activity" [131]. Another systemic review explored home telemedicine interventions for treating older adults with diabetes, finding six of 1,274 articles that met inclusion criteria. This article review showed that motivational interviewing as well as case management, education, closed-loop feedback communication, home telemonitoring devices or units, and coaching could significantly decrease the cost per person per year, decrease hospital admissions, improve mortality, and decrease the cognitive decline in older adults with diabetes [132].

MI is a technique focused on eliciting patient's own reasons for change as well as empowering them rather than dictate treatment plans. It is an approach worth applying to build a stronger relationship with one's patients, understanding their barriers to self-care, and eliciting change.

CONCLUSION

The rising prevalence of diabetes and its complications impose a significant health burden on the United States and the world. The main cause of diabetes is the combination of non-modifiable risk factors, such as age, family history, and genetics. However, the greater influence is due to modifiable risk factors. Many adults in the United States lead a sedentary lifestyle. More people are overweight and obese. People either have poor access to healthy food or make poor dietary choices. In combination, there is much that can be done to prevent the onset of this debilitating condition.

The best way to prevent diabetes is through lifestyle change. In addition to preventing diabetes, it is just as important to mitigate complications of patients who already have the disease. This requires efforts to reduce obesity and promotion of an active lifestyle in the general population. It may be difficult to encourage or empower patients to make such changes. Motivational Interviewing is one approach that should be utilized by physicians and health educators to support patients in their endeavors to a healthier life.

Although nonmedical approaches are highly advised, a growing population of patients living with diabetes requires better glycemic control. With the increasing incidence of T2D, the search for ideal therapies has become a high priority. Several therapeutic options have become available and include the use of SGLT2 and DDP-4 inhibitors and GPR40 agonists. Insulin Degludec offers a more user-friendly means of providing glycemic control for patients who require more units of insulin.

Focused research has opened avenues to merge diabetes care with technology. The artificial pancreas or closed-loop systems are being optimized to improve hyperglycemia, while minimizing episodes of hypoglycemia in a way that does not require the user's constant participation. Researchers are further delving into promising therapeutic options, such as pancreatic, islet cell, and stem cell transplantations. Further investigations are necessary to focus on understanding the mechanisms contributing to diabetes and its complications. As our knowledge of this condition expands, so can the treatment options. Perhaps we will one day live in a world where diabetes is curable and, by the very least, would be easier to manage successfully.

CONSENT FOR PUBLICATION

Not applicable.

CONFLICT OF INTEREST

The authors declare no conflict of interest, financial or otherwise.

ACKNOWLEDGEMENTS

Declared none.

REFERENCES

[1]   Kassab E, McFarlane SI, Sower JR. Vascular complications in diabetes and their prevention. Vasc Med 2001; 6(4): 249-55.
[http://dx.doi.org/10.1177/1358836X0100600409] [PMID: 11958392]

[2]   Lovic D, Piperidou A, Zografou I, Grassos H, Pittaras A, Manolis A. The growing epidemic of diabetes mellitus. Curr Vasc Pharmacol 2020; 18(2): 104-9.
[http://dx.doi.org/10.2174/1570161117666190405165911] [PMID: 30961501]

[3]   Chaturvedi N. The burden of diabetes and its complications: trends and implications for intervention. Diabetes Res Clin Pract 2007; 76 (Suppl. 1): S3-S12.
[http://dx.doi.org/10.1016/j.diabres.2007.01.019] [PMID: 17343954]

[4]   Diabetes Mellitus: A Major Risk Factor for Cardiovascular Disease. A Joint Editorial Statement by the American Diabetes Association; the National Heart, Lung, and Blood Institute; the Juvenile Diabetes Foundation International; the National Institute of Diabetes and Digestive and Kidney Diseases; and the American Heart Association 1999; 100(10): 1132-3.

[5]   Wu Y, Ding Y, Tanaka Y, Zhang W. Risk factors contributing to type 2 diabetes and recent advances in the treatment and prevention. Int J Med Sci 2014; 11(11): 1185-200.
        [http://dx.doi.org/10.7150/ijms.10001] [PMID: 25249787]

[6]   Prevention. CfDCa. National Diabetes Statistics Report: Estimates of Diabetes and Its Burden in the United States. US Department of Health and Human Services 2014.

[7]   Braveman PA, Kumanyika S, Fielding J, *et al.* Health disparities and health equity: the issue is justice. Am J Public Health 2011; 101 (Suppl. 1): S149-55.
        [http://dx.doi.org/10.2105/AJPH.2010.300062] [PMID: 21551385]

[8]   Towne SD, Bolin J, Ferdinand A, Nicklett EJ, Smith ML, Ory MG. Assessing diabetes and factors associated with foregoing medical care among persons with diabetes: disparities facing American Indian/Alaska native, black, hispanic, low income, and Southern adults in the U.S. (2011-2015). Int J Environ Res Public Health 2017; 14(5)E464
        [http://dx.doi.org/10.3390/ijerph14050464] [PMID: 28445431]

[9]   Standards of medical care in diabetes-2017: summary of revisions. Diabetes Care 2017; 40 (Suppl. 1): S4-5.
        [http://dx.doi.org/10.2337/dc17-S003] [PMID: 27979887]

[10]   Sanghera DK, Blackett PR. Type 2 diabetes genetics: beyond GWAS. J Diabetes Metab 2012; 3(198): 6948.
        [PMID: 23243555]

[11]   Jia H, Yu L, Jiang Z, Ji Q. Association between IGF2BP2 rs4402960 polymorphism and risk of type 2 diabetes mellitus: a meta-analysis. Arch Med Res 2011; 42(5): 361-7.
        [http://dx.doi.org/10.1016/j.arcmed.2011.08.001] [PMID: 21839790]

[12]   Sladek R, Rocheleau G, Rung J, *et al.* A genome-wide association study identifies novel risk loci for type 2 diabetes. Nature 2007; 445(7130): 881-5.
        [http://dx.doi.org/10.1038/nature05616] [PMID: 17293876]

[13]   Hu FB, Manson JE, Stampfer MJ, *et al.* Diet, lifestyle, and the risk of type 2 diabetes mellitus in women. N Engl J Med 2001; 345(11): 790-7.
        [http://dx.doi.org/10.1056/NEJMoa010492] [PMID: 11556298]

[14]   van Dam RM, Willett WC, Rimm EB, Stampfer MJ, Hu FB. Dietary fat and meat intake in relation to risk of type 2 diabetes in men. Diabetes Care 2002; 25(3): 417-24.
        [http://dx.doi.org/10.2337/diacare.25.3.417] [PMID: 11874924]

[15]   Schulze MB, Manson JE, Ludwig DS, *et al.* Sugar-sweetened beverages, weight gain, and incidence of type 2 diabetes in young and middle-aged women. JAMA 2004; 292(8): 927-34.
        [http://dx.doi.org/10.1001/jama.292.8.927] [PMID: 15328324]

[16]   Pamidi S, Tasali E. Obstructive sleep apnea and type 2 diabetes: is there a link? Front Neurol 2012; 3: 126.
        [http://dx.doi.org/10.3389/fneur.2012.00126] [PMID: 23015803]

[17]   Yoshida M, Booth SL, Meigs JB, Saltzman E, Jacques PF. Phylloquinone intake, insulin sensitivity, and glycemic status in men and women. Am J Clin Nutr 2008; 88(1): 210-5.
        [http://dx.doi.org/10.1093/ajcn/88.1.210] [PMID: 18614743]

[18]   Mathieu C, Badenhoop K. Vitamin D and type 1 diabetes mellitus: state of the art. Trends Endocrinol Metab 2005; 16(6): 261-6.
        [http://dx.doi.org/10.1016/j.tem.2005.06.004] [PMID: 15996876]

[19]   Giulietti A, Gysemans C, Stoffels K, *et al.* Vitamin D deficiency in early life accelerates Type 1 diabetes in non-obese diabetic mice. Diabetologia 2004; 47(3): 451-62.
[http://dx.doi.org/10.1007/s00125-004-1329-3] [PMID: 14758446]

[20]   van Halteren AGS, van Etten E, de Jong EC, Bouillon R, Roep BO, Mathieu C. Redirection of human autoreactive T-cells Upon interaction with dendritic cells modulated by TX527, an analog of 1,25 dihydroxyvitamin D(3). Diabetes 2002; 51(7): 2119-25.
[http://dx.doi.org/10.2337/diabetes.51.7.2119] [PMID: 12086941]

[21]   Mathieu C, Waer M, Laureys J, Rutgeerts O, Bouillon R. Prevention of autoimmune diabetes in NOD mice by 1,25 dihydroxyvitamin D3. Diabetologia 1994; 37(6): 552-8.
[http://dx.doi.org/10.1007/BF00403372] [PMID: 7926338]

[22]   Musso G, Gambino R, Cassader M. Interactions between gut microbiota and host metabolism predisposing to obesity and diabetes. Annu Rev Med 2011; 62: 361-80.
[http://dx.doi.org/10.1146/annurev-med-012510-175505] [PMID: 21226616]

[23]   Farag A, Karam J, Nicasio J, McFarlane SI. Prevention of type 2 diabetes: an update. Curr Diab Rep 2007; 7(3): 200-7.
[http://dx.doi.org/10.1007/s11892-007-0032-4] [PMID: 17547837]

[24]   Pappachan JM, Varughese GI, Sriraman R, Arunagirinathan G. Diabetic cardiomyopathy: Pathophysiology, diagnostic evaluation and management. World J Diabetes 2013; 4(5): 177-89.
[http://dx.doi.org/10.4239/wjd.v4.i5.177] [PMID: 24147202]

[25]   Kannel WB, McGee DL. Diabetes and cardiovascular disease. The Framingham study. JAMA 1979; 241(19): 2035-8.
[http://dx.doi.org/10.1001/jama.1979.03290450033020] [PMID: 430798]

[26]   Nishikawa T, Edelstein D, Du XL, *et al.* Normalizing mitochondrial superoxide production blocks three pathways of hyperglycaemic damage. Nature 2000; 404(6779): 787-90.
[http://dx.doi.org/10.1038/35008121] [PMID: 10783895]

[27]   Cai L, Li W, Wang G, Guo L, Jiang Y, Kang YJ. Hyperglycemia-induced apoptosis in mouse myocardium: mitochondrial cytochrome C-mediated caspase-3 activation pathway. Diabetes 2002; 51(6): 1938-48.
[http://dx.doi.org/10.2337/diabetes.51.6.1938] [PMID: 12031984]

[28]   Petrova R, Yamamoto Y, Muraki K, *et al.* Advanced glycation endproduct-induced calcium handling impairment in mouse cardiac myocytes. J Mol Cell Cardiol 2002; 34(10): 1425-31.
[http://dx.doi.org/10.1006/jmcc.2002.2084] [PMID: 12393002]

[29]   Vigersky RA. An overview of management issues in adult patients with type 2 diabetes mellitus. J Diabetes Sci Technol 2011; 5(2): 245-50.
[http://dx.doi.org/10.1177/193229681100500207] [PMID: 21527089]

[30]   Schoen RE, Weissfeld JL, Kuller LH, *et al.* Insulin-like growth factor-I and insulin are associated with the presence and advancement of adenomatous polyps. Gastroenterology 2005; 129(2): 464-75.
[http://dx.doi.org/10.1016/j.gastro.2005.05.051] [PMID: 16083703]

[31]   Sandhu MS, Dunger DB, Giovannucci EL. Insulin, insulin-like growth factor-I (IGF-I), IGF binding proteins, their biologic interactions, and colorectal cancer. J Natl Cancer Inst 2002; 94(13): 972-80.
[http://dx.doi.org/10.1093/jnci/94.13.972] [PMID: 12096082]

[32]   Giovannucci E, Harlan DM, Archer MC, *et al.* Diabetes and cancer: a consensus report. CA Cancer J Clin 2010; 60(4): 207-21.
[http://dx.doi.org/10.3322/caac.20078] [PMID: 20554718]

[33]   Sima AA. Encephalopathies: the emerging diabetic complications. Acta Diabetol 2010; 47(4): 279-93.
[http://dx.doi.org/10.1007/s00592-010-0218-0] [PMID: 20798963]

[34]   Ergul A, Kelly-Cobbs A, Abdalla M, Fagan SC. Cerebrovascular complications of diabetes: focus on

stroke. Endocr Metab Immune Disord Drug Targets 2012; 12(2): 148-58.
[http://dx.doi.org/10.2174/187153012800493477] [PMID: 22236022]

[35]   Stiles MC, Seaquist ER. Cerebral structural and functional changes in type 1 diabetes. Minerva Med 2010; 101(2): 105-14.
[PMID: 20467409]

[36]   Tomassoni D, Bellagamba G, Postacchini D, Venarucci D, Amenta F. Cerebrovascular and brain microanatomy in spontaneously hypertensive rats with streptozotocin-induced diabetes. Clinical and experimental hypertension (New York, NY : 1993) 2004; 26(4): 305-21.
[http://dx.doi.org/10.1081/CEH-120034136]

[37]   Criqui MH. Peripheral arterial disease--epidemiological aspects. Vascular medicine (London, England) 2001; 6(3 Suppl): 3-7.

[38]   Diabetes Care 2003; 26(12): 3333-41.
[http://dx.doi.org/10.2337/diacare.26.12.3333] [PMID: 14633825]

[39]   Weitz JI, Byrne J, Clagett GP, *et al.* Diagnosis and treatment of chronic arterial insufficiency of the lower extremities: a critical review. Circulation 1996; 94(11): 3026-49.
[http://dx.doi.org/10.1161/01.CIR.94.11.3026] [PMID: 8941154]

[40]   Dormandy JA, Rutherford RB. Management of peripheral arterial disease (PAD). TASC Working Group. TransAtlantic Inter-Society Consensus (TASC). J Vasc Surg 2000; 31(1 Pt 2): S1-S296.
[PMID: 10666287]

[41]   Zatalia SR, Sanusi H. The role of antioxidants in the pathophysiology, complications, and management of diabetes mellitus. Acta Med Indones 2013; 45(2): 141-7.
[PMID: 23770795]

[42]   Fong DS, Aiello L, Gardner TW, *et al.* Retinopathy in diabetes. Diabetes Care 2004; 27 (Suppl. 1): S84-7.
[http://dx.doi.org/10.2337/diacare.27.2007.S84] [PMID: 14693935]

[43]   Toth-Manikowski S, Atta MG. Diabetic Kidney Disease: Pathophysiology and Therapeutic Targets. J Diabetes Res 2015; 2015697010
[http://dx.doi.org/10.1155/2015/697010] [PMID: 26064987]

[44]   Diabetic cardiomyopathy: where we are and where we are going FAU - Lee, Wang-Soo FAU - Kim, Jaetaek. Korean J Intern Med (Korean Assoc Intern Med) 2017; 32(3): 404-21.
[http://dx.doi.org/10.3904/kjim.2016.208]

[45]   Perkovic V, Heerspink HL, Chalmers J, *et al.* Intensive glucose control improves kidney outcomes in patients with type 2 diabetes. Kidney Int 2013; 83(3): 517-23.
[http://dx.doi.org/10.1038/ki.2012.401] [PMID: 23302714]

[46]   Inzucchi SE, Bergenstal RM, Buse JB, Diamant M, Ferrannini E, Nauck M, *et al.* Management of Hyperglycemia in Type 2 Diabetes: A Patient-Centered Approach. Position Statement of the American Diabetes Association (ADA) and the European Association for the Study of Diabetes (EASD) 2012; 35(6): 1364-79.

[47]   Wu M-S, Johnston P, Sheu W-H, *et al.* Effect of metformin on carbohydrate and lipoprotein metabolism in NIDDM patients. Diabetes Care 1990; 13(1): 1-8.
[http://dx.doi.org/10.2337/diacare.13.1.1] [PMID: 2404714]

[48]   United Kingdom Prospective Diabetes Study (UKPDS). 13: Relative efficacy of randomly allocated diet, sulphonylurea, insulin, or metformin in patients with newly diagnosed non-insulin dependent diabetes followed for three years. BMJ 1995; 310(6972): 83-8.
[http://dx.doi.org/10.1136/bmj.310.6972.83] [PMID: 7833731]

[49]   Shaw RJ, Lamia KA, Vasquez D, *et al.* The kinase LKB1 mediates glucose homeostasis in liver and therapeutic effects of metformin. Science 2005; 310(5754): 1642-6.
[http://dx.doi.org/10.1126/science.1120781] [PMID: 16308421]

[50]   Turner RC, Cull CA, Frighi V, Holman RR. Glycemic control with diet, sulfonylurea, metformin, or insulin in patients with type 2 diabetes mellitus: progressive requirement for multiple therapies (UKPDS 49). JAMA 1999; 281(21): 2005-12.
[http://dx.doi.org/10.1001/jama.281.21.2005] [PMID: 10359389]

[51]   Davis TM, Clifford RM, Davis WA. Effect of insulin therapy on quality of life in Type 2 diabetes mellitus: The Fremantle Diabetes Study. Diabetes Res Clin Pract 2001; 52(1): 63-71.
[http://dx.doi.org/10.1016/S0168-8227(00)00245-X] [PMID: 11182217]

[52]   Antoniades C, Tousoulis D, Marinou K, *et al.* Effects of insulin dependence on inflammatory process, thrombotic mechanisms and endothelial function, in patients with type 2 diabetes mellitus and coronary atherosclerosis. Clin Cardiol 2007; 30(6): 295-300.
[http://dx.doi.org/10.1002/clc.20101] [PMID: 17551966]

[53]   Association AD. Standards of medical care in diabetes—2016. Diabetes Care 2016; 39 (Suppl. 1): s1-s106.

[54]   Inzucchi SE, Bergenstal RM, Buse JB, *et al.* Management of hyperglycemia in type 2 diabetes, 2015: a patient-centered approach: update to a position statement of the American Diabetes Association and the European Association for the Study of Diabetes. Diabetes Care 2015; 38(1): 140-9.
[http://dx.doi.org/10.2337/dc14-2441] [PMID: 25538310]

[55]   Belsey J, Krishnarajah G. Glycaemic control and adverse events in patients with type 2 diabetes treated with metformin + sulphonylurea: a meta-analysis. Diabetes Obes Metab 2008; 10 (Suppl. 1): 1-7.
[http://dx.doi.org/10.1111/j.1463-1326.2008.00884.x] [PMID: 18435668]

[56]   Nathan DM, Buse JB, Davidson MB, *et al.* Medical management of hyperglycemia in type 2 diabetes: a consensus algorithm for the initiation and adjustment of therapy: a consensus statement of the American Diabetes Association and the European Association for the Study of Diabetes. Diabetes Care 2009; 32(1): 193-203.
[http://dx.doi.org/10.2337/dc08-9025] [PMID: 18945920]

[57]   Anderson SL, Marrs JC. Dapagliflozin for the treatment of type 2 diabetes. Ann Pharmacother 2012; 46(4): 590-8.
[http://dx.doi.org/10.1345/aph.1Q538] [PMID: 22433611]

[58]   Taskinen MR, Rosenstock J, Tamminen I, *et al.* Safety and efficacy of linagliptin as add-on therapy to metformin in patients with type 2 diabetes: a randomized, double-blind, placebo-controlled study. Diabetes Obes Metab 2011; 13(1): 65-74.
[http://dx.doi.org/10.1111/j.1463-1326.2010.01326.x] [PMID: 21114605]

[59]   Gallwitz B, Rosenstock J, Rauch T, *et al.* 2-year efficacy and safety of linagliptin compared with glimepiride in patients with type 2 diabetes inadequately controlled on metformin: a randomised, double-blind, non-inferiority trial. Lancet 2012; 380(9840): 475-83.
[http://dx.doi.org/10.1016/S0140-6736(12)60691-6] [PMID: 22748821]

[60]   Ekström N, Svensson A-M, Miftaraj M, *et al.* Cardiovascular safety of glucose-lowering agents as add-on medication to metformin treatment in type 2 diabetes: report from the Swedish National Diabetes Register. Diabetes Obes Metab 2016; 18(10): 990-8.
[http://dx.doi.org/10.1111/dom.12704] [PMID: 27282621]

[61]   Zinman B, Wanner C, Lachin JM, *et al.* EMPA-REG outcome investigators. Empagliflozin, cardiovascular outcomes, and mortality in type 2 diabetes. N Engl J Med 2015; 373(22): 2117-28.
[http://dx.doi.org/10.1056/NEJMoa1504720] [PMID: 26378978]

[62]   Roumie CL, Greevy RA, Grijalva CG, *et al.* Association between intensification of metformin treatment with insulin *vs* sulfonylureas and cardiovascular events and all-cause mortality among patients with diabetes. JAMA 2014; 311(22): 2288-96.
[http://dx.doi.org/10.1001/jama.2014.4312] [PMID: 24915260]

[63]   Garber AJ, Abrahamson MJ, Barzilay JI, Blonde L, Bloomgarden ZT, Bush MA, *et al.* Consensus statement by the american association of clinical endocrinologists and american college of endocrinology on the comprehensive type 2 diabetes management algorithm--2016 executive summarY. Endocrine practice : Official Journal of the American College of Endocrinology and the American Association of Clinical Endocrinologists 2016; 22(1): 84-113.

[64]   Amiel SA, Dixon T, Mann R, Jameson K. Hypoglycaemia in Type 2 diabetes. Diabet Med 2008; 25(3): 245-54.
[http://dx.doi.org/10.1111/j.1464-5491.2007.02341.x] [PMID: 18215172]

[65]   Abbatecola AM, Paolisso G, Corsonello A, Bustacchini S, Lattanzio F. Antidiabetic oral treatment in older people: does frailty matter? Drugs Aging 2009; 26 (Suppl. 1): 53-62.
[http://dx.doi.org/10.2165/11534660-000000000-00000] [PMID: 20136169]

[66]   Risk of hypoglycaemia in types 1 and 2 diabetes: effects of treatment modalities and their duration. Diabetologia 2007; 50(6): 1140-7.
[http://dx.doi.org/10.1007/s00125-007-0599-y] [PMID: 17415551]

[67]   Gerich JE. Oral hypoglycemic agents. N Engl J Med 1989; 321(18): 1231-45.
[http://dx.doi.org/10.1056/NEJM198911023211805] [PMID: 2677730]

[68]   Crasto W, Jarvis J, Hackett E, *et al.* Insulin U-500 in severe insulin resistance in type 2 diabetes mellitus. Postgrad Med J 2009; 85(1002): 219-22.
[http://dx.doi.org/10.1136/pgmj.2008.073379] [PMID: 19417173]

[69]   Claxton AJ, Cramer J, Pierce C. A systematic review of the associations between dose regimens and medication compliance. Clin Ther 2001; 23(8): 1296-310.
[http://dx.doi.org/10.1016/S0149-2918(01)80109-0] [PMID: 11558866]

[70]   Rodbard HW, Gough S, Lane W, Korsholm L, Bretler DM, Handelsman Y. Reduced risk of hypoglycemia with insulin degludec *versus* insulin glargine in patients with type 2 diabetes requiring high doses of basal insulin: a meta-analysis of 5 randomized begin trials. Endocrine practice : official journal of the American College of Endocrinology and the American Association of Clinical Endocrinologists 2014; 20(4): 285-92.
[http://dx.doi.org/10.4158/EP13287.OR]

[71]   Lane WS, Cochran EK, Jackson JA, Scism-Bacon JL, Corey IB, Hirsch IB, *et al.* High-dose insulin therapy: is it time for U-500 insulin? Endocrine practice : official journal of the American College of Endocrinology and the American Association of Clinical Endocrinologists 2009; 15(1): 71-9.

[72]   Tim Heise UH. Leszek Nosek, Susanne Bøttcher, Charlotte Granhall, Hanne Haahr. Insulin degludec has a two-fold longer half-life and a more consistent pharmacokinetic profile compared with insulin glargine. Endocrine Absracts 2012; 28: 188.

[73]   Warren ML, Chaykin LB, Jabbour S, Sheikh-Ali M, Hansen CT, Nielsen TSS, *et al.* Insulin Degludec 200 Units/mL Is Associated With Lower Injection Frequency and Improved Patient-Reported Outcomes Compared With Insulin Glargine 100 Units/mL in Patients With Type 2 Diabetes Requiring High-Dose Insulin. Clinical diabetes : a publication of the American Diabetes Association 2017; 35(2): 90-5.

[74]   Peyrot M, Barnett AH, Meneghini LF, Schumm-Draeger PM. Insulin adherence behaviours and barriers in the multinational Global Attitudes of Patients and Physicians in Insulin Therapy study. Diabet Med 2012; 29(5): 682-9.
[http://dx.doi.org/10.1111/j.1464-5491.2012.03605.x] [PMID: 22313123]

[75]   Gough SCL, Bhargava A, Jain R, Mersebach H, Rasmussen S, Bergenstal RM. Low-Volume Insulin Degludec 200 Units/mL Once Daily Improves Glycemic Control Similarly to Insulin Glargine With a Low Risk of Hypoglycemia in Insulin-Naïve Patients With Type 2 Diabetes. A 26-week, randomized, controlled, multinational, treat-to-target trial: The BEGIN LOW VOLUME trial 2013; 36(9): 2536-42.

[76]   Mancini AD, Poitout V. GPR40 agonists for the treatment of type 2 diabetes: life after 'TAKing' a hit.

Diabetes Obes Metab 2015; 17(7): 622-9.
[http://dx.doi.org/10.1111/dom.12442] [PMID: 25604916]

[77]   Tanaka H, Yoshida S, Oshima H, *et al.* Chronic treatment with novel GPR40 agonists improve whole-body glucose metabolism based on the glucose-dependent insulin secretion. J Pharmacol Exp Ther 2013; 346(3): 443-52.
[http://dx.doi.org/10.1124/jpet.113.206466] [PMID: 23853170]

[78]   Bain SC. The clinical development program of lixisenatide: a once-daily glucagon-like Peptide-1 receptor agonist. Diabetes Ther 2014; 5(2): 367-83.
[http://dx.doi.org/10.1007/s13300-014-0073-z] [PMID: 25027491]

[79]   Larsen CM, Faulenbach M, Vaag A, *et al.* Interleukin-1-receptor antagonist in type 2 diabetes mellitus. N Engl J Med 2007; 356(15): 1517-26.
[http://dx.doi.org/10.1056/NEJMoa065213] [PMID: 17429083]

[80]   Carlström M, Larsen FJ, Nyström T, *et al.* Dietary inorganic nitrate reverses features of metabolic syndrome in endothelial nitric oxide synthase-deficient mice. Proc Natl Acad Sci USA 2010; 107(41): 17716-20.
[http://dx.doi.org/10.1073/pnas.1008872107] [PMID: 20876122]

[81]   Ghasemi A, Zahediasl S. Potential therapeutic effects of nitrate/nitrite and type 2 diabetes mellitus. Int J Endocrinol Metab 2013; 11(2): 63-4.
[http://dx.doi.org/10.5812/ijem.9103] [PMID: 23825974]

[82]   Singh VP, Bali A, Singh N, Jaggi AS. Advanced glycation end products and diabetic complications. Korean J Physiol Pharmacol 2014; 18(1): 1-14.
[http://dx.doi.org/10.4196/kjpp.2014.18.1.1] [PMID: 24634591]

[83]   Ceriello A, Testa R. Antioxidant anti-inflammatory treatment in type 2 diabetes. Diabetes Care 2009; 32 (Suppl. 2): S232-6.
[http://dx.doi.org/10.2337/dc09-S316] [PMID: 19875557]

[84]   Heitzer T, Schlinzig T, Krohn K, Meinertz T, Münzel T. Endothelial dysfunction, oxidative stress, and risk of cardiovascular events in patients with coronary artery disease. Circulation 2001; 104(22): 2673-8.
[http://dx.doi.org/10.1161/hc4601.099485] [PMID: 11723017]

[85]   Rahimi R, Nikfar S, Larijani B, Abdollahi M. A review on the role of antioxidants in the management of diabetes and its complications. Biomedicine & pharmacotherapy = Biomedecine & pharmacotherapie 2005; 59(7): 365-73.
[http://dx.doi.org/10.1016/j.biopha.2005.07.002]

[86]   Jia W. Continuous glucose monitoring in China: Then, now and in the future. J Diabetes Investig 2017; 8(1): 3-5.
[http://dx.doi.org/10.1111/jdi.12521] [PMID: 27178651]

[87]   Clarke SF, Foster JR. A history of blood glucose meters and their role in self-monitoring of diabetes mellitus. Br J Biomed Sci 2012; 69(2): 83-93.
[http://dx.doi.org/10.1080/09674845.2012.12002443] [PMID: 22872934]

[88]   Ruan Y, Thabit H, Leelarathna L, *et al.* Variability of Insulin Requirements Over 12 Weeks of Closed-Loop Insulin Delivery in Adults With Type 1 Diabetes. Diabetes Care 2016; 39(5): 830-2.
[http://dx.doi.org/10.2337/dc15-2623] [PMID: 26965717]

[89]   Thabit H, Hovorka R. Coming of age: the artificial pancreas for type 1 diabetes. Diabetologia 2016; 59(9): 1795-805.
[http://dx.doi.org/10.1007/s00125-016-4022-4] [PMID: 27364997]

[90]   Hovorka R. Closed-loop insulin delivery: from bench to clinical practice. Nat Rev Endocrinol 2011; 7(7): 385-95.
[http://dx.doi.org/10.1038/nrendo.2011.32] [PMID: 21343892]

[91]   Hovorka R. Continuous glucose monitoring and closed-loop systems. Diabet Med 2006; 23(1): 1-12.
[http://dx.doi.org/10.1111/j.1464-5491.2005.01672.x] [PMID: 16409558]

[92]   Kumareswaran K, Evans ML, Hovorka R. Closed-loop insulin delivery: towards improved diabetes care. Discov Med 2012; 13(69): 159-70.
[PMID: 22369975]

[93]   Phillip M, Battelino T, Atlas E, *et al.* Nocturnal glucose control with an artificial pancreas at a diabetes camp. N Engl J Med 2013; 368(9): 824-33.
[http://dx.doi.org/10.1056/NEJMoa1206881] [PMID: 23445093]

[94]   Brown SA, Kovatchev BP, Breton MD, *et al.* Multinight "bedside" closed-loop control for patients with type 1 diabetes. Diabetes Technol Ther 2015; 17(3): 203-9.
[http://dx.doi.org/10.1089/dia.2014.0259] [PMID: 25594434]

[95]   Thabit H, Tauschmann M, Allen JM, *et al.* Home Use of an Artificial Beta Cell in Type 1 Diabetes. N Engl J Med 2015; 373(22): 2129-40.
[http://dx.doi.org/10.1056/NEJMoa1509351] [PMID: 26379095]

[96]   Leelarathna L, Dellweg S, Mader JK, *et al.* Day and night home closed-loop insulin delivery in adults with type 1 diabetes: three-center randomized crossover study. Diabetes Care 2014; 37(7): 1931-7.
[http://dx.doi.org/10.2337/dc13-2911] [PMID: 24963110]

[97]   Haidar A, Legault L, Matteau-Pelletier L, *et al.* Outpatient overnight glucose control with dual-hormone artificial pancreas, single-hormone artificial pancreas, or conventional insulin pump therapy in children and adolescents with type 1 diabetes: an open-label, randomised controlled trial. Lancet Diabetes Endocrinol 2015; 3(8): 595-604.
[http://dx.doi.org/10.1016/S2213-8587(15)00141-2] [PMID: 26066705]

[98]   Jones MC. Therapies for diabetes: pramlintide and exenatide. Am Fam Physician 2007; 75(12): 1831-5.
[PMID: 17619527]

[99]   Renukuntla VS, Ramchandani N, Trast J, Cantwell M, Heptulla RA. Role of glucagon-like peptide-1 analogue *versus* amylin as an adjuvant therapy in type 1 diabetes in a closed loop setting with ePID algorithm. J Diabetes Sci Technol 2014; 8(5): 1011-7.
[http://dx.doi.org/10.1177/1932296814542153] [PMID: 25030181]

[100]   Trevitt S, Simpson S, Wood A. Artificial pancreas device systems for the closed-loop control of type 1 diabetes: what systems are in development? J Diabetes Sci Technol 2016; 10(3): 714-23.
[http://dx.doi.org/10.1177/1932296815617968] [PMID: 26589628]

[101]   O'Keeffe DT, Maraka S, Basu A, Keith-Hynes P, Kudva YC. Cybersecurity in artificial pancreas experiments. Diabetes Technol Ther 2015; 17(9): 664-6.
[http://dx.doi.org/10.1089/dia.2014.0328] [PMID: 25923544]

[102]   Hampson FA, Freeman SJ, Ertner J, *et al.* Pancreatic transplantation: surgical technique, normal radiological appearances and complications. Insights Imaging 2010; 1(5-6): 339-47.
[http://dx.doi.org/10.1007/s13244-010-0046-3] [PMID: 22347927]

[103]   Pancreas Transplantation for Patients With Type 1 Diabetes. Diabetes Care 2003; 26(suppl 1): s120-.

[104]   Ojo AO, Meier-Kriesche HU, Hanson JA, *et al.* The impact of simultaneous pancreas-kidney transplantation on long-term patient survival. Transplantation 2001; 71(1): 82-90.
[http://dx.doi.org/10.1097/00007890-200101150-00014] [PMID: 11211201]

[105]   Sutherland DE, Gruessner RW, Dunn DL, *et al.* Lessons learned from more than 1,000 pancreas transplants at a single institution. Ann Surg 2001; 233(4): 463-501.
[http://dx.doi.org/10.1097/00000658-200104000-00003] [PMID: 11303130]

[106]   Lombardo C, Perrone VG, Amorese G, *et al.* Update on pancreatic transplantation on the management of diabetes. Minerva Med 2017; 108(5): 405-18.

[PMID: 28466634]

[107] Tatum JA, Meneveau MO, Brayman KL. Single-donor islet transplantation in type 1 diabetes: patient selection and special considerations. Diabetes Metab Syndr Obes 2017; 10: 73-8.
[http://dx.doi.org/10.2147/DMSO.S105692] [PMID: 28280376]

[108] Sakata N, Hayes P, Tan A, *et al.* MRI assessment of ischemic liver after intraportal islet transplantation. Transplantation 2009; 87(6): 825-30.
[http://dx.doi.org/10.1097/TP.0b013e318199c7d2] [PMID: 19300184]

[109] Ryan EA, Paty BW, Senior PA, *et al.* Five-year follow-up after clinical islet transplantation. Diabetes 2005; 54(7): 2060-9.
[http://dx.doi.org/10.2337/diabetes.54.7.2060] [PMID: 15983207]

[110] Bennet W, Sundberg B, Groth CG, *et al.* Incompatibility between human blood and isolated islets of Langerhans: a finding with implications for clinical intraportal islet transplantation? Diabetes 1999; 48(10): 1907-14.
[http://dx.doi.org/10.2337/diabetes.48.10.1907] [PMID: 10512353]

[111] Wang C, Du X, He S, *et al.* A preclinical evaluation of alternative site for islet allotransplantation. PLoS One 2017; 12(3)e0174505
[http://dx.doi.org/10.1371/journal.pone.0174505] [PMID: 28358858]

[112] Tekin Z, Garfinkel MR, Chon WJ, *et al.* Outcomes of Pancreatic Islet Allotransplantation Using the Edmonton Protocol at the University of Chicago. Transplant Direct 2016; 2(10)e105
[http://dx.doi.org/10.1097/TXD.0000000000000609] [PMID: 27795987]

[113] Chhabra P, Brayman KL. Stem cell therapy to cure type 1 diabetes: from hype to hope. Stem Cells Transl Med 2013; 2(5): 328-36.
[http://dx.doi.org/10.5966/sctm.2012-0116] [PMID: 23572052]

[114] Kroon E, Martinson LA, Kadoya K, *et al.* Pancreatic endoderm derived from human embryonic stem cells generates glucose-responsive insulin-secreting cells *in vivo*. Nat Biotechnol 2008; 26(4): 443-52.
[http://dx.doi.org/10.1038/nbt1393] [PMID: 18288110]

[115] Jeon K, Lim H, Kim JH, *et al.* Differentiation and transplantation of functional pancreatic beta cells generated from induced pluripotent stem cells derived from a type 1 diabetes mouse model. Stem Cells Dev 2012; 21(14): 2642-55.
[http://dx.doi.org/10.1089/scd.2011.0665] [PMID: 22512788]

[116] Couri CE, Oliveira MC, Stracieri AB, *et al.* C-peptide levels and insulin independence following autologous nonmyeloablative hematopoietic stem cell transplantation in newly diagnosed type 1 diabetes mellitus. JAMA 2009; 301(15): 1573-9.
[http://dx.doi.org/10.1001/jama.2009.470] [PMID: 19366777]

[117] Voltarelli JC, Couri CE, Stracieri AB, *et al.* Autologous hematopoietic stem cell transplantation for type 1 diabetes. Ann N Y Acad Sci 2008; 1150: 220-9.
[http://dx.doi.org/10.1196/annals.1447.048] [PMID: 19120300]

[118] Leventhal J, Abecassis M, Miller J, *et al.* Chimerism and tolerance without GVHD or engraftment syndrome in HLA-mismatched combined kidney and hematopoietic stem cell transplantation. Sci Transl Med 2012; 4(124)124ra28
[http://dx.doi.org/10.1126/scitranslmed.3003509] [PMID: 22399264]

[119] Gir P, Oni G, Brown SA, Mojallal A, Rohrich RJ. Human adipose stem cells: current clinical applications. Plast Reconstr Surg 2012; 129(6): 1277-90.
[http://dx.doi.org/10.1097/PRS.0b013e31824ecae6] [PMID: 22634645]

[120] Fan CG, Zhang QJ, Zhou JR. Therapeutic potentials of mesenchymal stem cells derived from human umbilical cord. Stem Cell Rev Rep 2011; 7(1): 195-207.
[http://dx.doi.org/10.1007/s12015-010-9168-8] [PMID: 20676943]

[121] Mizuno H, Tobita M, Uysal AC. Concise review: Adipose-derived stem cells as a novel tool for future

regenerative medicine. Stem Cells 2012; 30(5): 804-10.
[http://dx.doi.org/10.1002/stem.1076] [PMID: 22415904]

[122] Chandra V, Swetha G, Muthyala S, *et al.* Islet-like cell aggregates generated from human adipose tissue derived stem cells ameliorate experimental diabetes in mice. PLoS One 2011; 6(6)e20615
[http://dx.doi.org/10.1371/journal.pone.0020615] [PMID: 21687731]

[123] Li G, Zhang P, Wang J, *et al.* The long-term effect of lifestyle interventions to prevent diabetes in the China Da Qing Diabetes Prevention Study: a 20-year follow-up study. Lancet 2008; 371(9626): 1783-9.
[http://dx.doi.org/10.1016/S0140-6736(08)60766-7] [PMID: 18502303]

[124] The Diabetes Prevention Program (DPP): description of lifestyle intervention. Diabetes Care 2002; 25(12): 2165-71.
[http://dx.doi.org/10.2337/diacare.25.12.2165] [PMID: 12453955]

[125] Salas-Salvadó J, Bulló M, Babio N, *et al.* Reduction in the incidence of type 2 diabetes with the Mediterranean diet: results of the PREDIMED-Reus nutrition intervention randomized trial. Diabetes Care 2011; 34(1): 14-9.
[http://dx.doi.org/10.2337/dc10-1288] [PMID: 20929998]

[126] Knowler WC, Barrett-Connor E, Fowler SE, *et al.* Reduction in the incidence of type 2 diabetes with lifestyle intervention or metformin. N Engl J Med 2002; 346(6): 393-403.
[http://dx.doi.org/10.1056/NEJMoa012512] [PMID: 11832527]

[127] Devlin JT. Effects of exercise on insulin sensitivity in humans. Diabetes Care 1992; 15(11): 1690-3.
[http://dx.doi.org/10.2337/diacare.15.11.1690] [PMID: 1468302]

[128] Jeon CY, Lokken RP, Hu FB, van Dam RM. Physical activity of moderate intensity and risk of type 2 diabetes: a systematic review. Diabetes Care 2007; 30(3): 744-52.
[http://dx.doi.org/10.2337/dc06-1842] [PMID: 17327354]

[129] Tuomilehto J, Lindström J, Eriksson JG, *et al.* Prevention of type 2 diabetes mellitus by changes in lifestyle among subjects with impaired glucose tolerance. N Engl J Med 2001; 344(18): 1343-50.
[http://dx.doi.org/10.1056/NEJM200105033441801] [PMID: 11333990]

[130] M S. Clinical perspectives on motivational interviewing in diabetes care. Diabetes Spectr 2011; 24(3): 179-81.
[http://dx.doi.org/10.2337/diaspect.24.3.179]

[131] Thepwongsa I, Muthukumar R, Kessomboon P. Motivational interviewing by general practitioners for Type 2 diabetes patients: a systematic review. Fam Pract 2017; 34(4): 376-83.
[http://dx.doi.org/10.1093/fampra/cmx045] [PMID: 28486622]

[132] Walker CL, Kopp M, Binford RM, Bowers CJ. Home telehealth interventions for older adults with diabetes. Home Healthc Now 2017; 35(4): 202-10.
[http://dx.doi.org/10.1097/NHH.0000000000000522] [PMID: 28353510]

CHAPTER 3

Blurred Vision in the Diabetic Patient – Reversible and Non-reversible Causes – General Classification of Diabetic Eye Disease

Rony Gelman*

Department of Ophthalmology, State University of New York, Downstate Medical Center, NY, USA

Abstract: In this chapter, we review the established classification system of diabetic retinopathy and diabetic macular edema. Reversible and non-reversible causes of vision loss in diabetic patients are discussed with illustrative clinical examples.

Keywords: Diabetic retinopathy, Epiretinal membrane, Macular edema, Macular ischemia, Neovascular glaucoma, Tractional retinal detachment, Vitreomacular traction.

INTRODUCTION

Diabetic eye disease may be characterized by the location of involvement within the eye, specifically the anterior or posterior segment. Anterior segment changes may involve the cornea, aqueous fluid drainage angle, or the natural crystalline lens, resulting in poor corneal epithelial wound healing, neovascular glaucoma (NVG), or cataract formation, respectively.

Certain causes of vision loss due to anterior segment changes may be reversible, assuming no concomitant irreversible posterior segment damage. Cataract secondary to diabetes mellitus (DM), for example, maybe successfully treated with surgery. On the other hand, certain anterior segment changes may result in irreversible vision loss. NVG, for example, is due to occlusion of the trabecular meshwork from angle neovascularization and may lead to irreversible optic neuropathy and vision loss despite treatment with glaucoma filtration surgery [1].

Diabetic eye disease involving the anterior segment is fully discussed in chapters 5 ("Diabetes and the Cornea") and 6 ("Diabetes, Cataract, and Glaucoma"). In this

* **Corresponding author Rony Gelman:** Department of Ophthalmology, State University of New York, Downstate Medical Center, NY, USA; E-mail: rony.gelman@downstate.edu

Douglas R. Lazzaro and Samy I. McFarlane (Eds.)

chapter, we review the classification system of diabetic retinopathy and focus on reversible and non-reversible causes of vision loss secondary to involvement of the posterior segment.

CLASSIFICATION SYSTEM

Diabetic eye disease involving the posterior segment may be classified based on structural changes observed on clinical examination, fluorescein angiography, and optical coherence tomography (OCT). A well-established classification system divides diabetic retinopathy into non-proliferative diabetic retinopathy (NPDR) and proliferative diabetic retinopathy (PDR) [2].

NPDR is characterized by vascular changes confined to the intraretinal space: microaneurysms, dilation of retinal venules, intraretinal hemorrhages, and cotton-wool spots, which are vascular infarctions at the level of the retinal nerve fiber layer. A severity scale subdivides NPDR into mild, moderate, and severe forms. Mild NPDR includes microaneurysms only, while moderate NPDR is characterized by more than solely microaneurysms but less severe changes than seen in severe NPDR. Severe NPDR is classically described as following the "4-2-1" rule, where presence of any of the following indicates severe NPDR: severe intraretinal hemorrhages and microaneurysms in each of the four quadrants of the retina, beading of the retinal venous blood vessels in two or more quadrants, or a prominent intraretinal microvascular abnormality (IRMA) in one or more quadrant. If two or more characteristics of severe NPDR are present, then it is characterized as very severe NPDR.

Progression of diabetic retinopathy from NPDR leads to PDR. Neovascularization is the hallmark of PDR and may occur at the optic disc (neovascularization of the disc [NVD]) or elsewhere on the retinal surface (neovascularization elsewhere [NVE]). A severity scale subdivides PDR into an early non-high risk and a high-risk form. Early PDR is defined by the presence of neovascularization that does not meet high-risk PDR criteria.

Criteria for high-risk PDR include any of the following: neovascularization on or within one disc diameter of the optic disc measuring about one-quarter to one-third of the disc area with preretinal or vitreous hemorrhage, any NVD with preretinal or vitreous hemorrhage, or NVE at least one-quarter of disc area with preretinal or vitreous hemorrhage.

Lastly, diabetic retinopathy at any stage may lead to increased vascular permeability, resulting in retinal edema and intra-retinal deposition of lipids in the form of hard exudates (HE). A classification system of diabetic macular edema (DME) based on the location of edema and HE deposits subdivides macular edema into clinically significant macular edema (CSME) and non-CSME [2]. CSME is defined as presence of any of the following detected by biomicroscopic examination or stereoscopic fundus photography: thickening of the retina within 500 microns of the macular center, deposition of HE at or within 500 microns of the macular center with associated thickening of the adjacent retina, or retinal thickening measuring at least one disc area in size that is at least partly within one disc diameter of the macular center.

Spectral-domain OCT (SD-OCT) is a novel imaging modality that has supplemented clinical examination for the detection and monitoring of macular edema [3]. The use of OCT to study diabetic eye disease is fully discussed in chapter 7 ("OCT and fluorescein findings in the diabetic patient"). OCT enables the accurate detection of and quantitative measurements of center-involving DME (ci-DME) and its progression, which has been critical in anti-VEGF treatment strategies, established by several pivotal randomized clinical trials [4 - 6]. These are discussed further in chapters 8 and 10.

REVERSIBLE AND NON-REVERSIBLE CAUSES OF VISION LOSS IN DIABETIC RETINOPATHY

Reversible posterior segment causes of vision loss include DME, non-clearing vitreous hemorrhage (NCVH), vitreomacular traction (VMT) and epiretinal membrane (ERM), and tractional retinal detachment (TRD) without macular detachment. Non-reversible causes of vision loss include chronic DME, DME complicated by subfoveal HE or fibrosis, advanced TRD with the detachment of the macula, TRD complicated by rhegmatogenous retinal detachment (RRD), macular ischemia, and NVG. We discuss these etiologies with illustrative examples in the sections to follow.

Diabetic Macular Edema

DME is a spectrum of disease and clinically may present in mild, moderate or severe forms [2]. OCT enables precise quantitative metrics to assess the degree of DME.

Mild DME may present as mild thickening or cystic changes that maybe only appreciated by OCT with minimal to no effect on vision. Fig. (1) shows a patient with mild cystic changes on OCT and no visual complaints with 20/30 vision. Mild DME in such cases may cause minimal to no vision loss and may resolve after improvement of glycemic control.

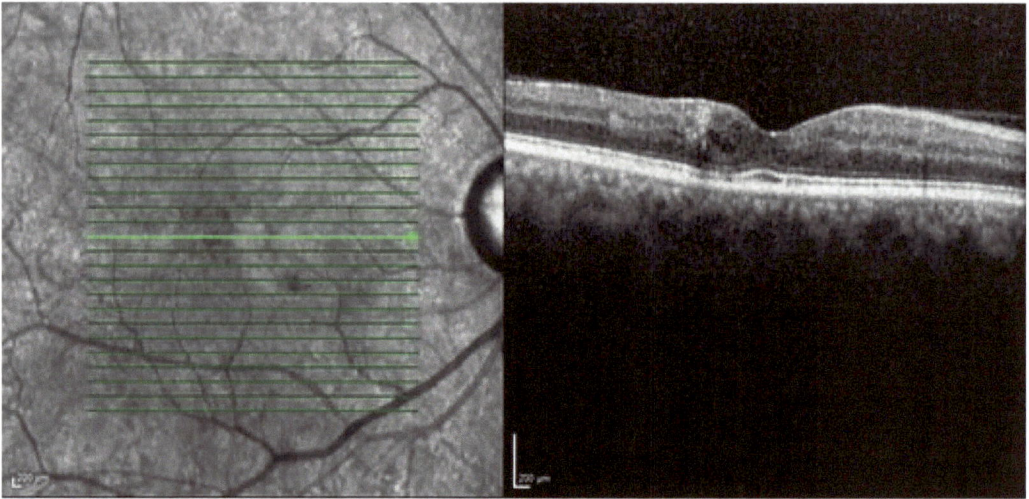

Fig. (1). SD-OCT of the right eye from a patient with type II DM showing mild parafoveal macular edema and microaneurysms. The patient was asymptomatic and vision was 20/30.

However, if systemic glycemic and lipid control worsens, DME may cause vision loss. Fig. (**2**) illustrates a case of CSME with macular thickening and HE deposition. FA and OCT (Figs. **3** and **4**) confirm the presence of DME. If attempts to optimize glycemic control fail, treatment options such as focal laser photocoagulation, intravitreal anti-VEGF agents, or intravitreal steroid injections or implants may improve the DME [4 - 9]. Fig. (**4**) illustrates improvement of ci-DME following intravitreal bevacizumab and intravitreal dexamethasone implant treatment.

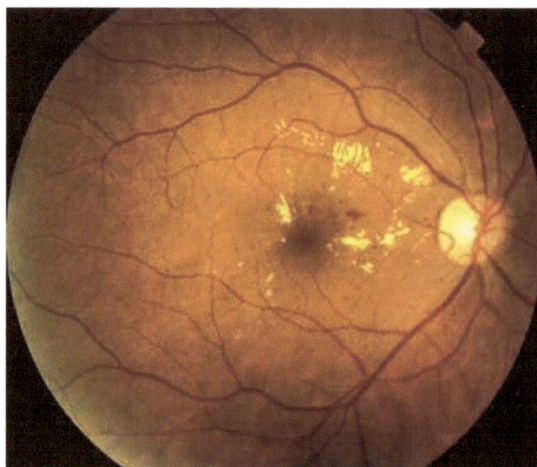

Fig. (2). Color fundus photograph of the right eye from a patient with poorly controlled DM and hyperlipidemia showing intra-retinal hard exudate deposition and macular edema consistent with CSME.

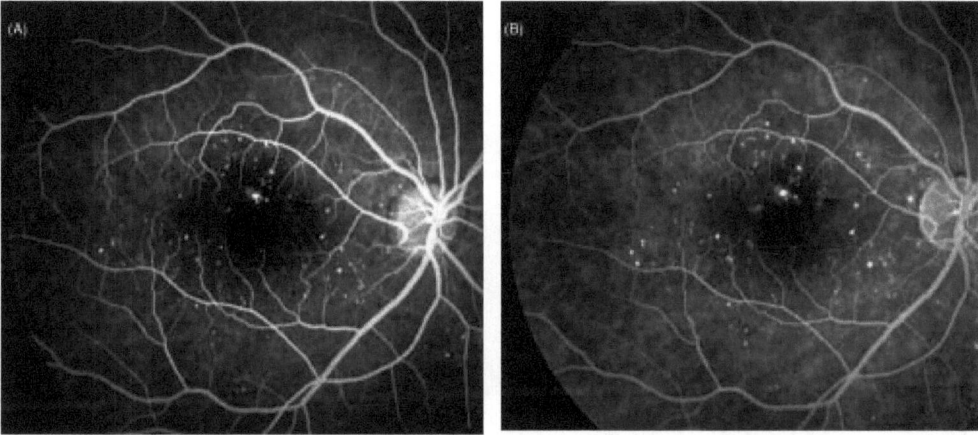

Fig. (3). Fluorescein angiogram from the same patient in Fig. (**2**) showing progressive leakage of microanuerysms from early (**a**) to late (**b**) frames of the study, indicating the presence of DME.

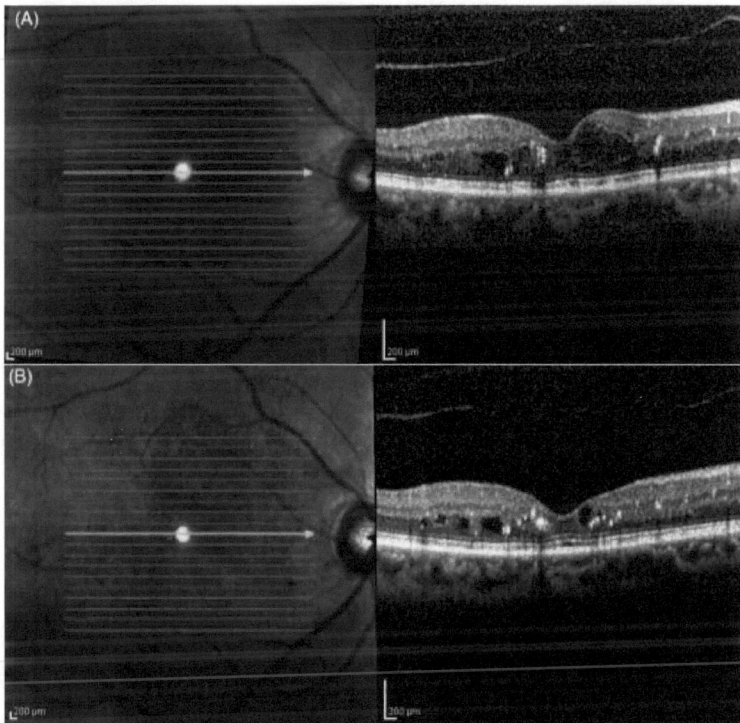

Fig. (4). OCT scans centered on the fovea (horizontal green arrow) from the same patient in Fig. (**2**). (**a**) At baseline ci-DME is present with intraretinal HE. (**b**) After several treatments with intravitreal bevacizumab injections and an intravitreal dexamethasone implant, there is an improvement of DME. Visual acuity improved from 20/70 to 20/40.

Moderate to severe cases of ci-DME that are chronic in duration may have minimal improvement of anatomic alterations assessed by OCT or to functional loss assessed by visual acuity. The patient in Fig. (**5**) presented with chronic CSME not responsive to prior focal laser treatment. FA (Fig. **6**) confirmed DME and NPDR changes, and SD-OCT (Fig. **7**) showed minimal improvement of the ci-DME after intravitreal anti-VEGF therapy.

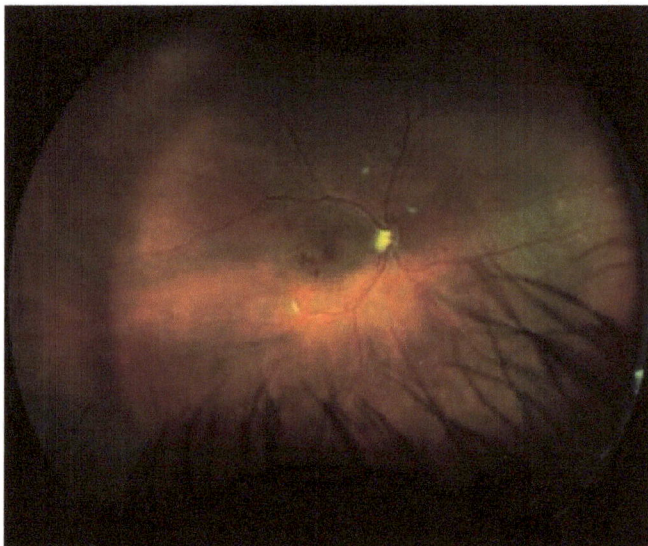

Fig. (5). Wide field Optos photograph of a patient with poorly controlled DM with CSME and severe NPDR. Shown are macular thickening, cotton wool spots, and intraretinal hemorrhage in the macula and all 4 quadrants. The patient had prior focal laser treatment.

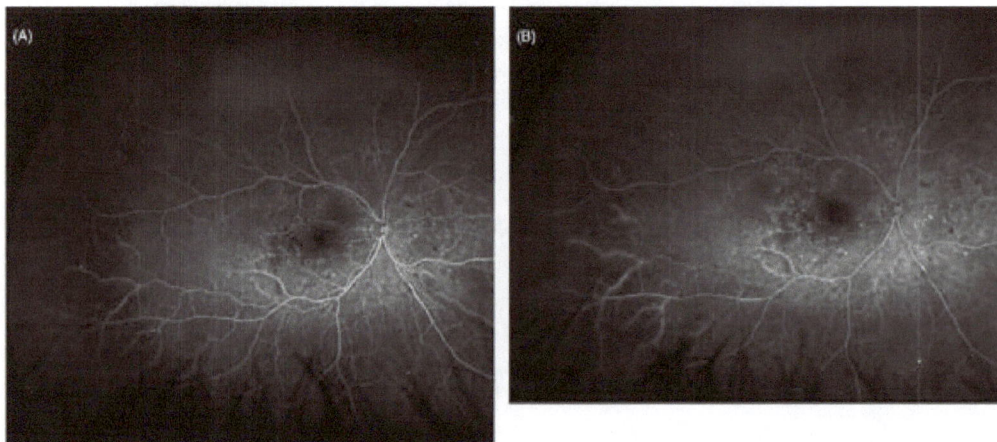

Fig. (6). Optos fluorescein angiogram from the same patient in Fig. (**6**) showing progressive leakage of microanuerysms from early (**a**) to late (**b**) frames of the study, indicating the presence of DME. Also present is an enlarged foveal avascular zone and staining of retinal venules. Staining of focal laser scars is present.

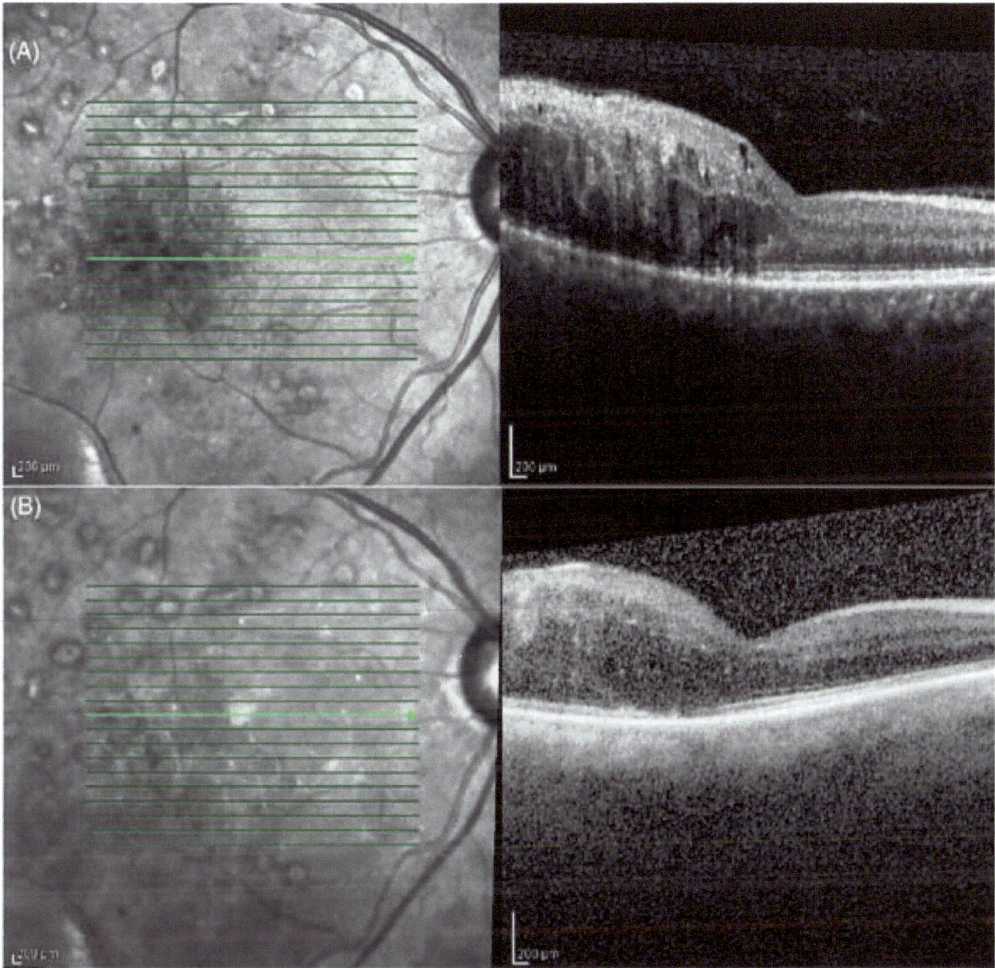

Fig. (7). OCT scans centered on the fovea (horizontal green arrow) from the same patient in Fig. (**5**). (**a**) At baseline ci-DME is present with HE. (**b**) After several treatments with intravitreal bevacizumab, and aflibercept, there is modest improvement of DME. Visual acuity improved from 20/50 to 20/40.

Very severe cases of CSME may fail all treatment modalities due to chronicity, or may altogether be poor candidates for treatment due to subfoveal HE deposits and/or fibrosis. Fig. (**8**) illustrates a patient with CSME with a circinate ring of HE complicated by subfoveal deposition. FA (Fig. **9**) shows damage to the foveal center and SD-OCT (Fig. **10**) clearly shows the disruption of retinal architecture due to the subfoveal HE. Although DME is present, this patient is a poor candidate for laser or pharmacologic therapy and vision loss is likely non-reversible.

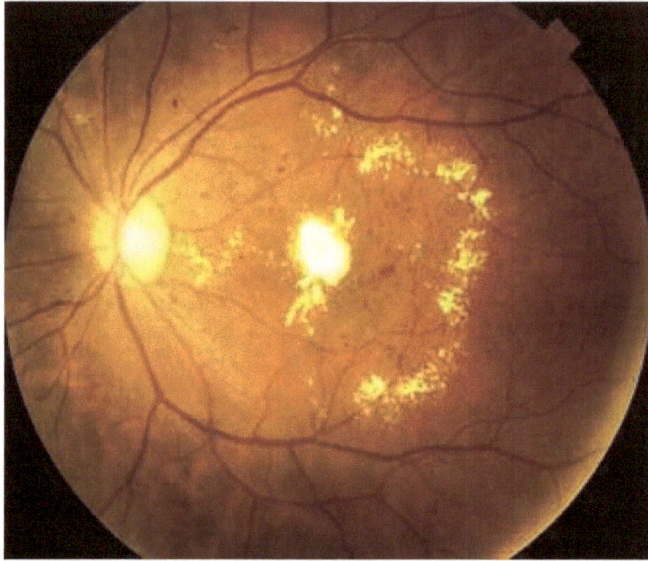

Fig. (8). Color fundus photograph of the left eye of a patient with poorly controlled DM and hyperlipidemia showing severe intra-retinal hard exudate deposition concentrated in the foveal center and macular edema consistent with CSME. Visual acuity was 20/800.

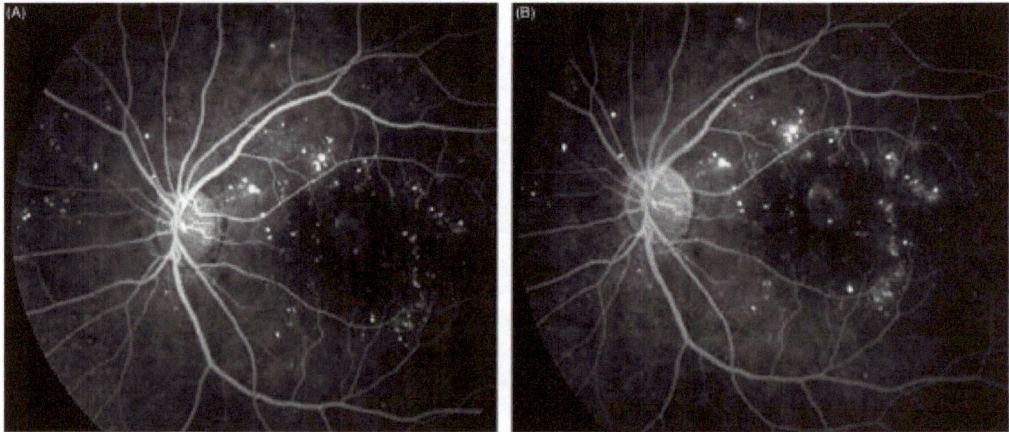

Fig. (9). Fluorescein angiogram from the same patient in Fig. (8) showing progressive leakage of microanuerysms from early **(a)** to late **(b)** frames of the study, indicating the presence of DME. There is also staining of the central hard exudates with capillary dropout and damage to the foveal avascular zone.

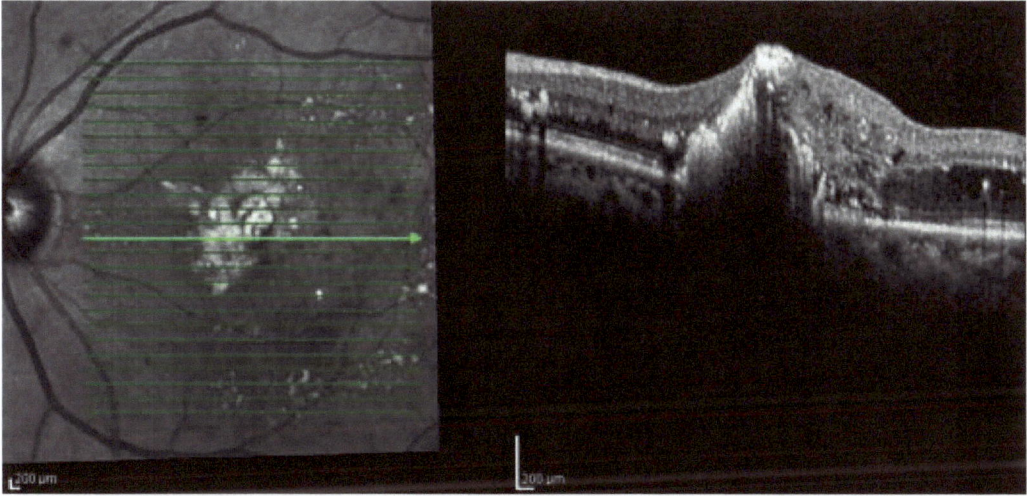

Fig. (10). SD-OCT scan centered on the fovea (horizontal green arrow) from the same patient in Fig. (**8**). There is a severe disruption of all retinal layers due to the subfoveal deposition of hard exudate.

Complications from Proliferative Diabetic Retinopathy

PDR can result in vitreous hemorrhage, which may lead to sudden and severe vision loss. A vitreous hemorrhage may not resolve with observation, and the resulting NCVH may require vitrectomy surgery. The risk of vision loss from NCVH may be reduced by application of pan-retinal laser photocoagulation treatment (PRP) once high-risk PDR develops [10], or at physician discretion at lower than high-risk PDR threshold if other factors indicate treatment. Fig. (**11**) shows wide field imaging of a 29-year-old patient with poorly controlled type I DM. Although the patient had no visual complaints and vision was 20/20 in both eyes, wide-field FA (Fig. **12**) showed extensive retinal ischemia and multiple points of NVE. The patient had a history of poor medical compliance and extensive loss to follow-up, and therefore recommendation was made to undergo PRP treatment to minimize risk of possibly non-reversible vision loss.

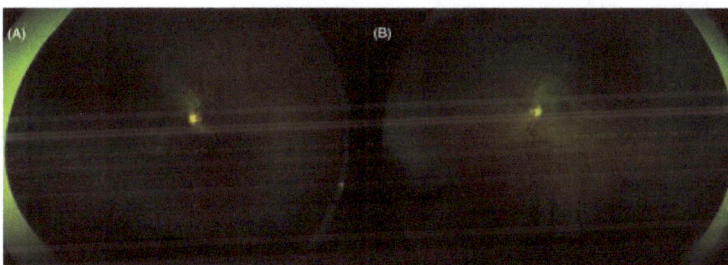

Fig. (11). Wide field Optos photographs of (**a**) right and (**b**) left eyes of a 29-year-old patient with poorly controlled type I DM. No DME is present but peripheral retinal ischemia and multiple points of NVE are seen in both eyes consistent with PDR.

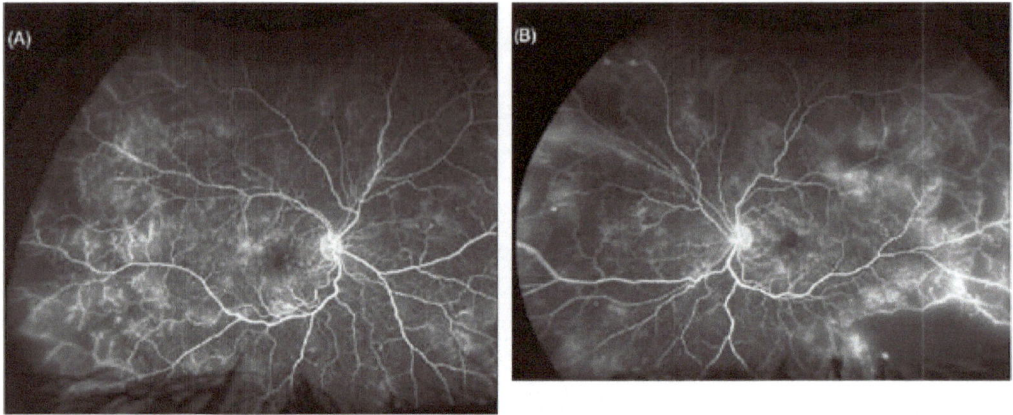

Fig. (12). Optos fluorescein angiogram of the **(a)** right and **(b)** left eyes from the same patient in Fig. **(11)** showing PDR with extensive peripheral retinal ischemia.

Another complication of high-risk PDR is fibrovascular membrane proliferation, which may progress to TRD and ultimately irreversible vision loss if not treated. Prompt treatment with PRP before macular detachment ensues from traction may halt the proliferative process and stabilize vision. An example is illustrated in Fig. **(13)** of a patient with poorly controlled DM who received PRP laser treatment in both eyes for high-risk PDR. Although FA (Fig. **14**) shows extensive peripheral ischemia, the tractional membrane proliferation ceased after laser treatment and vision remained stable during several years of follow up.

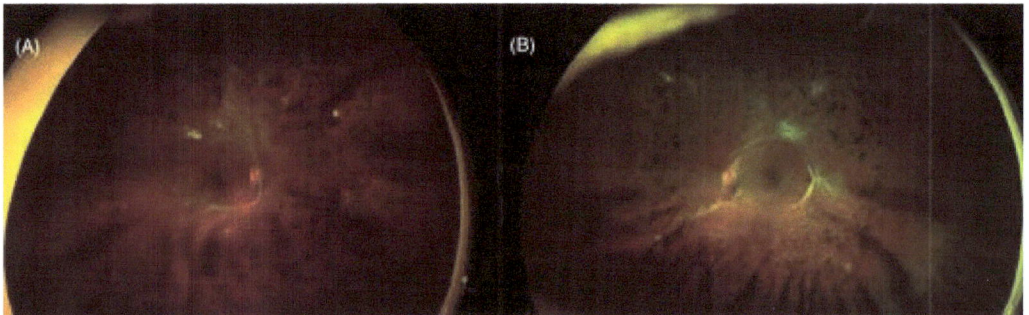

Fig. (13). Wide field Optos photographs of **(a)** right and **(b)** left eyes of a patient with poorly controlled DM. The patient received dense PRP treatment in both eyes for high-risk PDR. Noted in both eyes are tractional membranes emanating from the optic nerves with proliferation along the arcades into the temporal macular regions. After PRP treatment, the fibrovascular membrane proliferation halted and the traction and visual acuity remained stable for several years.

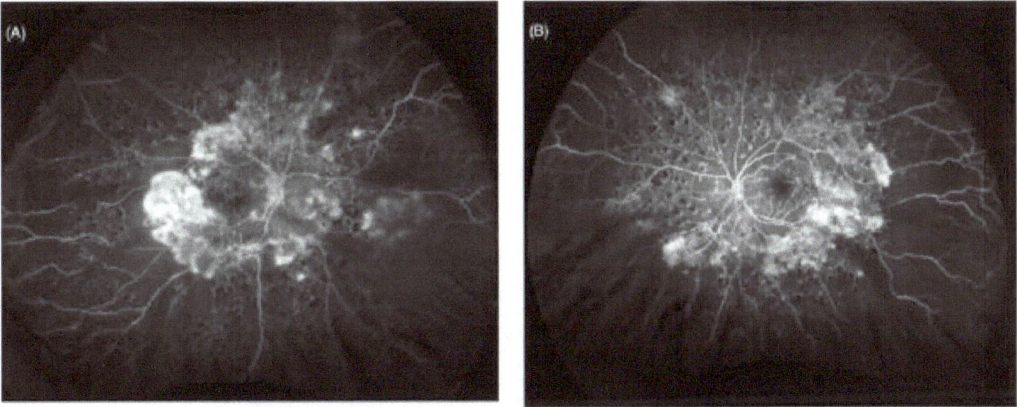

Fig. (14). Wide field Optos fluorescein angiogram of **(a)** right and **(b)** left eyes of the patient from Fig. (13) showing staining of the fibrovascular membranes, peripheral retinal ischemia, and PRP laser scars in both eyes.

A not uncommon clinical finding in patients with newly diagnosed PDR is that of asymmetric vision loss. Fig. **(15)** shows two examples of poorly controlled diabetic patients who presented after irreversible vision loss developed in their left eyes from macular ischemia and NVG. PRP laser treatment stabilized PDR disease in the left eyes in anticipation of vitrectomy, while PRP prevented vision loss from high-risk PDR in their right eyes.

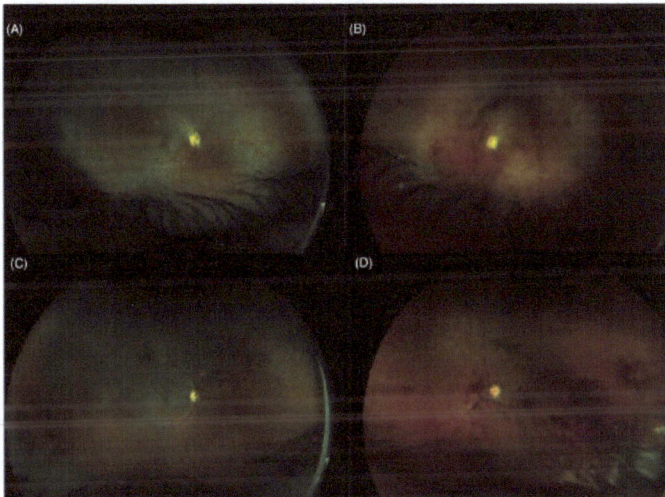

Fig. (15). Wide field Optos photographs of two patients with poorly controlled DM and PDR. Patient #1: **(a)** right eye showed regressed PDR after PRP treatment and **(b)** left eye showed stabilization of VH and NVG following PRP. Patient #2: similar to the patient #1, this patient's PDR in the right eye was stabilized following PRP treatment (c), while PRP stabilized the VH and NVG in the left eye (d) in anticipation for vitrectomy surgery.

Prompt treatment with PRP is especially critical in monocular patients, who sustained irreversible vision loss from diabetic eye disease in one eye. The patient in Fig. (**16**) previously lost vision to no light perception level in his right eye from TRD and NVG secondary to PDR. He presented with active PDR in his left eye, which was stabilized with PRP treatment and retained useful vision, although there was moderate irreversible visual impairment from macular ischemia (Fig. **17**).

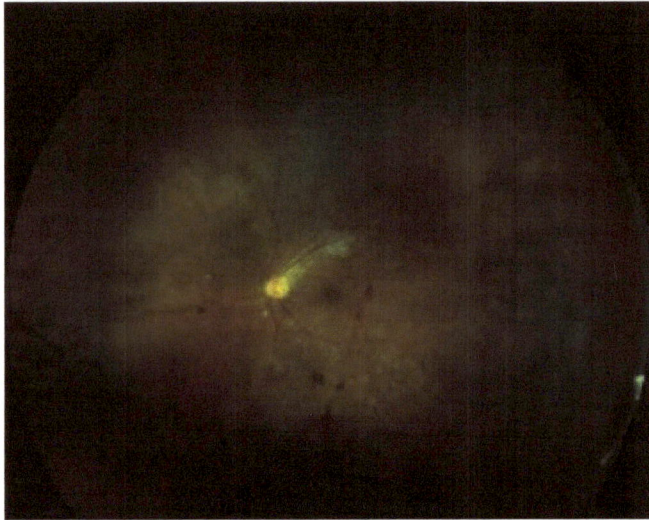

Fig. (16). Wide field Optos photograph of the left eye from a monocular patient with poorly controlled DM and PDR, stabilized after PRP treatment. Vision in the right eye was completely lost from TRD and NVG.

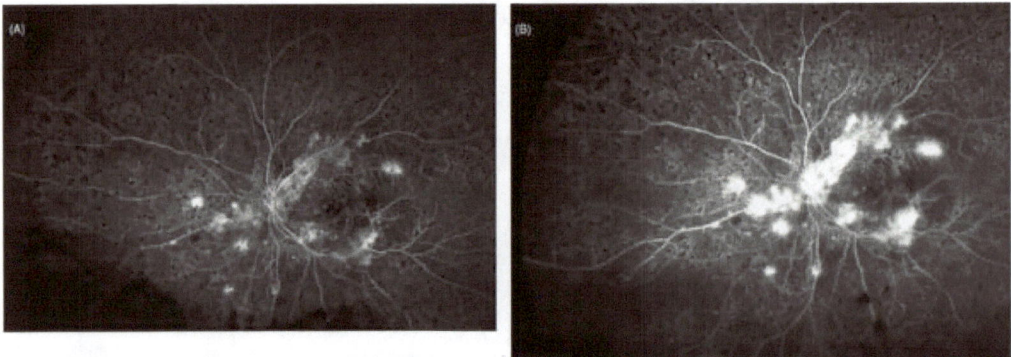

Fig. (17). Wide field Optos fluorescein angiogram of the patient from Fig. (**16**). (**a**) Early and (**b**) late frames show leakage from fibrovascular proliferation along the vascular arcades and peripheral NVE. There is also marked ischemia of the macula and peripheral retina. PRP laser treatment stabilized the PDR and vision remained stable, but limited to 20/100 due to macular ischemia.

Further complication from PDR is fibrovascular proliferation causing anterior-to-posterior vitreoretinal traction, ultimately resulting in a TRD. The TRD may be complicated by progressive traction resulting in a retinal tear or retinal hole, leading to a combined TRD and RRD. Visual prognosis in such cases is invariably poor and reversibility of vision loss after retinal surgery is usually unlikely due to the severe underlying retinal pathology.

TRD located outside of the macula (extramacular) may have little or no visual impact and may be monitored closely if adequate PRP treatment halts the proliferative process. Cases of TRD with limited visualization secondary to NCVH may require vitrectomy surgery. Ultimate visual outcome and reversibility of visual loss following vitrectomy depends on several factors: (1) the extent of TRD involvement, specifically extramacular *vs.* extension of involvement resulting in macular detachment; (2) degree of macular ischemia, which may cause irreversible vision loss; and (3) concomitant or post-surgical CME. Fig. (**18**) shows a case of a 36-year-old patient with poorly controlled DM, who received PRP treatment, but progressed to NCVH and extramacular TRD. Following vitrectomy surgery with membrane peeling and endolaser, the VH was removed, tractional membrane forces were relieved and vision improved from 20/400 preoperatively to 20/25 postoperatively.

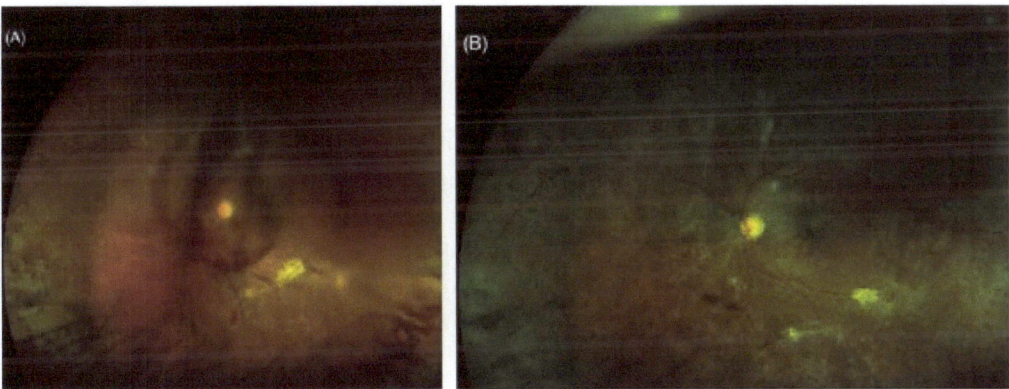

Fig. (18). Wide field Optos photographs of **(a)** left eye from a patient with poorly controlled DM and PDR, NCVH and TRD threatening to detach the macula, despite prior PRP treatment. Visual acuity was 20/400. **(b)** After pars plana vitrectomy with membrane peeling and endolaser, the VH was removed, tractional membranes were isolated, and fill in laser treatment was completed. Visual acuity improved to 20/25.

Synchysis scintillans, sometimes referred to as cholesterolosis bulbi, is an opacification of the vitreous which may occur after chronic VH and is due to deposition of cholesterol crystals within liquefied vitreous. Vision can be variably affected and vision loss is usually reversible after vitrectomy assuming no other concomitant sources for irreversible vision loss. Fig. (**19**) shows an example of a patient with long-standing DM who was found to have crystalline deposits in the vitreous, consistent with synchysis scintillans. The patient was visually asymptomatic with the acuity of 20/50. These deposits obscured clinical fundus examination, but wide-field FA clearly demonstrated PDR with extensive peripheral ischemia (Fig. **19**).

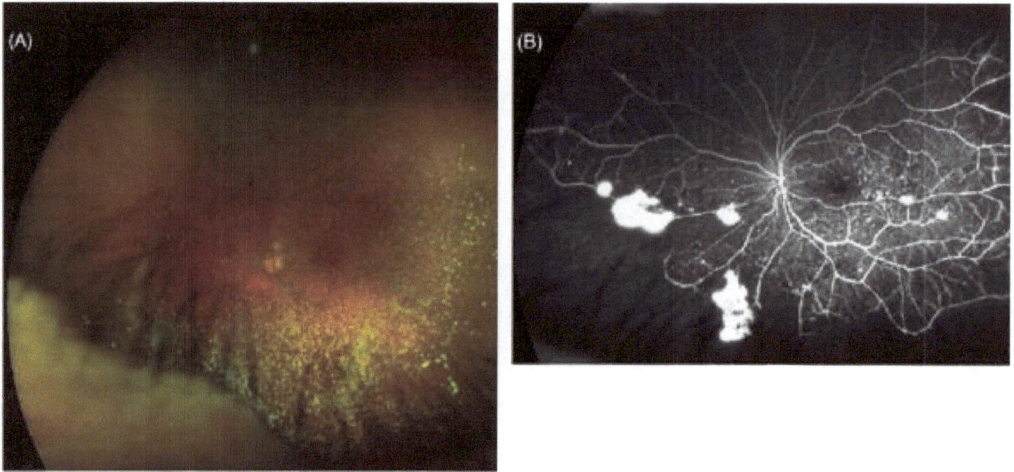

Fig. (19). Wide field Optos imaging of **(a)** left eye from a patient with poorly controlled DM and PDR. Crystalline deposits from synchysis scintillans scattered throughout the vitreous interfered with clear visualization of the retina. **(b)** Fluorescein angiography helped to clearly visualize severe peripheral retinal ischemia with multiple points of NVE.

Macular ischemia is an etiology of irreversible vision loss in diabetic patients, however, the vision loss can be variable depending on the extent of ischemia. Common features across the spectrum of macular ischemia are capillary dropout and increased size of the foveal avascular zone detected by FA. Fig. (**17**) illustrated an FA from a diabetic patient with moderate vision loss from macular ischemia, while in Fig. (**20**) we see a patient with severe macular ischemia causing profound blindness.

PDR is an etiology for NVG, which is an optic neuropathy that clinically exhibits cupping and pallor of the optic nerve (Fig. **21**). NVG is fully discussed in chapter 6 ("Diabetes, Cataract, and Glaucoma"), we briefly highlight NVG in this section as an etiology for variable irreversible vision loss, which may range from peripheral visual field defects to loss of central fixation and blindness with advanced disease. An example of optic disc changes from NVG is shown in Fig. (**21**).

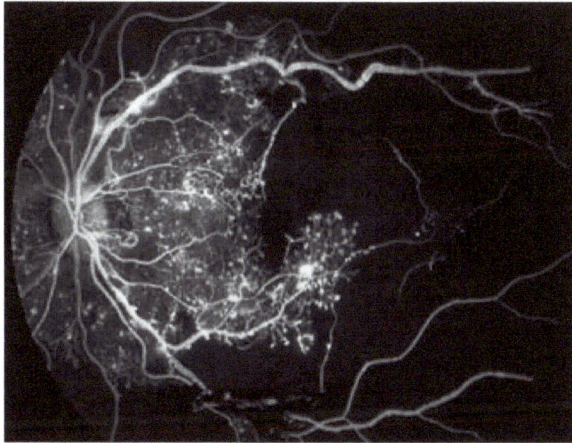

Fig. (20). An example of severe macular ischemia. Shown is a FA from a patient with poorly controlled DM and profound vision loss reduced to the ability to only count fingers at one foot.

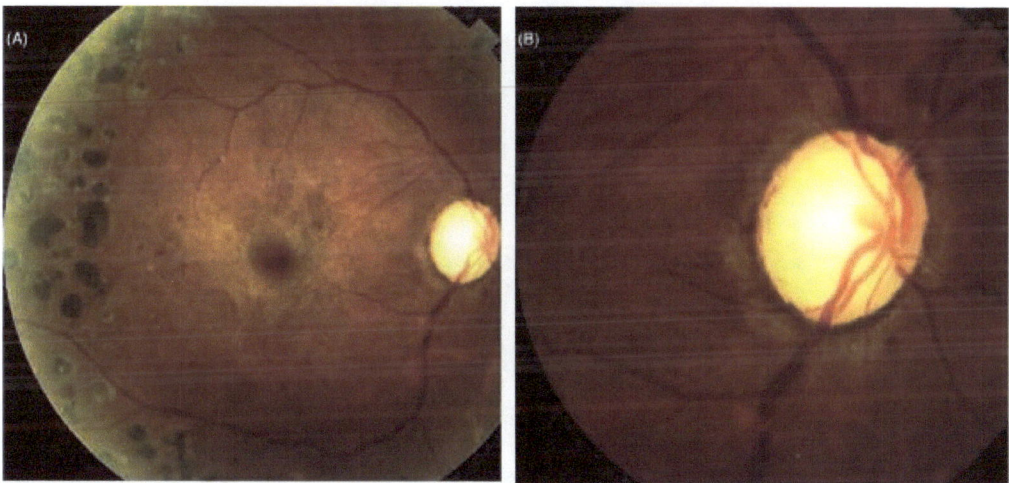

Fig. (21). An example of NVG secondary to PDR in a patient with poorly controlled DM. **(a)** Color fundus photograph shows marked optic nerve cupping and pallor, macular ischemia with an epiretinal membrane and PRP laser scars. **(b)** Higher magnification photograph of the optic nerve details the extensive cupping and pallor.

Vitreomacular Traction and Epiretinal Membrane

NCVH caused by PDR may induce formation of an epiretinal membrane (ERM), which is a sheet of fibrous tissue covering the macular surface. ERM can be mild and have no effect on vision or visual symptoms, or can cause macular pucker, which may reduce vision and cause metamorphopsia. SD-OCT has greatly enhanced our understanding of the morphology and progression of vitreomacular traction and tractional detachments in patients with diabetic retinopathy [11].

Mild cases of ERM may be observed, while moderate to severe cases can be treated surgically with vitrectomy and membrane peeling maneuvers. Metamorphosia usually improves after surgery, while visual improvement will depend on presence of concomitant irreversible causes of vision loss, such as macular ischemia. Fig. (**22**) illustrates an example of severe ERM with macular pucker induced by NCVH from PDR, with the recovery of vision and improvement of metamorphopsia after vitrectomy with membrane peeling surgery.

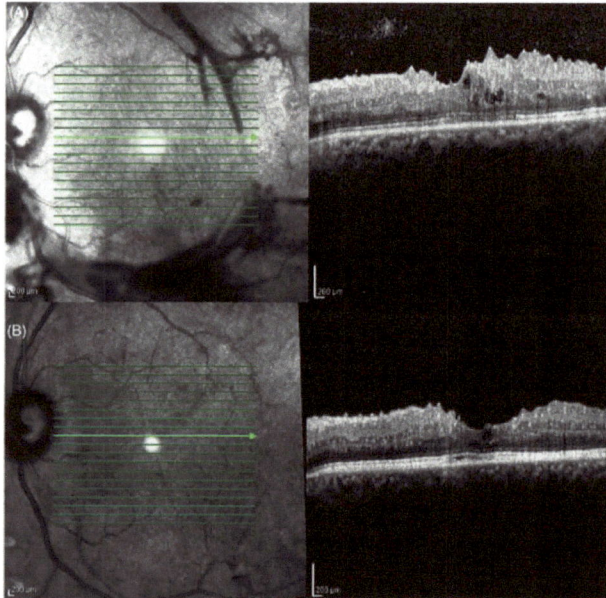

Fig. (22). SD-OCT scans centered on the fovea (horizontal green arrows) of the left eye from a patient with poorly controlled DM. **(a)** Vitreous hemorrhage is present with mild CME and a severe ERM resulting in macular pucker. **(b)** After vitrectomy with membrane peeling, the macular pucker improved and vision improved from 20/200 to 20/60.

VMT can cause severe vision loss that may be limited in recovery if traction causes detachment of the macula. Surgical intervention is invariably required [12] and recovery of vision after surgery will depend on: (1) the chronicity and severity of the TRD; (2) if the retinal detachment was exacerbated by a rhegmatogenous component; and (3) the severity of macular ischemia. Fig. (**23**) illustrates a case of a poorly controlled diabetic with a history of extensive loss to follow up, which resulted in a TRD that detached the macula. Despite anatomically successful surgery, there was some irreversible vision loss secondary to the TRD and macular ischemia (Fig. **23**).

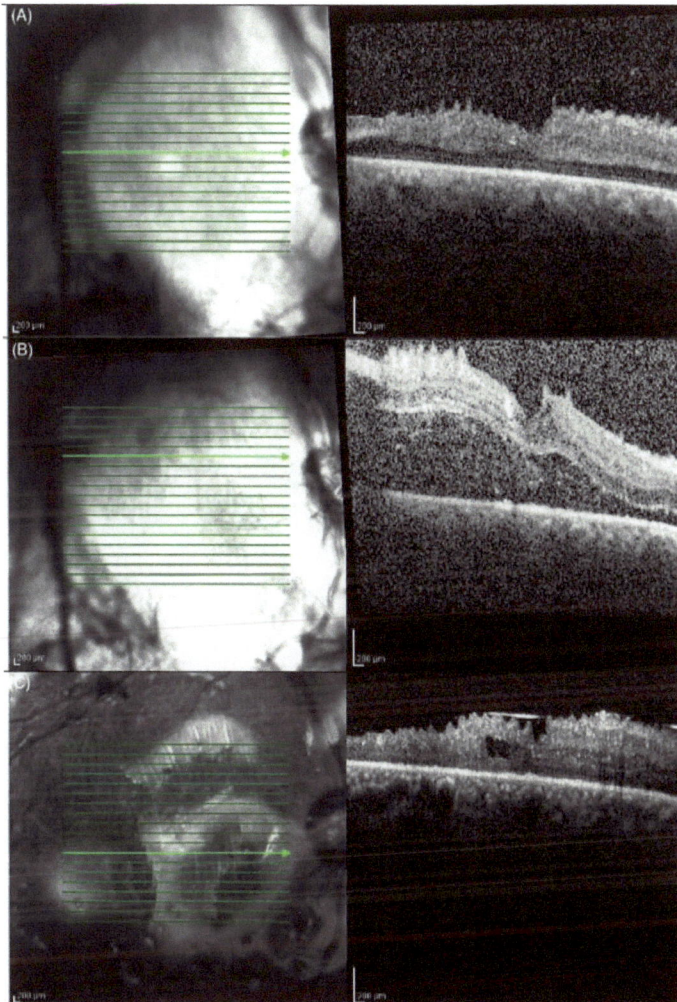

Fig. (23). SD-OCT scans centered on the fovea (horizontal green arrows) of the right eye from a patient with poorly controlled DM. **(a)** At presentation, the patient had severe macular puckering, NCVH, and a TRD threatening to detach the macula. Vision was 20/200. As there was an inadequate view to perform PRP secondary to hemorrhage, the patient was advised to proceed with surgery, but was lost to follow up. **(b)** When the patient returned 6 months later, vision dropped to hand motion and the TRD progressed to detach the macula. **(c)** After vitrectomy with membrane peeling and silicone oil tamponade, the retina was reattached but vision was limited at 20/400 due to severe macular ischemia.

VMT can cause vision loss and metamorphopsia, which can be stabilized after adequate treatment of PDR. Fig. (**13**) showed an example of a diabetic patient with PDR who developed fibrovascular proliferation and VMT, which stabilized after PRP treatment. In Fig. (**24**), we see the corresponding SD-OCT of the right eye, and serial tracked OCT scans over several years of follow up showed stable VMT.

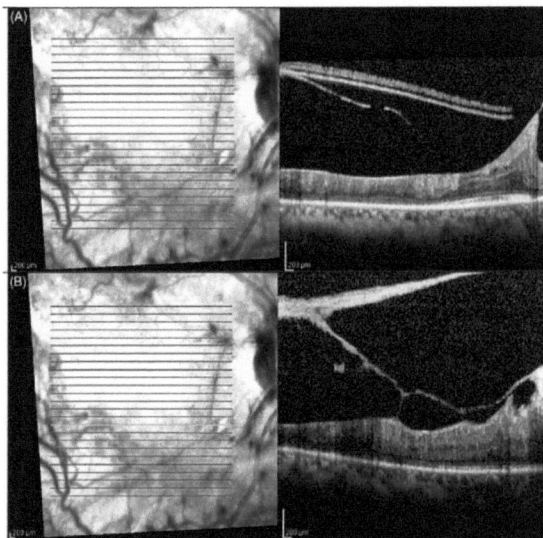

Fig. (24). SD-OCT scans of the right eye from the same patient as in Fig. **(13)**. **(a)** Scan is centered through the foveal region (green arrow), showing focal peripapillary VMT. **(b)** Scan taken inferior to the fovea shows severe VMT. PDR was stabilized by PRP treatment and the patient elected to monitor the VMT, which remained stable during several years of follow up.

CONCLUSION

In this chapter, we reviewed the well-established classification system for grading diabetic retinopathy and criteria for CSME. We highlight the use of SD-OCT to detect ci-DME, which has been pivotal for treatment with various pharmacologic agents. Etiologies of reversible and non-reversible vision loss in the diabetic patient were reviewed with illustrative cases to highlight key features of each process.

CONSENT FOR PUBLICATION

Not applicable.

CONFLICT OF INTEREST

The author declares no conflict of interest, financial or otherwise.

ACKNOWLEDGEMENTS

Declared none.

REFERENCES

[1]   Rodrigues GB, Abe RY, Zangalli C, *et al.* Neovascular glaucoma: a review. Int J Retina Vitreous 2016; 2: 26.

[http://dx.doi.org/10.1186/s40942-016-0051-x] [PMID: 27895936]

[2]   Wilkinson CP, Ferris FL III, Klein RE, *et al.* Proposed international clinical diabetic retinopathy and diabetic macular edema disease severity scales. Ophthalmology 2003; 110(9): 1677-82.
[http://dx.doi.org/10.1016/S0161-6420(03)00475-5] [PMID: 13129861]

[3]   Ruia S, Saxena S, Gemmy Cheung CM, Gilhotra JS, Lai TY. Spectral domain optical coherence tomography features and classification systems for diabetic macular edema: a review. Asia Pac J Ophthalmol (Phila) 2016; 5(5): 360-7.
[http://dx.doi.org/10.1097/APO.0000000000000218] [PMID: 27632028]

[4]   Wells JA, Glassman AR, Ayala AR, *et al.* Aflibercept, bevacizumab, or Ranibizumab for diabetic macular edema: two-year results from a comparative effectiveness randomized clinical trial. Ophthalmology 2016; 123(6): 1351-9.
[http://dx.doi.org/10.1016/j.ophtha.2016.02.022] [PMID: 26935357]

[5]   Brown DM, Schmidt-Erfurth U, Do DV, *et al.* Intravitreal aflibercept for diabetic macular edema: 100-week results from the VISTA and VIVID studies. Ophthalmol 2015; 122(10): 2044-52.
[http://dx.doi.org/10.1016/j.ophtha.2015.06.017] [PMID: 26198808]

[6]   Nguyen QD, Brown DM, Marcus DM, *et al.* Ranibizumab for diabetic macular edema: results from 2 phase III randomized trials: RISE and RIDE. Ophthalmology 2012; 119(4): 789-801.
[http://dx.doi.org/10.1016/j.ophtha.2011.12.039] [PMID: 22330964]

[7]   Photocoagulation for diabetic macular edema. Early Treatment Diabetic Retinopathy Study report number 1. Early Treatment Diabetic Retinopathy Study research group. Arch Ophthalmol 1985; 103(12): 1796-806.
[http://dx.doi.org/10.1001/archopht.1985.01050120030015] [PMID: 2866759]

[8]   Boyer DS, Yoon YH, Belfort R Jr, *et al.* Three-year, randomized, sham-controlled trial of dexamethasone intravitreal implant in patients with diabetic macular edema. Ophthalmology 2014; 121(10): 1904-14.
[http://dx.doi.org/10.1016/j.ophtha.2014.04.024] [PMID: 24907062]

[9]   Campochiaro PA, Brown DM, Pearson A, *et al.* Sustained delivery fluocinolone acetonide vitreous inserts provide benefit for at least 3 years in patients with diabetic macular edema. Ophthalmology 2012; 119(10): 2125-32.
[http://dx.doi.org/10.1016/j.ophtha.2012.04.030] [PMID: 22727177]

[10]   Photocoagulation treatment of proliferative diabetic retinopathy. Clinical application of Diabetic Retinopathy Study (DRS) findings, DRS Report Number 8. Ophthalmology 1981; 88(7): 583-600.
[PMID: 7196564]

[11]   Kim YC, Shin JP. Spectral-domain optical coherence tomography findings of tractional retinal elevation in patients with diabetic retinopathy. Graefes Arch Clin Exp Ophthalmol 2016; 254(8): 1481-7.
[http://dx.doi.org/10.1007/s00417-015-3206-9] [PMID: 26542121]

[12]   Berrocal MH, Acaba LA, Acaba A. Surgery for diabetic eye complications. Curr Diab Rep 2016; 16(10): 99.
[http://dx.doi.org/10.1007/s11892-016-0787-6] [PMID: 27612846]

CHAPTER 4

Diabetes and Ocular Infections

Jennifer Lopez and **Allison E. Rizzuti**[*]

Medical Center, NYU Langone, NY, United States

Abstract: This chapter will review some of the infections that can be seen in and around the eye in diabetic patients. Specifically, six cases of infection will be highlighted and discussed.

Keywords: Cerebral, Cellulitis, Cornea, Endophthalmitis, Infection, Mucor, Preseptal, Ulcer, Vitritis.

INTRODUCTION

Infection is a well-known complication of diabetes, and most commonly involves the skin, lower respiratory tract and genitourinary tract. Patients with diabetes are also prone to ocular infection, and studies have found that diabetics are at an increased risk of conjunctivitis [1, 2] However, there is limited research examining the association between diabetes and other ocular infections, such as keratitis, endophthalmitis and orbital cellulitis. It is well established that diabetics are particularly susceptible to infections involving staphylococcus, pneumococcus, mycobacteria and candida; organisms which can cause devastating consequences in the eye. Not only can these infections be vision threatening, but because of the eye's close proximity to the cavernous sinus and brain, they can be life threatening as well. In this chapter, we will examine the topic of ocular infection in diabetes with a series of case reports.

RHINO-ORBITAL-CEREBRAL MUCORMYCOSIS

Case 1

A 27-year-old man with a history of poorly controlled diabetes presented with 5 days of left eyelid swelling and vision loss. He had a mildly elevated temperature at 38.4°C, but otherwise stable vital signs. His physical examination on presentation was remarkable for eyelid edema resulting in the inability to open his

---

[*] **Corresponding author Allison Rizzuti:** Medical Center, NYU Langone, NY, United States;
E-mail: Allison.Rizzuti@nyumc.org

Douglas R. Lazzaro and Samy I. McFarlane (Eds.)

left eye and loss of his left light pupillary reflex. His labs were significant for a white blood cell count of 21,100 cells/μL with a left shift and decreased hemoglobin of 10.9g/dL. He had a blood glucose level of 22.4mmol/L and hemoglobin A1c of 15.7%. The patient was admitted to the hospital with diabetic ketoacidosis and treated with intravenous insulin and fluids. One day after the presentation, his eyelid and facial edema worsened, his left eye became ophthalmoplegic and his left pupil was noted to be mid-dilated. Funduscopic examination revealed a pale optic disc, a cherry-red spot in his macula, and narrow retinal arteries consistent with a retinal artery occlusion (Fig. **1**). He was also noted to have areas of necrosis and purulent discharge within his nasal cavity which rapidly destroyed his nasal architecture. Cultures from the purulent discharge revealed mucormycosis and he was treated with intravenous amphotericin B.

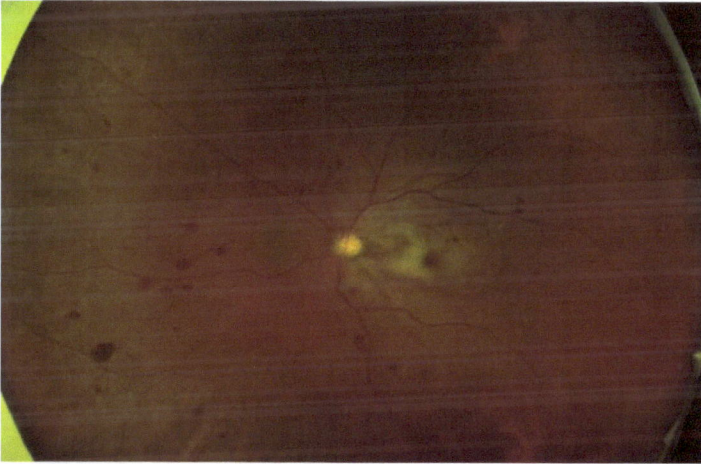

Fig. (1). Left fundus showing a pale optic disc and cherry-red spot on macula consistent with retinal artery occlusion.

Diabetic patients are at an increased risk of developing rhino-orbito-cerebral mucormycosis, an infection caused by a fungal pathogen that causes rapid tissue necrosis. Patients with uncontrolled hyperglycemia are most susceptible, particularly patients with diabetic ketoacidosis due to the resulting acidosis which creates a favorable environment for the growth of *Rhizopus* [4]. The infection occurs after the inhalation of spores into the paranasal sinuses and the orbit may become involved when the infection spreads laterally. Irreversible vision loss can occur due to the compressive effect on the optic nerve and the central retinal artery. If not treated promptly, the infection can spread to the brain *via* the cavernous sinus and can ultimately result in death. Patients typically present with signs and symptoms of orbital cellulitis and so the suspicion of mucormycosis must be high in order to institute the appropriate management. Mucormycosis is initially treated with surgical debridement and intravenous amphotericin B as well as treating the underlying predisposing factor such as hyperglycemia.

PRE-SEPTAL & ORBITAL CELLULITIS

Case 2

A 58-year-old male with uncontrolled diabetes presented with one week of redness and swelling of the left eye (Fig. **2**). Physical examination of his left eye was significant for periorbital edema and erythema with a round and reactive pupil and full extraocular muscle movements. On presentation, his best corrected visual acuity was 20/30 in the left eye. Slit lamp examination of his left eye was significant for 1+ injection with decreased tear film and superficial punctate epithelial erosions. His glucose on admission was 210mg/dL and labs revealed a hemoglobin A1C of 11.9%. He received intravenous Vancomycin and Unasyn that was transitioned to oral Augmentin along with erythromycin ointment. Cultures eventually grew *streptococcus anginosus.* At the time of discharge, his visual acuity improved to 20/20 -1 bilaterally.

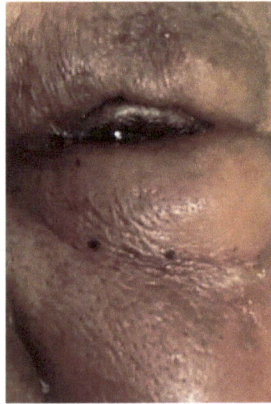

Fig. (2). Pre-septal cellulitis.

Case 3

A 46 year old man with no known past medical history presented with pain and swelling of his right eye for three days. On presentation, he was found to be febrile with an exam remarkable for right periorbital erythema, edema and discharge. Physical examination of his right eye revealed decreased visual acuity, chemosis, and evidence of severe non-proliferative diabetic retinopathy. He was diagnosed with Type 2 Diabetes after his labs revealed a glucose level of 277mg/dL and a hemoglobinA1c of 9.8%. CT scan of the orbit showed post septal inflammation consistent with orbital cellulitis and he was admitted for empiric intravenous ceftriaxone, ampicillin-sulbactam and amphotericin. Cultures of the discharge grew *K. Pneumoniae* (Fig. **3**). Three days after presentation, he complained of persistent pain and worsening vision. Repeat CT scan revealed worsening right orbital cellulitis with a subperiosteal abscess adjacent to the ethmoid sinus, displacing the medial rectus muscle (Fig. **4**). The patient underwent drainage of the abscess as well as an extended course of intravenous antibiotics.

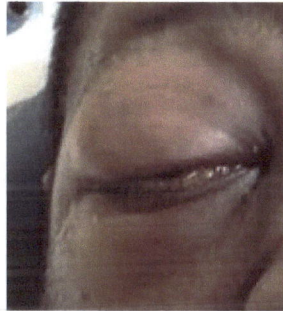

Fig. (3). Orbital cellulitis.

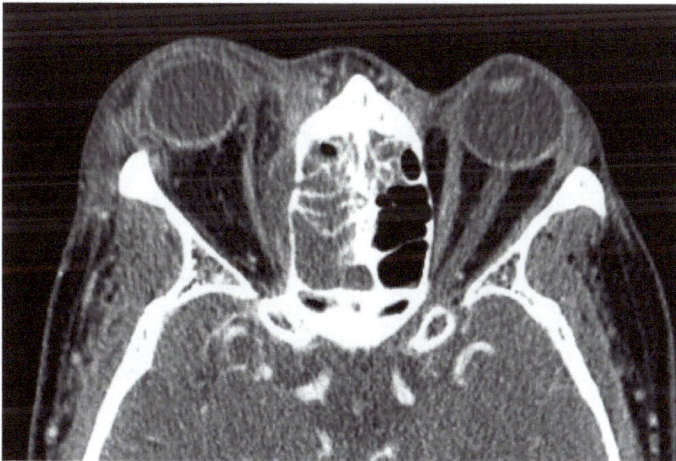

Fig. (4). CT scan showing right subperiosteal abscess.

Preseptal cellulitis is defined as an infection involving the superficial soft tissue structures anterior to the orbital septum. Generally, preseptal cellulitis is more common than orbital cellulitis and carries a more favorable prognosis, however, prompt diagnosis and treatment is crucial in order to prevent further spread of the infection [6, 7]. Clinically, preseptal cellulitis manifests as eyelid edema and erythema, usually with normal visual acuity and pupillary exam and intact extraocular movements.

Orbital cellulitis is an infection of the soft tissues posterior to the orbital septum. Urgent recognition and treatment of orbital cellulitis is required due to the risk of compression of the optic nerve and central retinal artery which can result in permanent vision loss. Furthermore, orbital cellulitis can be life threatening as it may result in a cavernous sinus thrombosis, brain abscesses or meningitis. Clinically, it is distinguished from preseptal cellulitis by the presence of ophthalmoplegia, proptosis, pupillary abnormalities and vision loss [7, 8].

In both preseptal and orbital cellulitis, sinusitis represents the most common source of infection. A study examining orbital complications of paranasal sinusitis found diabetes was a common preexisting disease. Diabetes may also be associated with a more severe presentation of orbital disease [9]. Although the most common organisms are typically staphylococcal and streptococcal species, it is important to consider fungal etiologies in these patients. Treatment is with systemic antibiotics, and surgical drainage is often required in cases of abscess formation.

INFECTIOUS KERATITIS

Case 4

A 41-year-old male with poorly controlled diabetes presented with left eye pain associated with erythema, eyelid swelling and mild photophobia for three days [10]. At presentation, his visual acuity in the left eye was 20/25 and there was no relative afferent pupillary defect. Slit lamp examination of the left eye revealed an epithelial defect with stromal infiltrate and sectoral pannus (Fig. **5**). His labs revealed a blood glucose level of 17mmol/l with glucose and ketones present in his urine. Of note, he denied any previous contact lens use or trauma. Subsequently, he was diagnosed with infectious keratitis and treated with fortified vancomycin and tobramycin eye drops. Corneal scrapings ultimately revealed *S. Maltophilia.*

Infectious keratitis, or corneal ulcer, is a defect in the corneal epithelium with inflammation from a microbial infection. A study identifying the risk factors associated with corneal ulcers found diabetes to be the third most common risk factor after contact lens wear and trauma, and diabetics were found to have worse visual outcomes [11].

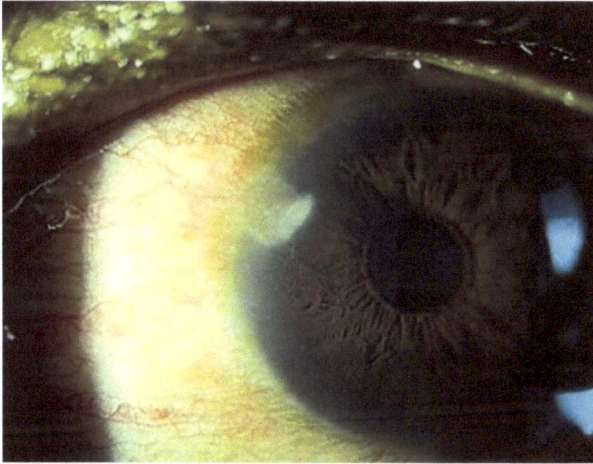

Fig. (5). Underlying corneal infiltrate and pannus at presentation.

The innate immune system is the primary barrier to corneal infections. Diabetics have impaired immune function with a weakened epithelial barrier and so are at a higher risk for developing corneal infections. This risk is significantly correlated with hemoglobin A1c [12]. The weakening of the corneal epithelial layer is in part due to a reduced number of hemi-desmosomes in diabetics, impairing the adhesion of the corneal epithelium to the underlying stroma. Diabetics also have increased erythrocyte aldose reductase activity which causes sorbitol to accumulate and damage the corneal epithelium [13]. Because of the microvascular complications of diabetes, patients are at risk for diabetic neurotrophic keratopathy, neuropathy of the ophthalmic division of the trigeminal nerve. These patients have decreased corneal sensation resulting in ulcers that are often refractory to treatment [14].

ENDOPHTHALMITIS

Case 5

A 64-year-old male with poorly controlled diabetes presented with pain and swelling of his right thumb associated with fever for one day. He was admitted to the hospital with a diagnosis of tenosynovitis complicated by bacteremia and treated with cloxacillin. One day after presentation, he complained of blurry vision in both eyes and purulent discharge. On examination, his visual acuity was counting fingers in his right eye and 20/100 in his left eye. Slit lamp examination was significant for 2+ anterior chamber cells and hypopyon in the right eye and vitritis bilaterally. Dilated funduscopic examination revealed a Roth spot in the left eye. He was ultimately diagnosed with endogenous endophthalmitis secondary to tenosynovitis with blood cultures revealing methicillin sensitive *Staphylococcus aureus*. After appropriate treatment including intravenous cloxacillin, levofloxacin eye drops and intravitreal vancomycin and ceftazidime, he recovered to 20/20 visual acuity [15].

Endophthalmitis is defined as infection and inflammation of the internal parts of the eye and is often sight-threatening. Patients present with pain and decreased vision and physical examination may reveal eyelid edema, conjunctival injection, hypopyon and inflammation in the vitreous cavity. A tap of the vitreous cavity may identify the offending organisms, which can be bacterial, fungal or viral. Treatment typically involves intravitreal antibiotics or pars plana vitrectomy.

Endogenous endophthalmitis occurs from hematogenous microbial spread from a distant infection, and is often associated with states of immunodeficiency [16 - 18]. Diabetes is the most common predisposing risk factor associated with endogenous endophthalmitis [17, 19, 20]. Visual outcome is highly dependent on the underlying microbial organism with gram-positive bacteria and Aspergillus associated with the worst outcomes [18].

Because cataracts are often associated with diabetes, many diabetic patients undergo cataract surgery and while the outcomes for cataract surgery are generally excellent, diabetic patients have poorer visual outcomes as well as an increased risk of developing post-operative endophthalmitis [2, 13]. As in endogenous endophthalmitis, treatment is with intravitreal antibiotics or pars plana vitrectomy.

CONCLUSION

Diabetes can be a cause of mild infections in and around the eye, as well as sight and life threatening ones. Just as diabetics have an increased risk of systemic infection, eye infections are at increased rates as well in the diabetic patient. Prompt diagnosis and management must be instituted quickly to reduce morbidity and mortality.

CONSENT FOR PUBLICATION

Not applicable.

CONFLICT OF INTEREST

The authors confirm that consent from the patients is not necessary due to the nature of figures (cropped and unidentifiable).

ACKNOWLEDGEMENTS

Declared none.

REFERENCES

[1]   Ansari AS, de Lusignan S, Hinton W, Munro N, McGovern A. The association between diabetes, level of glycaemic control and eye infection: Cohort database study. Prim Care Diabetes 2017; 11(5): 421-9.
        [http://dx.doi.org/10.1016/j.pcd.2017.05.009] [PMID: 28648963]

[2]   Skarbez K, Priestley Y, Hoepf M, Koevary SB, Hoepf M, Koevary SB. Comprehensive review of the effects of diabetes on ocular health. Expert Rev Ophthalmol 2010; 5(4): 557-77.
        [http://dx.doi.org/10.1586/eop.10.44] [PMID: 21760834]

[3]   Chen YX, He YX, Zhou H, Wang M, Su SO. Rapidly progressive rhino-orbito-cerebral mucormycosis in a patient with type 2 diabetes: A case report. Exp Ther Med 2017; 13(3): 1054-6.
        [http://dx.doi.org/10.3892/etm.2017.4074] [PMID: 28450941]

[4]   Chow V, Khan S, Balogun A, Mitchell D, Mühlschlegel FA. Invasive rhino-orbito-cerebral mucormycosis in a diabetic patient - the need for prompt treatment. Med Mycol Case Rep 2014; 8: 5-9.
        [http://dx.doi.org/10.1016/j.mmcr.2014.12.002] [PMID: 25750854]

[5]   Yang SJ, Park SY, Lee YJ, *et al.* Klebsiella pneumoniae orbital cellulitis with extensive vascular occlusions in a patient with type 2 diabetes. Korean J Intern Med (Korean Assoc Intern Med) 2010; 25(1): 114-7.
        [http://dx.doi.org/10.3904/kjim.2010.25.1.114] [PMID: 20195414]

[6]   Ambati BK, Ambati J, Azar N, Stratton L, Schmidt EV. Periorbital and orbital cellulitis before and after the advent of Haemophilus influenzae type B vaccination. Ophthalmol 2000; 107(8): 1450-3.
        [http://dx.doi.org/10.1016/S0161-6420(00)00178-0] [PMID: 10919886]

[7]   Lee S, Yen MT. Management of preseptal and orbital cellulitis. Saudi J Ophthalmol 2011; 25(1): 21-9.
        [http://dx.doi.org/10.1016/j.sjopt.2010.10.004] [PMID: 23960899]

[8]   Colapinto P, Aslam SA, Frangouli O, Joshi N. Undiagnosed type 2 diabetes mellitus presenting with orbital cellulitis. Orbit 2008; 27(5): 380-2.
        [http://dx.doi.org/10.1080/01676830802328519] [PMID: 18836938]

[9]   Chang Y, Chen P, Hung J, Chen H, Tseng S. Orbital complications of paranasal sinusitis in Taiwan , 1988 through 2015 : Acute ophthalmological manifestations , diagnosis , and management 2017; 1-14.

[10]   Holifield K, Lazzaro DR. Case report: spontaneous Stenotrophomonas maltophilia keratitis in a diabetic patient. Eye Contact Lens 2011; 37(5): 326-7.
        [http://dx.doi.org/10.1097/ICL.0b013e3182146e26] [PMID: 21617538]

[11]   Jin H, Parker WT, Law NW, *et al.* Evolving risk factors and antibiotic sensitivity patterns for microbial keratitis at a large county hospital. Br J Ophthalmol 2017; 101(11): 1483-7.
        [http://dx.doi.org/10.1136/bjophthalmol-2016-310026] [PMID: 28336675]

[12]   Gekka M, Miyata K, Nagai Y, *et al.* Corneal epithelial barrier function in diabetic patients. Cornea 2004; 23(1): 35-7.
        [http://dx.doi.org/10.1097/00003226-200401000-00006] [PMID: 14701955]

[13]   Jeganathan VSE, Wang JJ, Wong TY. Ocular associations of diabetes other than diabetic retinopathy. Diabetes Care 2008; 31(9): 1905-12.
        [http://dx.doi.org/10.2337/dc08-0342] [PMID: 18753669]

[14]   Lockwood A, Hope-Ross M, Chell P. Neurotrophic keratopathy and diabetes mellitus. Eye (Lond) 2006; 20(7): 837-9.
        [http://dx.doi.org/10.1038/sj.eye.6702053] [PMID: 16215544]

[15]   Agrawal RV, Teoh SC, Yong V. Bilateral endogenous endophthalmitis associated with methicillin sensitive Staphylococcus aureus (MSSA) related tenosynovitis: case report. Ocul Immunol Inflamm 2012; 20(3): 224-6.
[http://dx.doi.org/10.3109/09273948.2012.676702] [PMID: 22512341]

[16]   Mavrakanas TA, de Haller R, Philippe J. Endogenous endophthalmitis in a patient with diabetes and foot osteomyelitis. Can J Diabetes 2015; 39(1): 18-20.
[http://dx.doi.org/10.1016/j.jcjd.2014.05.011] [PMID: 25444679]

[17]   Zhang H, Liu Z. Endogenous endophthalmitis: a 10-year review of culture-positive cases in northern China. Ocul Immunol Inflamm 2010; 18(2): 133-8.
[http://dx.doi.org/10.3109/09273940903494717] [PMID: 20370344]

[18]   Ness T, Pelz K, Hansen LL. Endogenous endophthalmitis: microorganisms, disposition and prognosis. Acta Ophthalmol Scand 2007; 85(8): 852-6.
[http://dx.doi.org/10.1111/j.1600-0420.2007.00982.x] [PMID: 17725616]

[19]   Bjerrum SS, la Cour M. 59 eyes with endogenous endophthalmitis- causes, outcomes and mortality in a Danish population between 2000 and 2016. Graefes Arch Clin Exp Ophthalmol 2017; 255(10): 2023-7.
[http://dx.doi.org/10.1007/s00417-017-3760-4] [PMID: 28791473]

[20]   Vaziri K, Pershing S, Albini TA, Moshfeghi DM, Moshfeghi AA. Risk factors predictive of endogenous endophthalmitis among hospitalized patients with hematogenous infections in the United States. Am J Ophthalmol 2015; 159(3): 498-504.
[http://dx.doi.org/10.1016/j.ajo.2014.11.032] [PMID: 25486541]

CHAPTER 5

Neuro-Ophthalmic Complications of Diabetes Mellitus

Julie DeBacker[1,*] and **Alessandro Albano**[2]

¹ NYU School of Medicine, NYU Langone Health, NY, USA
² SUNY Downstate College of Medicine, Brooklyn, NY, USA

Abstract: Eye disease attributed to Diabetes can have devastating effects on all aspects of vision as all parts of the eyes are subject to damage including the optic nerve and cranial nerves. In this chapter, we will discuss the most common neuro-ophthalmic problems seen in diabetic patients.

Keywords: Cataract, Cranial Nerve, Diplopia, Neuro-Ophthalmology, Neuropathy, Optic, Pupil.

INTRODUCTION

DIABETES AND NEURO-OPHTHALMOLOGIC COMPLICATIONS

Cranial Nerve Palsies in Diabetes

Double vision greatly limits a person's daily activities, and diabetes mellitus is one of the known culprits affecting cranial nerves innervating eye muscles leading to symptomatic ocular misalignment and thus binocular diplopia. Nerves are damaged by microvascular injury of small blood vessels that supply nerves, a common serious complication of diabetes. Endothelial cells lining blood vessels are not insulin-dependent and therefore take in greater than normal amounts of glucose when glucose levels are high in diabetes. The excess glucose causes abnormal thickening and weakening of the blood vessel basement membranes, leading to bleeding and slowing of blood flow. This poor blood flow to nerves and neurons causes neuronal ischemia, leading to loss of function [1].

Diabetes most commonly affects the third cranial nerve (III) followed by the sixth cranial nerve (VI), which control eye muscles affecting ocular movements. Crani-

* Corresponding author Julie DeBacker: NYU School of Medicine, NYU Langone Health, NY, USA;
E-mail: julie.debacker@nyumc.org

al nerve four (IV), also involved in eye movement, is much less commonly affected. Isolated palsies of CN III and CN VI secondary to diabetes occur significantly more frequently than palsies of multiple nerves at the same time [2]. And, the nerve palsies typically occur unilaterally. Ischemic injury of two nerves simultaneously is very rare, and bilateral ischemic injury of the same ocular motor nerve is even rarer [3]. Multiple cranial nerve involvement and/or bilateral cranial nerve involvement warrants further workup for an alternative cause.

The oculomotor nerve (CN III) innervates the medial rectus which adducts the eye, the superior rectus which elevates the eye while in the abducted position, the inferior oblique which elevates the eye while in the adducted position, and the inferior rectus which depresses the eye. It also innervates the levator palpebrae superioris muscle, which elevates the superior eyelid. CN III also carries parasympathetic nerve fibers to the ciliary body for accommodation and to the pupillary constrictor muscle to constrict the pupil [3]. The abducens nerve (CN VI) controls only the lateral rectus muscle, which abducts the eye [4]. Both cranial nerve palsies may cause significant binocular diplopia, and again, this can be quite debilitating and have negative impacts on the lives of affected patients. Diabetic cranial nerve palsies are significantly linked to poor glycemic control and are shown to recover with the improvement of hyperglycemia [4, 5]. Three patient cases are presented here to discuss common clinical presentations of oculomotor and abducens nerve palsies caused by diabetes along with a treatment option to shorten the recovery time from an abducens nerve palsy.

Case 1: Diabetic Patient Presents with an Oculomotor Nerve Palsy

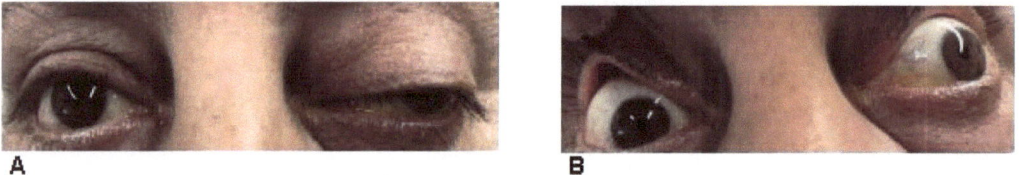

Fig. (1). Patient showing exotropic strabismus with a downward and outward position of the left eye (A and B) with left ptosis (A).

A 65-year-old male patient of the NYU Medical Center's Department of Ophthalmology with a past medical history of diabetes mellitus type 2 presented with a left partial pupil-sparing CN III palsy with which progressed to include ptosis within one week. The patient displayed limitations of left adduction, elevation and depression of the eye, and left ptosis (Figs. **1**, **2**, and **3**).

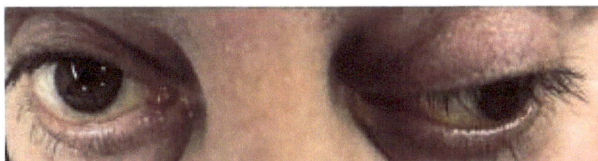

Fig. (2). Patient showing limited adduction and elevation of the left eye.

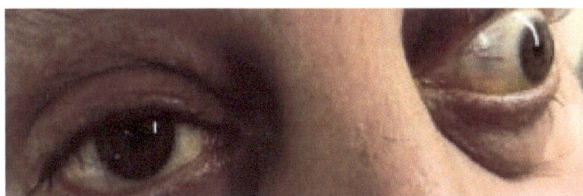

Fig. (3). Patient showing limited elevation of the left eyelid.

In diabetes, a CN III palsy is pupil-sparing, whereas a complete, isolated oculomotor nerve palsy results in ophthalmoplegia, ptosis, and mydriasis. The oculomotor nerve has a branched structure, with the parasympathetic fibers controlling pupil constriction running superficial to the nerve [5]. Partial oculomotor nerve palsies may have varied presentations based on the muscles affected downstream of the nerve damage. Typically, the eye movement abnormalities cause exotropic strabismus (diverging crossed eyes) leading to binocular diplopia. The affected eye will be displaced inferiorly and laterally ("down and out"). An isolated CN III palsy leaves the action of the other two cranial nerves, CN IV and VI, unopposed: The lateral rectus pulls the eye laterally without opposition from the medial rectus, and the superior oblique muscle (innervated by CN IV—the trochlear nerve) pushes the eye downward without opposition from the superior rectus and inferior oblique muscles. With control of a diabetic patient's hyperglycemia, the oculomotor nerve function is expected to return with symptoms self-resolving over three to six months but may take up to or over one year.

Less common but more serious causes of oculomotor nerve palsies should always be considered and ruled out with neuroimaging, especially compression of CN III by an aneurysm of the posterior communicating artery or the posterior cerebral artery in the brain.[7] Of note, oculomotor nerve palsy due to compression by an aneurysmal lesion typically presents with pupil dilation, which is a distinguishing feature from oculomotor nerve palsy caused by diabetes [6].

Cases 2 and 3: Botulinum Toxin A as a Treatment of Diplopia from Diabetic Abducens Nerve Palsy

A 52-year-old female patient with a 15-year history of diabetes mellitus type 2 and glycated hemoglobin (HbA$_{1C}$) of 8.7% (normal 4% - 5.6%, diabetes > 6.4%) presented with diplopia, squinting, and visible esotropic strabismus with a medially rotated left eye that started several days earlier. She was diagnosed with CN VI palsy in the left eye. The patient had a career as a computer operator and was unable to work as a result of her diplopia. Although nerve function typically restores itself after glycemic control, it usually takes several months to over a year for the symptoms to resolve. Botulinum toxin A was injected into the medial rectus muscle of her left eye the same day and her strabismus and diplopia completely resolved. Fig. (**4**) [9]. Injection of botulinum toxin A into the ipsilateral medial rectus muscle has been used as a treatment for CN VI palsy since the early 1980s. Injection as early as possible after symptoms are noticed is recommended to achieve complete resolution of diplopia [10].

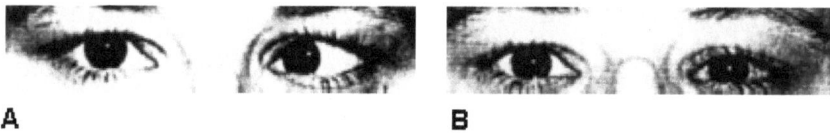

A   **B**

Fig. (4). (A) The female patient before injection of botulinum toxin A displaying esotropic strabismus with a medially rotated left eye. **(B)** The patient after injection showing complete resolution of strabismus and associated diplopia.

A second patient was a 50-year-old male with an 8-year history of diabetes mellitus type 2 and HbA$_{1C}$ of 8.7% presenting with severe diplopia, squinting, visible esotropic strabismus with a medially rotated left eye, and diagnosis of a left abducens nerve palsy persisting for 3 months. This patient worked as a taxi driver and had been unable to work due to his diplopia. Botulinum toxin A was injected into the left medial rectus muscle resulting in improved but not complete resolution of the diplopia. The use of corrective lenses achieved complete resolution Fig. (**5**) [9]. Treatment with botulinum toxin A sooner after his abducens nerve palsy symptoms started would have likely resulted in better resolution of his diplopia without corrective lenses.

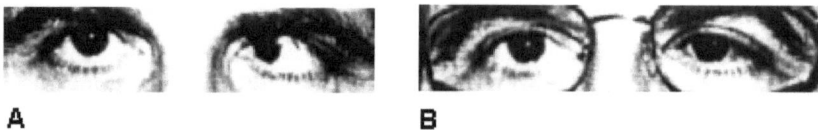

A   **B**

Fig. (5). (A) The male patient before injection of botulinum toxin A displaying esotropic strabismus with a medially rotated left eye. **(B)** The patient after injection showing incomplete resolution of strabismus, with diplopia resolving only after the addition of corrective lenses.

An isolated abducens nerve palsy results in the inability of the lateral rectus muscle to abduct the eye leading to esotropia, or strabismus with the affected eye turned inward, and manifesting as binocular horizontal diplopia. Diabetes is a common cause of acquired unilateral abducens nerve palsy. If a patient presents with a CN VI palsy of unknown etiology, he or she has a 6-fold increase in odds of having coexistent diabetes [7]. Since an isolated abducens nerve palsy has such a high likelihood of having a microvascular ischemic etiology, especially when due to diabetes mellitus, use of high-cost MRI to rule out more serious etiologies including tumors, intracranial hemorrhage, subdural hematoma, or brainstem infarction is controversial [8].

Non-Arteritic Anterior Ischemic Optic Neuropathy

Non-arteritic anterior ischemic optic neuropathy (NAION) is a potential cause of vision loss in patients with diabetes. There are several other causes of NAION, and this type of ischemic optic neuropathy should be distinguished from arteritic anterior ischemic optic neuropathy which is usually due to giant cell arteritis and posterior ischemic optic neuropathy; neither will be discussed here. Patients with NAION are typically over the age of 50 years old, are more likely to be Caucasian, more likely to be women in those with diabetes, and they present with sudden painless monocular vision loss [11]. On exam, initial visual acuity is 20/20 in about one third, better than 20/40 in about half, and 20/200 or worse in about 20% [12]. Formal visual field testing often reveals an altitudinal defect. A relative afferent pupillary defect in the affected eye is observed, and there is almost always optic disc edema that later self-resolves, but may be longer-lasting in those with diabetes [11, 13]. Telangiectatic dilated vessels overlying the optic disc is characteristically seen in patients with diabetes rather than in patients without diabetes [13]. In cases where there is a question about the diagnosis, viewing the cup to disc ratio of the contralateral eye may point to the correct diagnosis: A small disc with a small or absent optic disc cup has been associated with NAION and is often referred to as a "disc at risk." [11]. About 42% of patients improve and stabilize in their vision at six months. Recurrence in the same eye is rare; however, there is a 15-20% risk of occurrence in the contralateral eye [12].

In NAION, ischemia occurs to the anterior portion of the optic nerve, an area supplied by posterior ciliary arteries. The pathophysiology of NAION is incompletely understood and believed to be related to autoregulation of blood flow which is equal to perfusion pressure divided by resistance to blood flow [11].

Several treatments have been tried, including steroids, and there is no evidence to suggest an effective therapy.

Optic Neuropathy in Young Patients with Diabetes

In children to young adults with diabetes who present with optic neuropathy,

Wolfram Syndrome type I should be considered. Wolfram syndrome is a rare condition comprised of diabetes mellitus, diabetes insipidus, progressive optic nerve atrophy, and sensorineural deafness. It is an autosomal recessive syndrome and genetic testing reveals mutations in the WFS1 gene. The condition has been shown to affect the visual pathway from the retinal nerve fiber layer through the optic radiations (pre-geniculate to post-geniculate pathway). Patients tend to present with various levels of severity, but usually more severe in the young, and it is often bilateral. Visual acuity progressively declines and corresponds to the thinning of the retinal nerve fiber layer on optical coherence tomography. Visual field defects, dyschromatopsia, optic nerve pallor, and an afferent pupillary defect may be seen [14].

Pupils in Diabetes

Pupils may also be affected in patients with diabetes, specifically leading to diminished accommodative amplitude. Accommodation relies on integration from sensory, neuromuscular, and other biophysical input to change the lens of the eye in order to automatically adjust the eye's focus on objects at near and far distances [16]. Age, having diabetes, and duration of diabetes have been shown to be risk factors in decreased accommodative amplitude [15].

CONCLUSION

Diabetes Mellitus can cause cranial nerve palsies, optic neuropathies, and pupillary abnormalities. A single cranial nerve may be involved (more commonly), but diabetes can also cause multiple simultaneous cranial neuropathies as well. NAION can also be a result of systemic disease. All patients with diabetes presenting with cranial nerve problems must be evaluated thoroughly by the ophthalmologist and neuro-ophthalmologist.

CONSENT FOR PUBLICATION

Not applicable.

CONFLICT OF INTEREST

The authors confirm that consent from the patients is not necessary due to the nature of figures (cropped and unidentifiable).

ACKNOWLEDGEMENTS

Declared none.

REFERENCES

[1]   Cameron NE, Eaton SEM, Cotter MA, Tesfaye S. Vascular factors and metabolic interactions in the pathogenesis of diabetic neuropathy. Diabetologia 2001; 44(11): 1973-88.
[http://dx.doi.org/10.1007/s001250100001] [PMID: 11719828]

[2]   Greco D, Gambina F, Maggio F. Ophthalmoplegia in diabetes mellitus: a retrospective study. Acta Diabetol 2009; 46(1): 23-6.
[http://dx.doi.org/10.1007/s00592-008-0053-8] [PMID: 18758685]

[3]   Lajmi H, Hmaied W, Ben Jalel W, *et al.* Oculomotor palsy in diabetics. J Fr Ophtalmol 2018; 41(1): 45-9.
[http://dx.doi.org/10.1016/j.jfo.2017.06.010] [PMID: 29290461]

[4]   Agarwal A, Eisenberg A, Woods SK. A common cause of cranial nerve VI palsy-hidden in plain sight: a teachable moment. JAMA Intern Med 2016; 176(8): 1066-7.
[http://dx.doi.org/10.1001/jamainternmed.2016.2661] [PMID: 27367021]

[5]   Chou PY, Wu KH, Huang P. Ptosis as the only manifestation of diabetic superior division oculomotor nerve palsy: A case report. Medicine (Baltimore) 2017; 96(46)e8739
[http://dx.doi.org/10.1097/MD.0000000000008739] [PMID: 29145322]

[6]   Jo YS, Kim SK, Kim DH, Kim JH, Na SJ. Complete oculomotor nerve palsy caused by direct compression of the posterior cerebral artery. J Stroke Cerebrovasc Dis 2015; 24(7): e189-90.
[http://dx.doi.org/10.1016/j.jstrokecerebrovasdis.2015.04.010] [PMID: 25939862]

[7]   Patel SV, Holmes JM, Hodge DO, Burke JP. Diabetes and hypertension in isolated sixth nerve palsy: a population-based study. Ophthalmol 2005; 112(5): 760-3.
[http://dx.doi.org/10.1016/j.ophtha.2004.11.057] [PMID: 15878054]

[8]   Elder C, Hainline C, Galetta SL, Balcer LJ, Rucker JC. Isolated abducens nerve palsy: update on evaluation and diagnosis. Curr Neurol Neurosci Rep 2016; 16(8): 69.
[http://dx.doi.org/10.1007/s11910-016-0671-4] [PMID: 27306521]

[9]   Broniarczyk-Loba A, Czupryniak L, Nowakowska O, Loba J. Botulinum toxin A in the early treatment of sixth nerve palsy-induced diplopia in type 2 diabetes. Diabetes Care 2004; 27(3): 846-7.
[http://dx.doi.org/10.2337/diacare.27.3.846] [PMID: 14988321]

[10]   Murray ADN. Early botulinum toxin treatment of acute sixth nerve palsy. Eye (Lond) 1991; 5(Pt 1): 45-7.
[http://dx.doi.org/10.1038/eye.1991.9] [PMID: 2060670]

[11]   Hayreh SS. Ischemic optic neuropathy. Prog Retin Eye Res 2009; 28(1): 34-62.
[http://dx.doi.org/10.1016/j.preteyeres.2008.11.002] [PMID: 19063989]

[12]   Hayreh SS, Zimmerman MB. Nonarteritic anterior ischemic optic neuropathy: natural history of visual outcome. Ophthalmol 2008; 115(2): 298-305.e2.
[http://dx.doi.org/10.1016/j.ophtha.2007.05.027] [PMID: 17698200]

[13]   Hayreh SS, Zimmerman MB. Nonarteritic anterior ischemic optic neuropathy: clinical characteristics in diabetic patients *versus* nondiabetic patients. Ophthalmol 2008; 115(10): 1818-25.
[http://dx.doi.org/10.1016/j.ophtha.2008.03.032] [PMID: 18502511]

[14]   Hoekel J, Narayanan Λ, Rutlin J, *et al.* Visual pathway function and structure in Wolfram syndrome: patient age, variation and progression. BMJ Open Ophthalmol 2018; 3(1)e000081
[http://dx.doi.org/10.1136/bmjophth-2017-000081] [PMID: 29657975]

[15]   Braun CI, Benson WE, Remaley NA, Chew EY, Ferris FL III. Accommodative amplitudes in the Early Treatment Diabetic Retinopathy Study. Retina 1995; 15(4): 275-81.
[http://dx.doi.org/10.1097/00006982-199515040-00001] [PMID: 8545570]

[16]   Kaufman PL. Accommodation and Presbyopia: Neuromuscular and Biophysical Aspects.Adler's Physiology of the eye. 9th ed. St Louis: CV Mosby 1994; pp. 391-411.

CHAPTER 6

Overview of Anterior and Posterior Segment Complications

Steven Agemy[1], **Zaki Azam**[2] and **Eric Shrier**[2,*]

[1] *New York Eye and Ear Infirmary of Mount Sinai, NY, USA*

[2] *SUNY- Downstate College of Medicine, Brooklyn, NY, USA*

Abstract: Diabetic eye disease is a potential vision-threatening condition. The most well-known complication of uncontrolled diabetes is diabetic retinopathy, but diabetes can affect various structures of the globe other than the retina. Anterior segment complications include ocular surface disease, which includes Dry Eye Syndrome and diabetic keratopathy, cataracts, refractive changes, extraocular movement disorders, and neovascular glaucoma. Posterior segment complications include diabetic papillopathy and retinopathy. Diabetic retinopathy causes vision loss in multiple ways including macular edema and ischemia, vitreous hemorrhage, and retinal detachment. Tight glucose control can help to prevent these complications from occurring.

Keywords: Cataract, Dry Eye Syndrome, Diabetic keratopathy, Diabetic papillopathy, Diabetic retinopathy, Diabetic macular edema, Non-proliferative diabetic retinopathy, Neovascular glaucoma, Ocular surface disease, Proliferative diabetic retinopathy, Tractional retinal detachment.

INTRODUCTION

Diabetic eye disease is becoming an increasing problem, in part due to longer life expectancy and the change in diet and exercise habits in developed countries [1, 2]. The most well known ocular complication, diabetic retinopathy, is one of the leading causes of blindness worldwide [3]. In the eye, manifestations are found in almost every segment including the orbit and lids and the anterior and posterior segments of the globe [4]. As these complications can lead to permanent vision loss, it is imperative that they are promptly identified so that proper treatment can be initiated. The onset of these complications can vary depending on how well the blood glucose is controlled and the time since the development of diabetes. The following chapter will give a general overview of the diabetic ocular complications associated with the anterior and posterior segment of the globe.

---

* **Corresponding author Eric M. Shrier:** DO - State University of New York - SUNY - Downstate College of Medicine, NY, 11203, USA; E-mail: eric.shrier@downstate.edu

Douglas R. Lazzaro and Samy I. McFarlane (Eds.)

Anterior Segment Complications

Ocular Surface Diseases

Ocular Surface Diseases (OSD) can damage the interpalpebral ocular surface, including the conjunctiva and cornea. Mechanisms related to diabetic OSD include decreased tear production, reduced corneal sensitivity, and impaired corneal re-epithelialization [5 - 7]. This process can lead to signs and symptoms of damage to ocular surface structures, including noticeable irritation from corneal epitheliopathy, decline of visual function, and even chronic tissue disruption. Dry eye syndrome (DES) and diabetic keratopathy are two forms of OSD for which diabetes is a risk factor [8].

Dry Eye Syndrome (DES)

DM is a known risk factor for DES. The prevalence of DES in diabetes has been reported to be as high as 54.3% [9]. That number increases with aging and is 50% more common among women than men. The incidence has a positive correlation with the level of glycated hemoglobin [8]. 20% of dry eye syndrome may occur in individuals with Type 2 diabetes aged between 43 and 86 years [10]. Additionally, there is a significant correlation between DES and the duration of diabetes [8].

The connection between diabetes mellitus and dry eye syndrome is complex and multifactorial. Sustained hyperglycemia triggers an inflammatory cascade leading to corneal epithelial dysfunction, lacrimal gland dysfunction, decreased mucin production, and diabetic keratopathy. These issues lead to decreased tear formation and tear film instability causing the dry eye syndrome [11 - 14].

Diabetic patients with dry eye syndrome typically have the same symptoms as non-diabetics with DES. The common presenting symptoms include foreign body sensation, burning, itching, excessive tearing, discharge, redness, light-sensitivity, and intermittent blurring of vision [15]. On slit lamp examination, various stains can be used to visualize damaged or absent conjunctival/corneal epithelium. In more severe cases, slit lamp examination may identify corneal filaments, neovascularization, and scarring [16]. Additional diagnostic testing includes tear break up time (TBUT), Schirmer's test, matrix metalloproteinase-9 (MMP-9) testing, tear osmolarity, and tear film interferometry [17].

The early diagnosis and treatment of dry eye are pivotal to prevent complications. Other than strict glycemic control, the current treatments for diabetic and non-diabetic dry eye patients are largely the same. The mainstay of mild to moderate disease is supplemental lubrication using artificial tears and longer-acting agents such as artificial tear ointments. Tear conserving interventions such as punctual plugs are also helpful. Concomitant lid disease must also be treated using warm compresses and eyelash scrubs. For more severe disease, prescribing anti-inflammatory agents such as cyclosporine and lifitegrast may enhance the production of the aqueous component of the tear layer and decrease inflammatory mediators [18 - 20]. Diet supplementation with oral flaxseed oil or fish oil has also been found to be useful in alleviating symptoms [21, 22].

Diabetic Keratopathy

Keratopathy is a well-known ocular manifestation of DM, presenting in more than 70% of the DM patients [23]. Abnormalities of the corneal epithelium and diminished corneal sensitivity increase the risk of developing corneal erosions, persistent epithelial defects, and/or corneal ulcers [23, 24]. Not only do diabetics have a higher incidence of these conditions, but they also tend to have more severe disease that may recur and be unresponsive to standard treatment options [25, 26].

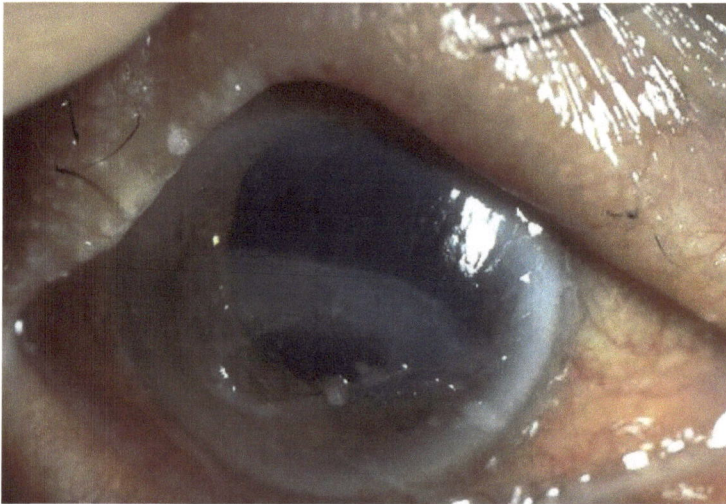

Fig. (1). Neurotrophic ulcer in a poorly controlled diabetic patient. An epithelial defect is noted centrally with surrounding whitening indicating stromal infiltrate. © 2017 American Academy of Ophthalmology.

Similar to dry eye syndrome in diabetics, the cause of diabetic keratopathy is multifactorial. The corneas of patients with diabetic keratopathy show pathologic changes including abnormally thickened basement membranes, abnormal adhesion between the stroma and basement membrane, and a reduction in hemidesmosomes, contributing to weak adhesions between the epithelium and underlying stroma [27 - 29]. In addition to structural changes, the loss of corneal sensation leads to numerous problems including delayed epithelial healing, decreased tear production, tear film instability, predisposition to corneal trauma, and susceptibility to develop neurotrophic ulcers [30, 31] (Fig. **1**).

The treatment of diabetic keratopathy depends on its presentation. For mild diseases, such as punctate keratopathy, artificial tears and lubricating ointments are the mainstay of the treatment. More advanced disease may include recurrent corneal erosions, persistent epithelial defects, and/or corneal ulcers. These conditions may require topical antibiotics to prevent or treat infections, a bandage contact lens or tarsorrhaphy to help with re-epithelialization, or surgical procedures to treat unresponsive conditions.

Refractive Changes

The swings from hypoglycemia to hyperglycemia in diabetic patients can cause transient refractive changes. Both myopic and hyperopic shifts are possible following several days or weeks of hyperglycemia, particularly in diabetic patients [32]. The refractive changes are thought to arise from alterations in the shape and thickness of the lens secondary to osmotic gradients created by abnormal blood glucose levels [33, 34]. The treatment for these refractive changes is normalization and sustained control of blood glucose levels with a return to baseline refraction, typically after a few weeks.

In addition to transient refractive changes, diabetics have been shown to develop presbyopia at an earlier age as compared to age-matched non-diabetics. Lens and zonule changes, loss of ciliary muscle tone, and a deficit in neural input to the ciliary muscle are thought to contribute to this early loss of accommodation [35].

Cataracts

Cataracts present 2-5 times more frequently in patients with diabetes and are associated with an earlier age of onset compared to the general population [36]. This risk can increase to 15-25 times in diabetic patients less than 40 years of age [37]. An estimated 20% of cataract procedures are performed on diabetic patients and epidemiological studies suggest that cataracts are the most common cause of visual impairment among older onset diabetic patients [38]. The ten-year cumulative incidence of cataract surgery is estimated to be 27% in patients with early-onset diabetes and 44% in cases of older-onset diabetes [36].

Cataracts can create cloudy or double vision and increase sensitivity to light; as such, it is a major cause of visual impairment [39]. The inciting mechanism of cataract formation in diabetics has been proposed to be through the generation of polyols from glucose by aldose reductase [40]. This results in a rise in osmotic stress on lens fibers causing them to swell with subsequent rupture [41]. Posterior subcapsular and cortical cataracts (Fig. **2**) are more common in diabetics than non-diabetics while there has been no association found between diabetes and nuclear sclerotic cataracts [42, 43]. Although conflicting evidence exists, cataract surgery may result in adverse effects post-operatively including progression of diabetic retinopathy, diabetic macular edema, vitreous hemorrhage, iris neovascularization, endophthalmitis and loss of vision [44 - 46]. Considering these potential adverse effects, it is important for the retina specialist and cataract surgeon to discuss the risk *versus* benefit of cataract surgery for a diabetic patient. These discussions should also include whether or not pre- and/or post-operative anti-VEGF treatment may be beneficial.

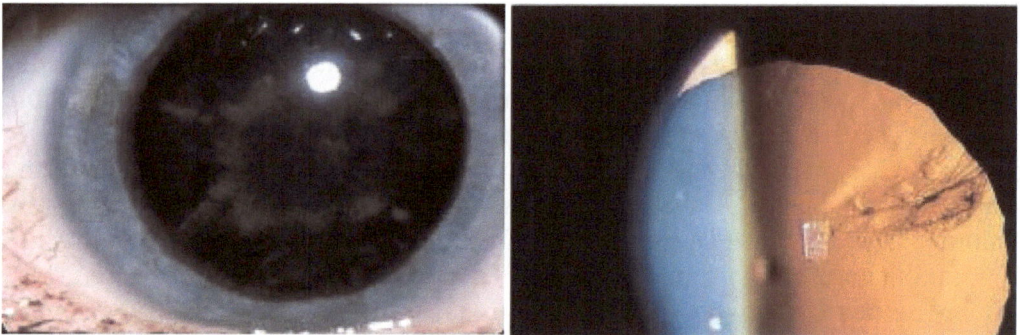

Fig. (2). Posterior capsular cataract (left) and focal cortical cataract (right). © 2017 American Academy of Ophthalmology.

Ocular Movement Disorders

Ocular movement disorders comprise a group of disorders causing impairment in eye movements. Cranial nerve mononeuropathies are one cause of ocular movement disorders, which are known to be a complication of diabetes. More specifically, diabetes is a known risk factor for the development of a microvascular cranial nerve palsy involving the third, fourth, or sixth cranial nerves [47, 48]. Rush found 25-30% of acute extraocular muscle palsy cases in patients 45 years and older [49]. The incidence of cranial nerve palsies in diabetic patients is higher than non-diabetic patients. Watanabe *et al*. found that among 1,961 diabetic patients, 19 (0.97%) demonstrated cranial nerve palsies while the incidence of cranial nerve palsies in 3,841 non-diabetic patients was 0.13% [47]. A more recent study by Greco *et al*. showed the incidence to be 0.40% in diabetic patients. The same study found that the most common cranial nerve palsy among diabetics was a cranial nerve III (oculomotor) palsy (59.3%) followed by a cranial nerve VI (abducens) palsy (29.6%) [50]. Cranial nerve ischemia secondary to microvascular changes is thought to be the cause of cranial nerve palsies in diabetic patients.

Patients with microvascular cranial nerve III, IV, or VI palsies present with binocular diplopia, and ophthalmoparesis may be present on examination. A microvascular third nerve palsy may also present with ptosis. Typically, microvascular third nerve palsies are "pupil-sparing" although Jacobsen reported that 20% of these palsies have mild pupillary involvement [51]. Recovery of extraocular muscle function typically occurs within three months in diabetic related palsies [52].

Neovascular Glaucoma

Patients with longstanding, uncontrolled diabetes are at risk of developing a form of secondary glaucoma termed neovascular glaucoma. Neovascular glaucoma is characterized by proliferation of fibrovascular tissue in the anterior chamber angle causing either a secondary open-angle or secondary closed-angle mechanism that can lead to vision loss from optic nerve damage [53]. Proliferative diabetic retinopathy and central retinal vein occlusions account for nearly two thirds of all cases of neovascular glaucoma [54].

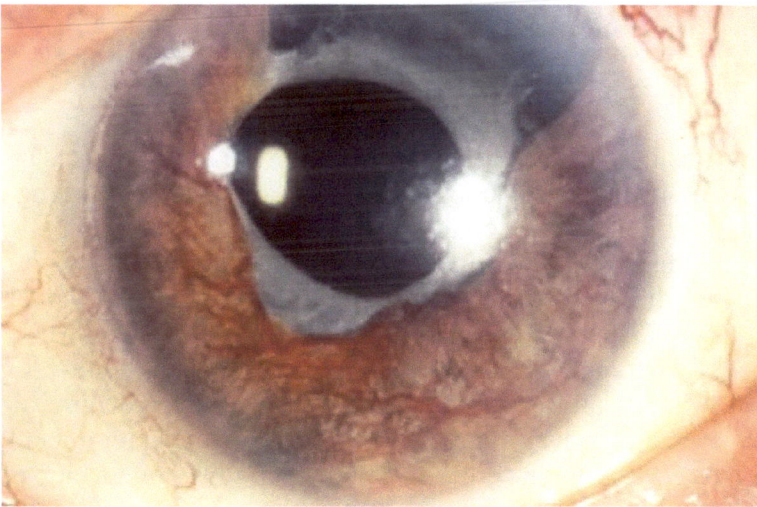

Fig. (3). Neovascularization of the iris secondary to proliferative diabetic disease. The new blood vessels can be seen on the surface of the iris extending from the pupillary margin to the iris periphery. © 2017 American Academy of Ophthalmology.

The development of neovascular glaucoma is most commonly related to retinal ischemia. As stated previously, proliferative diabetic retinopathy and central retinal vein occlusion are the two most common causes of this condition [54]. Retinal ischemia causes production of angiogenesis factors, the most commonly discussed being vascular endothelial growth factor (VEGF). The angiogenesis factors lead to growth of abnormal blood vessels in various structures of the globe including the iris (Fig. **3**) and angle structures. The abnormal blood vessels are accompanied by fibrovascular membrane formation into the angle structures causing trabecular meshwork dysfunction and a secondary open-angle glaucoma. Later in the disease process, these fibrovascular membranes can contract causing secondary closed-angle glaucoma [53].

The management of neovascular glaucoma is aimed at preventing disease progression and normalizing elevated intraocular pressure. Disease progression can be halted with reduction of anti-angiogenesis factors, which reverse and prevent new vessel proliferation. Panretinal photocoagulation and/or anti-VEGF intravitreal injections are used for this purpose. Panretinal photocoagulation reduces the amount of viable retina, which in turn reduces the release of pro-angiogenesis factors. Early stage anti-VEGF treatment has been shown to not only reverse angle neovascularization but also to reduce elevated intraocular pressure and prevent closure of the angle [55, 56]. Reduction of intraocular pressure can be accomplished in early stages using topical or oral medications while late stage disease may require a surgical approach [54].

Posterior Segment Complications

Diabetic Retinopathy

Diabetes is the leading cause of new blindness in the United States among adults aged 20-74 [57]. Its tendency to affect working age adults with long duration of expected survival, creates an economic and social burden. Any patient who has diabetes including ones who are "diet-controlled", or ones who have long-standing treated diabetes with new visual symptoms must be taken seriously. Complaints of visual distortion, "blurred vision" or "floaters" may be a sign of the development of what may be or may become irreversible blindness left untreated. Color vision changes and contrast sensitivity loss may be some of the earlier visual impairments noted by patients with early diabetic retinopathy [58, 59]. Furthermore, patients with diabetic retinopathy, are likely to develop other serious end-organ damage (*i.e.* chronic renal insufficiency, peripheral neuropathy and coronary artery disease) [60].

Significant and permanent visual decline that results from diabetes should be considered to be due to retinopathy until proven otherwise. Cataracts are often coincident to retinal damage and are far less critical to the long-term prospects for visual rehabilitation. Vision loss that is due to retinal problems (tractional or rhegmatogenous retinal detachment) may become permanent and even irreparable in a short period of time (days to months). Patients with diabetes well controlled on medications and even diabetics who are "diet-controlled" are still at risk of permanent vision loss from retinopathy.

Visual loss in diabetic retinopathy is best classified as moderate (a doubling of the visual angle (*i.e.* 20/20 to 20/40) (MVL) or severe (worse than 20/200) (SVL). Treatment goals in diabetic retinopathy historically is to lessen the chance of vision loss, be it moderate vision loss in the case of diabetic macular edema (DME) or severe vision loss in proliferative diabetic retinopathy (PDR). DME leads to moderate vision loss in a slower time frame. Highly- threatening retinopathy (PDR) leads to SVL, often acutely and can present with advanced disease.

Given the location of the retina and the experience needed for a proper fundus examination, the patient, primary care physician, and eyecare specialist may not make the diagnosis of diabetic retinopathy. Advanced means of examination (*i.e.* indirect ophthalmoscopy and slit-lamp biomicroscopy) are essential to diagnose the disease. It should be differentiated from the reversible previously mentioned causes of vision loss (*i.e.* refractive error or cataract), and should not be missed. It is also important to note that each case must be looked at individually as duration and severity of the systemic disease is not a reliable factor in differentiating permanent, severe eye-disease from that which is treatable and temporary.

There tends to be a subset of diabetic retinopathy patients who claim to "not have diabetes" but these patients can also have advanced, sight-threatening diabetic retinopathy on examination. Previously undiscovered genetic factors controlling retinal vascular perfusion, and development of neovascularization may provide an explanation for this occurrence. Patients have gone blind from mild and late-treated Type II DM and then soon thereafter developed renal failure.

Yearly eye examinations are an important tool assuming a qualified eye care physician provides them. An optical exam will not suffice, and patients are often unable to make this important distinction. Given the importance of early diagnosis and treatment, patients require lifelong follow-up by a qualified doctor (at least twice per year when there is a diagnosis of retinopathy).

Non-proliferative diabetic retinopathy (NPDR) (Fig. **4**) is classified as mild ("background"), moderate, and severe ("pre-proliferative"). It necessarily predates PDR, but can be variable in its manifestations and significance to vision. Often observation and observation are all that is recommended at this point, although its severity is occasionally under-estimated. If good glycemic and blood pressure control is maintained, anatomical and visual prognosis is fairly good. Interestingly, retinal disease may paradoxically worsen, however, when glycemic, blood pressure and serum lipid levels are controlled [60].

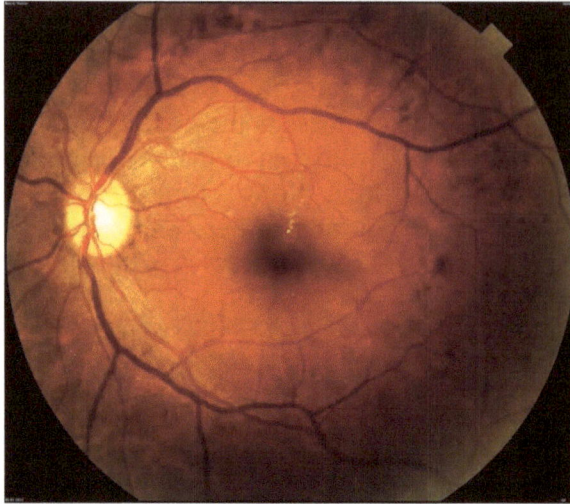

Fig. (4). Nonproliferative diabetic retinopathy (NPDR) with associated hard exudates, microaneurysms, and intraretinal hemorrhages.

Diabetic retinopathy is caused by abnormalities in the retinal vasculature similar to that occurring in the renal glomeruli. The accepted theory involves hyperglycemia induced thickening of the basement membrane, pericyte loss, and dysfunction of the vessel endothelium. Hypoxia, oxidative stress, inflammation and protein damage causes vascular endothelial growth factor (VEGF) and platelet-derived growth factor (PDGF) to be up regulated. During the early stages (non-proliferative diabetic retinopathy) damage to blood vessels can be identified as microaneurysmal saccular changes in capillaries and small intraretinal "dot-blot" hemorrhages. Cotton-wool spots, pointing to ischemia and infarction of the nerve-fiber layer, are also seen but not pathognomonic changes of diabetes. These nerve fiber layer infarcts can also be seen commonly in hypertension and collagen-vascular diseases [61].

Compensatory vascular anomalies due to vascular endothelial growth factor upregulation are typically seen just prior to proliferative diabetic retinopathy in the pre-proliferative retinopathy phase. These changes include intraretinal microvascular abnormalities (IRMA), venous beading, and extensive capillary non-perfusion. These retinal changes can be chronic and largely unnoticed for years, as vision abnormalities can be absent in this phase. As retinal ischemia worsens, levels of VEGF and inflammatory mediators increase in the vitreous cavity, which continues to cause dysfunction of the retinal capillaries. This may lead to leakage into the retina, which comes to exceed the resorptive capacity of the blood vessels and the underlying retinal pigment epithelium leading to diabetic macular edema (Fig. **5**). Retinal thickening and intraretinal lipid (exudate) eventually affect the macula causing vision changes. Severe vision loss can occur in untreated and/or late stage diabetic macular edema.

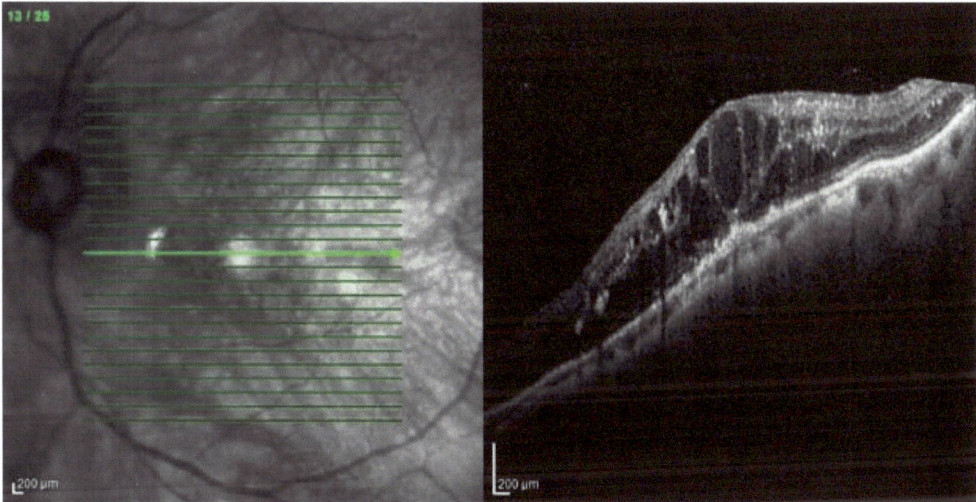

Fig. (5). Spectral-domain optical coherence tomography (OCT). The green arrow signifies a horizontal raster of the macula (left) showing diffuse intraretinal cystic spaces secondary to diabetic macular edema (right).

With the development of proliferative diabetic retinopathy, over-expression of VEGF causes new abnormal blood vessels to form in their attempt to recover the architecture of the retinal capillary network. These vessels are always pathologic, however, and can lead to bleeding into the vitreous cavity and traction on the retina with the possibility of severe, permanent vision loss. These new, tiny capillaries proliferate behind the body of the vitreous onto the optic disc and retina known respectively as neovascularization of the disc (NVD) and neovascularization elsewhere (NVE). These incompetent, fragile vessels tend to bleed which may occur spontaneously or as a result of vitreous traction. Involution of neovascularized fibrovascular tissue and the pulling effect of the vitreous body can lead to a tractional retinal detachment (TRD) (Fig. **6**). Separation of the vitreous from the optic nerve and retina may also induce bleeding and breaks in the retina.

The separation of the vitreous tends to occur later in diabetics due to altered proteins that make up the vitreous gel. This abnormal, stickier vitreous can lead to failure of separation from the macula possibly contributing to macular edema, and can itself distort the foveal pit. Distortion of the foveal pit by the vitreous is known as vitreo-macular traction syndrome (VMTS). This condition is best treated by pars-plana vitrectomy (PPV) where the traction is manually released.

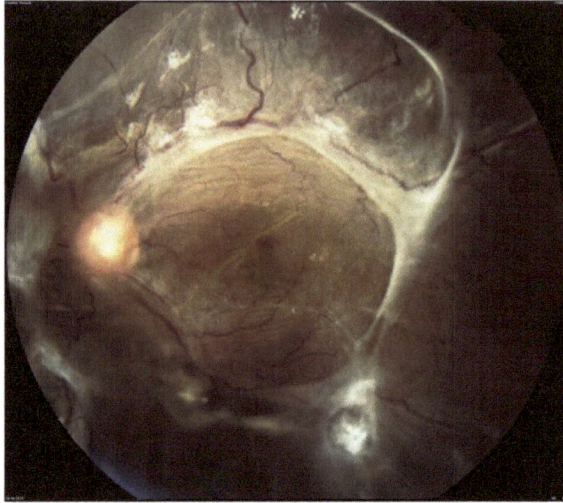

Fig. (6). Proliferative diabetic retinopathy (PDR) with fibrovascular proliferation on the surface of the retina extending from the optic nerve along the arcade vessels causing traction on the macula.

Diabetic retinopathy patients undergo PPV for a variety of indications. These include the aforementioned cases of VMTS, macular distortion from epiretinal membranes, non-clearing and significant vitreous hemorrhage, TRD threatening or involving the macula, and complex rhegmatogenous retinal detachments. As compared to earlier versions of PPV in the 1970s to 1990s, modern PPV is seen as faster and safer. Therefore, its indication and usage have somewhat expanded. Instruments range in size from 20 to 27-gauge. The goal of PPV in diabetics is to remove the vitreous body's posterior hyaloid membrane and most of the vitreous body substance thereby removing the "scaffold" for formation of tractional retinal detachments, vitreo-macular traction and recurrent vitreous hemorrhage. Even though modern pars plana vitrectomy has become safer than previous iterations, there are still risks involved with the surgery. These risks include bleeding, infection, retinal detachment, macular hole formation, glaucoma or optic neuropathy, which can result in permanent vision loss. Patients who were previously untreated with laser panretinal photocoagulation (PRP) may do especially poorly. In the earlier period of vitreoretinal surgery, vitrectomy for PDR carried higher risks-about a 10% chance of severe and permanent vision loss (NLP vision) [62].

Intravitreal anti-VEGF medications are now used frequently for PDR prior to surgery in cases where significant neovascularization exists. Caution must be exercised though, as involution and contraction of neovascularization occurs very rapidly and this may induce worsening TRD, retinal breaks and rhegmatogenous retinal detachment.

The treatment of CSDME based on results of the Early Treatment of Diabetic Retinopathy Study (ETDRS) is focal laser treatment. This treatment can decrease the chance of moderate vision loss by about 50% over several years [63, 64]. During the focal laser procedure, small spots of thermal laser are applied under direct visualization to leaking microaneurysms that are visible at the slit-lamp and further identified by intravenous fluorescein angiography (IVFA). IVFA is helpful in identifying areas of peripheral retinal non-perfusion and cases with co-existing macular ischemia. Focal laser is less useful in cases with diffuse macular edema and cases where microaneurysms are located within the foveal avascular zone.

Anti-VEGF intravitreal treatment is highly effective in treating diabetic macular edema, as VEGF is strongly implicated in vascular leakage from the abnormal diabetic capillaries [65, 66]. Multiple studies have shown anti-VEGF intravitreal treatment to be effective in treating diabetic macular edema and superior to focal laser [67 - 72]. Alternative treatments include intravitreal triamcinolone injection, which carries a high risk of ocular hypertension with possible glaucoma and cataract. The effects of triamcinolone on the retina are quite transitory and tachyphlaxis can be seen. Sustained-release intravitreal dexamethasone implant (Ozurdex®, Allergan, Inc., Irvine, California, USA) can be an effective treatment with a lower side effect profile compared to intravitreal triamcinolone [73] when considering steroid therapies.

Seriel optical coherence tomography (OCT) is invaluable for following the treatment response in diabetic macular edema. Spectral domain high resolution OCT is a great advance as it provides non-contact, quantification of the macular thickness, noting however, that IVFA is still needed to assess the retinal circulation.

Proliferative Diabetic Retinopathy (PDR) treatment is based on the results of the Diabetic Retinopathy Study (DRS). Pan-retinal photocoagulation (PRP) is beneficial in reducing the chance of severe vision loss over several years time [74, 75]. The decision to treat using PRP is based on the presence, location (on the disc or elsewhere) and extent of neovascularization along with the presence or absence of vitreous hemorrhage. Patients who are at high risk of progression, or non-compliance are usually offered earlier treatment. In PRP, large 300-500 micron spots of laser are applied under direct visualization to the peripheral retina. The effect of the laser is to "kill off" the dying, ischemic peripheral retina, thereby lowering the VEGF drive. This reduction in VEGF lowers the stimulus to develop neovascularization and macular edema formation.

In the setting of significant diabetic vitreous hemorrhage in PDR, properly applied PRP laser is always very helpful, as it directly reduces the load of VEGF delivered to the functioning retina. Patients treated with early PRP do quite well and typically maintain vision that will allow important life activities such as driving. In the diabetic patient with minimal prior laser or where significant laser cannot be safely applied through the vitreous hemorrhage, early treatment with vitrectomy is usually indicated [62]. For most patients who benefit from aggressive screening and treatment, vision loss may be reversed with very aggressive and appropriate treatment with a combination of laser, injections, and surgery.

Diabetic Papillopathy

Diabetic papillopathy (DP) is an uncommon, hyperemic optic disk swelling that occurs in patients with long-standing diabetes [76]. Its prevalence is 1.4% in diabetic patients and presents bilaterally in 50% of cases. DP is characterized by optic disk swelling resulting from vascular leakage and axonal edema in the area surrounding the optic nerve head, and may present with intra-retinal hemorrhages and exudates [77] (Fig. **7**).

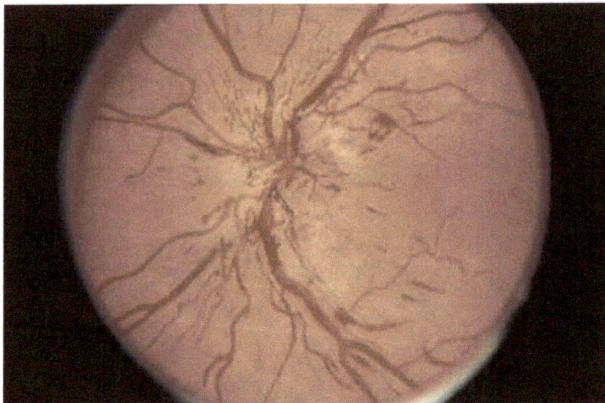

Fig. (7). Optic disc in diabetic papillopathy shows disc edema with prominent surface telangiectasia. © 2017 American Academy of Ophthalmology.

Although its pathogenesis remains unclear, DP may be associated with small cup/disc ratio and rapid glycemic/metabolic control [78]. As such, it is a diagnosis of exclusion [76], after alternative causes of optic disk swelling have been ruled out. DP is usually self-limited and has a good visual prognosis [77]. In fact, disc swelling often resolves spontaneously within 3–4 months [79]. However, in some cases, permanent visual damage can occur. Additionally, in eyes with DP, diabetic retinopathy tends to progress over time [77]. While there is no accepted therapy, intravitreal corticosteroids or anti-vascular endothelial growth factors such as bevacizumab have shown a beneficial effect on visual acuity while producing a rapid improvement of disc swelling [76].

CONCLUSION

Diabetes can cause both anterior and posterior segment manifestations in the eye. Dry eye, ocular surface disorders, refractive changes are all possible anterior issues. Ocular motility problems as well as an increased risk of glaucoma can also be seen in the diabetic. In the posterior segment, microvascular changes can lead to retinopathy, macular edema, and papillopathy. Anterior and posterior ocular issues are discussed in more detail in later chapters of the book.

CONSENT FOR PUBLICATION

Not applicable.

CONFLICT OF INTEREST

The author declares no conflict of interest, financial or otherwise.

ACKNOWLEDGEMENTS

Declared none.

REFERENCES

[1]   Wu Li teh, Fernandez-Loaiza P, Sauma J, *et al.* Classification of diabetic retinopathy and diabetic macular edema. World J Diabetes. 2013 Dec 15;4(6): 290–294.

[2]   Saaddine JB, Honeycutt AA, Narayan KM, Zhang X, Klein R, Boyle JP. Projection of diabetic retinopathy and other major eye diseases among people with diabetes mellitus: United States, 2005-2050. Arch Ophthalmol 2008; 126(12): 1740-7.
        [http://dx.doi.org/10.1001/archopht.126.12.1740] [PMID: 19064858]

[3]   Klein R, Klein BE, Moss SE, Davis MD, DeMets DL. The Wisconsin epidemiologic study of diabetic retinopathy. III. Prevalence and risk of diabetic retinopathy when age at diagnosis is 30 or more years. Arch Ophthalmol 1984; 102(4): 527-32.
        [http://dx.doi.org/10.1001/archopht.1984.01040030405011] [PMID: 6367725]

[4]   Jeganathan VSE, Wang JJ, Wong TY. Ocular associations of diabetes other than diabetic retinopathy. Diabetes Care 2008; 31(9): 1905-12.
        [http://dx.doi.org/10.2337/dc08-0342] [PMID: 18753669]

[5]   Cousen P, Cackett P, Bennett H, Swa K, Dhillon B. Tear production and corneal sensitivity in diabetes. J Diabetes Complications 2007; 21(6): 371-3.
        [http://dx.doi.org/10.1016/j.jdiacomp.2006.05.008] [PMID: 17967709]

[6]   Dogru M, Katakami C, Inoue M. Tear function and ocular surface changes in noninsulin-dependent diabetes mellitus. Ophthalmol 2001; 108(3): 586-92.
        [http://dx.doi.org/10.1016/S0161-6420(00)00599-6] [PMID: 11237914]

[7]   Rosenberg ME, Tervo TM, Immonen IJ, Müller LJ, Grönhagen-Riska C, Vesaluoma MH. Corneal structure and sensitivity in type 1 diabetes mellitus. Invest Ophthalmol Vis Sci 2000; 41(10): 2915-21.
        [PMID: 10967045]

[8]   Sayin N, Kara N, Pekel G. Ocular complications of diabetes mellitus. World J Diabetes 2015; 6(1): 92-108.
        [http://dx.doi.org/10.4239/wjd.v6.i1.92] [PMID: 25685281]

[9]   Achtsidis V, Eleftheriadou I, Kozanidou E, *et al.* Dry eye syndrome in subjects with diabetes and association with neuropathy. Diabetes Care 2014; 37(10): e210-1.
        [http://dx.doi.org/10.2337/dc14-0860] [PMID: 25249675]

[10]   Javadi M-A, Feizi S. Dry eye syndrome. J Ophthalmic Vis Res 2011; 6(3): 192-8.
        [PMID: 22454735]

[11]   Zhang X, Zhao L, Deng S, Sun X, Wang N. Dry eye syndrome in patients with diabetes mellitus: prevalence, etiology, and clinical characteristics. J Ophthalmol 2016; 20168201053
        [http://dx.doi.org/10.1155/2016/8201053] [PMID: 27213053]

[12]   Dias AC, Batista TM, Roma LP, *et al.* Insulin replacement restores the vesicular secretory apparatus in the diabetic rat lacrimal gland. Arq Bras Oftalmol 2015; 78(3): 158-63.
        [http://dx.doi.org/10.5935/0004-2749.20150041] [PMID: 26222104]

[13]   Módulo CM, Jorge AG, Dias AC, *et al.* Influence of insulin treatment on the lacrimal gland and ocular surface of diabetic rats. Endocrine 2009; 36(1): 161-8.
        [http://dx.doi.org/10.1007/s12020-009-9208-9] [PMID: 19551521]

[14]   Zhao Z, Liu J, Shi B, He S, Yao X, Willcox MD. Advanced glycation end product (AGE) modified proteins in tears of diabetic patients. Mol Vis 2010; 16: 1576-84.
        [PMID: 20806041]

[15]   Nichols KK, Nichols JJ, Mitchell GL. The lack of association between signs and symptoms in patients with dry eye disease. Cornea 2004; 23(8): 762-70.
        [http://dx.doi.org/10.1097/01.ico.0000133997.07144.9e] [PMID: 15502475]

[16]   Holland EJ, Mannis MJ, Lee WB. Ocular Surface Disease: Cornea, Conjunctiva and Tear Film Ocular Surface Disease: Cornea, Conjunctiva and Tear Film. London: Elsevier-Saunders 2013. Print

[17]   Zeev MS-B, Miller DD, Latkany R. Diagnosis of dry eye disease and emerging technologies. Clin Ophthalmol 2014; 8: 581-90.
        [PMID: 24672224]

[18]   Messmer EM. The pathophysiology, diagnosis, and treatment of dry eye disease. Dtsch Arztebl Int 2015; 112(5): 71-81.
        [http://dx.doi.org/10.3238/arztebl.2015.0071] [PMID: 25686388]

[19]   Kymionis GD, Bouzoukis DI, Diakonis VF, Siganos C. Treatment of chronic dry eye: focus on cyclosporine. Clin Ophthalmol 2008; 2(4): 829-36.
        [http://dx.doi.org/10.2147/OPTH.S1409] [PMID: 19668437]

[20]   Sheppard JD, Torkildsen GL, Lonsdale JD, *et al.* OPUS-1 Study Group. Lifitegrast ophthalmic solution 5.0% for treatment of dry eye disease: results of the OPUS-1 phase 3 study. Ophthalmology 2014; 121(2): 475-83.
        [http://dx.doi.org/10.1016/j.ophtha.2013.09.015] [PMID: 24289915]

[21]   Sheppard JD Jr, Singh R, McClellan AJ, *et al.* Long-term supplementation with n-6 and n-3 PUFAs improves moderate-to-severe keratoconjunctivitis sicca: A randomized double-blind clinical trial. Cornea 2013; 32(10): 1297-304.
        [http://dx.doi.org/10.1097/ICO.0b013e318299549c] [PMID: 23884332]

[22]   Brignole-Baudouin F, Baudouin C, Aragona P, *et al.* A multicentre, double-masked, randomized, controlled trial assessing the effect of oral supplementation of omega-3 and omega-6 fatty acids on a conjunctival inflammatory marker in dry eye patients. Acta Ophthalmol 2011; 89(7): e591-7.
        [http://dx.doi.org/10.1111/j.1755-3768.2011.02196.x] [PMID: 21834921]

[23]   Vieira-Potter VJ, Karamichos D, Lee DJ. Ocular complications of diabetes and therapeutic approaches. BioMed Res Int 2016; 20163801570
        [http://dx.doi.org/10.1155/2016/3801570] [PMID: 27119078]

[24]   Negi A, Vernon SA. An overview of the eye in diabetes. J R Soc Med 2003; 96(6): 266-72.

[http://dx.doi.org/10.1177/014107680309600603] [PMID: 12782689]

[25]   Yoon K-C, Im S-K, Seo M-S. Changes of tear film and ocular surface in diabetes mellitus. Korean J Ophthalmol 2004; 18(2): 168-74.
[http://dx.doi.org/10.3341/kjo.2004.18.2.168] [PMID: 15635831]

[26]   Friend J, Thoft RA. The diabetic cornea. Int Ophthalmol Clin 1984; 24(4): 111-23.
[http://dx.doi.org/10.1097/00004397-198402440-00011] [PMID: 6500867]

[27]   Tabatabay CA, Bumbacher M, Baumgartner B, Leuenberger PM. Reduced number of hemidesmosomes in the corneal epithelium of diabetics with proliferative vitreoretinopathy. Graefes Arch Clin Exp Ophthalmol 1988; 226(4): 389-92.
[http://dx.doi.org/10.1007/BF02172973] [PMID: 3169590]

[28]   Gipson IK, Spurr-Michaud SJ, Tisdale AS. Anchoring fibrils form a complex network in human and rabbit cornea. Invest Ophthalmol Vis Sci 1987; 28(2): 212-20.
[PMID: 8591898]

[29]   McDermott AM, Xiao TL, Kern TS, Murphy CJ. Non-enzymatic glycation in corneas from normal and diabetic donors and its effects on epithelial cell attachment *in vitro*. Optometry 2003; 74(7): 443-52.
[PMID: 12877277]

[30]   Hyndiuk RA, Kazarian EL, Schultz RO, Seideman S. Neurotrophic corneal ulcers in diabetes mellitus. Arch Ophthalmol 1977; 95(12): 2193-6.
[http://dx.doi.org/10.1001/archopht.1977.04450120099012] [PMID: 588113]

[31]   Araki K, Ohashi Y, Kinoshita S, Hayashi K, Kuwayama Y, Tano Y. Epithelial wound healing in the denervated cornea. Curr Eye Res 1994; 13(3): 203-11.
[http://dx.doi.org/10.3109/02713689408995778] [PMID: 8194368]

[32]   Wiemer NGM, Eekhoff EMW, Simsek S, *et al.* Refractive properties of the healthy human eye during acute hyperglycemia. Graefes Arch Clin Exp Ophthalmol 2008; 246(7): 993-8.
[http://dx.doi.org/10.1007/s00417-008-0810-y] [PMID: 18389272]

[33]   Okamoto F, Sone H, Nonoyama T, Hommura S. Refractive changes in diabetic patients during intensive glycaemic control. Br J Ophthalmol 2000; 84(10): 1097-102.
[http://dx.doi.org/10.1136/bjo.84.10.1097] [PMID: 11004091]

[34]   Furushima M, Imaizumi M, Nakatsuka K. Changes in refraction caused by induction of acute hyperglycemia in healthy volunteers. Jpn J Ophthalmol 1999; 43(5): 398-403.
[http://dx.doi.org/10.1016/S0021-5155(99)00098-2] [PMID: 10580662]

[35]   Adnan E, Efron N, Mathur A, *et al.* Amplitude of accommodation in type 1 diabetes. Invest Ophthalmol Vis Sci 2014; 55(10): 7014-8.
[http://dx.doi.org/10.1167/iovs.14-15376] [PMID: 25298413]

[36]   Klein BE, Klein R, Moss SE. Incidence of cataract surgery in the wisconsin epidemiologic study of diabetic retinopathy. Am J Ophthalmol 1995; 119(3): 295-300.
[http://dx.doi.org/10.1016/S0002-9394(14)71170-5] [PMID: 7872389]

[37]   Bernth-Petersen P, Bach E. Epidemiologic aspects of cataract surgery. III: Frequencies of diabetes and glaucoma in a cataract population. Acta Ophthalmol (Copenh) 1983; 61(3): 406-16.
[http://dx.doi.org/10.1111/j.1755-3768.1983.tb01439.x] [PMID: 6624407]

[38]   Hamilton AM, Ulbig MW, Polkinghorne P. Epidemiology of diabetic retinopathy. In: Ulbig MW, Polkinghorne P, Eds. Management of Diabetic Retinopathy london: BMJ Publishing G. Hamilton, AM 1996; pp. 1-15.

[39]   Harding JJ, Egerton M, van Heyningen R, Harding RS. Diabetes, glaucoma, sex, and cataract: analysis of combined data from two case control studies. Br J Ophthalmol 1993; 77(1): 2-6.
[http://dx.doi.org/10.1136/bjo.77.1.2] [PMID: 8435392]

[40]   Pollreisz Andreas. Diabetic cataract—pathogenesis, epidemiology and treatment. J Ophthalmology 2010; 2010: 8.

[41]   Kinoshita JH. Mechanisms initiating cataract formation. Proctor Lecture. Invest Ophthalmol 1974; 13(10): 713-24.
[PMID: 4278188]

[42]   Schäfer C, Lautenschläger C, Struck HG. Cataract types in diabetics and non-diabetics: a densitometric study with the Topcon-Scheimpflug camera. Klin Monatsbl Augenheilkd 2006; 223(7): 589-92.
[PMID: 16855942]

[43]   Saxena S, Mitchell P, Rochtchina E. Five-year incidence of cataract in older persons with diabetes and pre-diabetes. Ophthalmic Epidemiol 2004; 11(4): 271-7.
[http://dx.doi.org/10.1080/09286580490510733] [PMID: 15512989]

[44]   Varma SD, Mizuno A, Kinoshita JH. Diabetic cataracts and flavonoids. Science 1977; 195(4274): 205-6.
[http://dx.doi.org/10.1126/science.401544] [PMID: 401544]

[45]   Sebestyen JG. Intraocular lenses and diabetes mellitus. Am J Ophthalmol 1986; 101(4): 425-8.
[http://dx.doi.org/10.1016/0002-9394(86)90640-9] [PMID: 3963101]

[46]   Hayashi K, Igarashi C, Hirata A, Hayashi H. Changes in diabetic macular oedema after phacoemulsification surgery. Eye (Lond) 2009; 23(2): 389-96.
[http://dx.doi.org/10.1038/sj.eye.6703022] [PMID: 17962820]

[47]   Watanabe K, Hagura R, Akanuma Y, *et al.* Characteristics of cranial nerve palsies in diabetic patients. Diabetes Res Clin Pract 1990; 10(1): 19-27.
[http://dx.doi.org/10.1016/0168-8227(90)90077-7] [PMID: 2249603]

[48]   Acaroglu G, Akinci A, Zilelioglu O. Retinopathy in patients with diabetic ophthalmoplegia. Ophthalmologica 2008; 222(4): 225-8.
[http://dx.doi.org/10.1159/000130070] [PMID: 18463423]

[49]   Rush JA. Extraocular muscle palsies in diabetes mellitus. Int Ophthalmol Clin 1984; 24(4): 155-9.
[http://dx.doi.org/10.1097/00004397-198402440-00014] [PMID: 6500869]

[50]   Greco D, Gambina F, Maggio F. Ophthalmoplegia in diabetes mellitus: a retrospective study. Acta Diabetol 2009; 46(1): 23-6.
[http://dx.doi.org/10.1007/s00592-008-0053-8] [PMID: 18758685]

[51]   Jacobson DM. Relative pupil-sparing third nerve palsy: etiology and clinical variables predictive of a mass. Neurology 2001; 56(6): 797-8.
[http://dx.doi.org/10.1212/WNL.56.6.797] [PMID: 11274322]

[52]   Miller NR, Walsh FB, Hoyt WF. Walsh and Hoyt's Clinical Neuro-ophthalmology. Philadelphia: Lippincott Williams & Wilkins 2005. Print

[53]   Mansouri K. Shields Textbook of Glaucoma. 6th Edition., Shields Textbook of Glaucoma 2012.

[54]   Brown GC, Magargal LE, Schachat A, Shah H. Neovascular glaucoma. Etiologic considerations. Ophthalmology 1984; 91(4): 315-20.
[http://dx.doi.org/10.1016/S0161-6420(84)34293-2] [PMID: 6201791]

[55]   Sun Y, Liang Y, Zhou P, *et al.* Anti-VEGF treatment is the key strategy for neovascular glaucoma management in the short term. BMC Ophthalmol 2016; 16(1): 150.
[http://dx.doi.org/10.1186/s12886-016-0327-9] [PMID: 27576739]

[56]   Wakabayashi T, Oshima Y, Sakaguchi H, *et al.* Intravitreal bevacizumab to treat iris neovascularization and neovascular glaucoma secondary to ischemic retinal diseases in 41 consecutive cases 2008.
[http://dx.doi.org/10.1016/j.ophtha.2008.02.026]

[57]   57. National Society to Prevent Blindness. Vision problems in the U.S.: a statistical analysis. New York: National Society to Prevent Blindness, 1980. In, Retina, Ryan Volume 2. Mosby, 2002. 2002.

[58]   Arend O, Remky A, Evans D, Stüber R, Harris A. Contrast sensitivity loss is coupled with capillary dropout in patients with diabetes. Invest Ophthalmol Vis Sci 1997; 38(9): 1819-24.
[PMID: 9286271]

[59]   Feitosa-Santana C, Paramei GV, Nishi M, Gualtieri M, Costa MF, Ventura DF. Color vision impairment in type 2 diabetes assessed by the D-15d test and the Cambridge Colour Test. Ophthalmic Physiol Opt 2010; 30(5): 717-23.
[http://dx.doi.org/10.1111/j.1475-1313.2010.00776.x] [PMID: 20883359]

[60]   Diabetes Control and Complications Trial Research Group. The effect of intensive treatment of diabetes on the development and progression of ling-term complications in insulin-dependent diabetes mellitus. N Engl J Med 1993; 329: 936-77.

[61]   Engerman RL, Bloodworth JM Jr. Experimental diabetic retinopathy in dogs. Arch Ophthalmol 1965; 73: 205-10.
[http://dx.doi.org/10.1001/archopht.1965.00970030207013] [PMID: 14237790]

[62]   The Diabetic Retinopathy Vitrectomy Study Research Group. Early vitrectomy for severe vitreous hemorrhage in diabetic retinopathy. Two-year results of a randomized trial. Diabetic Retinopathy Vitrectomy Study report 2. Arch Ophthalmol 1985; 103(11): 1644-52.
[http://dx.doi.org/10.1001/archopht.1985.01050110038020] [PMID: 2865943]

[63]   Early Treatment of Diabetic Retinopathy Study Research Group. Photocoagulation for diabetic macular edema: ETDRS Study report number 1. Arch Ophthalmol 1985; 103: 1796-806.
[http://dx.doi.org/10.1001/archopht.1985.01050120030015]

[64]   Early Treatment Diabetic Retinopathy Study Research Group. Early photocoagulation for diabetic retinopathy. ETDRS report number 9. Ophthalmology 1991; 98(5) (Suppl.): 766-85.
[http://dx.doi.org/10.1016/S0161-6420(13)38011-7] [PMID: 2062512]

[65]   Aiello LP, Avery RL, Arrigg PG, *et al.* Vascular endothelial growth factor in ocular fluid of patients with diabetic retinopathy and other retinal disorders. N Engl J Med 1994; 331(22): 1480-7.
[http://dx.doi.org/10.1056/NEJM199412013312203] [PMID: 7526212]

[66]   Kim I, Ryan AM, Rohan R, *et al.* Constitutive expression of VEGF, VEGFR-1, and VEGFR-2 in normal eyes. Invest Ophthalmol Vis Sci 1999; 40(9): 2115-21.
[PMID: 10440268]

[67]   Nguyen QD, Shah SM, Khwaja AA, *et al.* READ-2 Study Group. Two-year outcomes of the ranibizumab for edema of the mAcula in diabetes (READ-2) study. Ophthalmology 2010; 117(11): 2146-51.
[http://dx.doi.org/10.1016/j.ophtha.2010.08.016] [PMID: 20855114]

[68]   Mitchell P, Bandello F, Schmidt-Erfurth U, *et al.* RESTORE study group. The RESTORE study: ranibizumab monotherapy or combined with laser *versus* laser monotherapy for diabetic macular edema. Ophthalmology 2011; 118(4): 615-25.
[http://dx.doi.org/10.1016/j.ophtha.2011.01.031] [PMID: 21459215]

[69]   Ishibashi T, Li X, Koh A, *et al.* REVEAL Study Group. The REVEAL Study: Ranibizumab monotherapy or combined with laser *versus* laser monotherapy in asian patients with diabetic macular edema. Ophthalmology 2015; 122(7): 1402-15.
[http://dx.doi.org/10.1016/j.ophtha.2015.02.006] [PMID: 25983216]

[70]   Nguyen QD, Brown DM, Marcus DM, *et al.* RISE and RIDE Research Group. Ranibizumab for diabetic macular edema: results from 2 phase III randomized trials: RISE and RIDE. Ophthalmology 2012; 119(4): 789-801.
[http://dx.doi.org/10.1016/j.ophtha.2011.12.039] [PMID: 22330964]

[71]   Korobelnik JF, Do DV, Schmidt-Erfurth U, *et al.* Intravitreal aflibercept for diabetic macular edema.

Ophthalmology 2014; 121(11): 2247-54.
[http://dx.doi.org/10.1016/j.ophtha.2014.05.006] [PMID: 25012934]

[72]   Soheilian M, Ramezani A, Bijanzadeh B, *et al.* Intravitreal bevacizumab (avastin) injection alone or combined with triamcinolone *versus* macular photocoagulation as primary treatment of diabetic macular edema. Retina 2007; 27(9): 1187-95.
[http://dx.doi.org/10.1097/IAE.0b013e31815ec261] [PMID: 18046223]

[73]   Boyer DS, Yoon YH, Belfort R Jr, *et al.* Ozurdex MEAD Study Group. Three-year, randomized, sham-controlled trial of dexamethasone intravitreal implant in patients with diabetic macular edema. Ophthalmology 2014; 121(10): 1904-14.
[http://dx.doi.org/10.1016/j.ophtha.2014.04.024] [PMID: 24907062]

[74]   The Diabetic Retinopathy Study Research Group. Preliminary report on effects of photocoagulation therapy. Am J Ophthalmol 1976; 81(4): 383-96.
[http://dx.doi.org/10.1016/0002-9394(76)90292-0] [PMID: 944535]

[75]   Diabetic Retinopathy Study Research Group. Photocoagulation treatment of proliferative diabetic retinopathy: the second report of diabetic retinopathy study findings. Ophthalmology 1978; 85(1): 82-106.
[http://dx.doi.org/10.1016/S0161-6420(78)35693-1] [PMID: 345173]

[76]   Al-Dhibi H, Khan AO. Response of diabetic papillopathy to intravitreal bevacizumab. Middle East Afr J Ophthalmol 2011; 18(3): 243-5.
[http://dx.doi.org/10.4103/0974-9233.84056] [PMID: 21887082]

[77]   Bayraktar Z, Alacali N, Bayraktar S. Diabetic papillopathy in type II diabetic patients. Retina 2002; 22(6): 752-8.
[http://dx.doi.org/10.1097/00006982-200212000-00011] [PMID: 12476102]

[78]   Ostri C, Lund-Andersen H, Sander B, Hvidt-Nielsen D, Larsen M. Bilateral diabetic papillopathy and metabolic control. Ophthalmology 2010; 117(11): 2214-7.
[http://dx.doi.org/10.1016/j.ophtha.2010.03.006] [PMID: 20557939]

[79]   Vaphiades MS. The disk edema dilemma. Surv Ophthalmol 2002; 47(2): 183-8.
[http://dx.doi.org/10.1016/S0039-6257(01)00301-0] [PMID: 11918898]

CHAPTER 7

Diabetes and the Cornea

Lucy Sun[1] and **Douglas R. Lazzaro**[2,*]

[1] *SUNY Downstate Medical Center, NY, USA*

[2] *Department of Ophthalmology, NYU Langone Health, NY, USA*

Abstract: Diabetes affects the eye in many ways. We most commonly think of posterior segment complications as the main problem causing loss of vision in diabetes which is certainly the most common way people suffer ocular damage. However, the anterior segment is not immune to diabetic complications, and the cornea can be affected in a variety of ways. The manifestations of the corneal disease will be discussed in detail in this chapter.

Keywords: Cornea, Cataract, Epithelial, Infection, Keratitis, Postoperative, Refractive, Ulcer.

The adult cornea is located in the outermost layer of the eye and functions to protect the eye from damage while also focusing on the entry of light. It contributes to approximately two-thirds of the eye's total focusing power, and is the most sensitive tissue of the body with the highest density of pain receptors. Therefore, damage to the cornea can lead to loss of vision, altered corneal sensation, and increased risk of infection. Structurally, the cornea is composed of 5 tissue layers organized into a transparent tissue containing immature resident immune cells and sensory nerve fibers. The 5 layers, from anterior to posterior are: corneal epithelium, bowman's layer, corneal stroma, Descemet's membrane, and corneal endothelium (Fig. **1**).

The cornea topography can be easily imaged by various methods and helps to determine normal *versus* abnormal layering of both anterior and posterior surfaces (Fig. **2**). Due to its transparent nature, the cornea is avascular and receives oxygen and nourishment *via* diffusion from the tear fluid of the outer surface, from the aqueous humor of the inner surface, and from the neurotrophins of the nerve fibers.

---

* **Corresponding author Douglas R. Lazzaro:** Department of Ophthalmology, NYU Langone Medical Center, USA; Email: Douglas.Lazzaro@nyulangone.org

Diabetes mellitus is a major systemic disease that can have marked effects and complications on all layers of the cornea. Corneal abnormalities as a result of diabetes have been termed diabetic keratopathy. This chapter reviews the pathophysiological, morphological, and clinical features of corneal changes secondary to diabetes.

CORNEAL EPITHELIUM

The corneal epithelium is an exceedingly active, self-renewing multicellular tissue layer composed of 5 to 7 layers of cells, with the outermost layer shedding constantly and the basal layer regenerating continuously to support the same thickness profile to maintain corneal power. It is extremely thin, measuring approximately 53um in thickness, with no statistically significant difference between the left and right eyes with respect to age, spherical equivalent refraction, or keratometry [1].

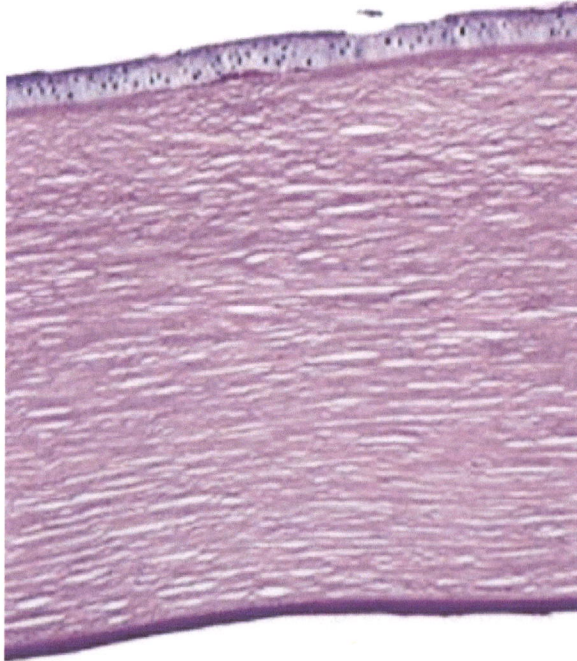

Fig. (1). -Cornea cross section-epithelium on top and endothelium on bottom.

Increase in Epithelial Thickness

In diabetic patients, an increase in central corneal epithelial thickness has been observed and may be one of the earliest detectable clinical changes in the diabetic eye [2]. The average corneal basement membrane (BM) thickness in non-diabetic patients is 54um, compared to 57um in diabetic patients [3]. The thickening is uniform along the length of the epithelial BM in the central cornea. No clear association has been found between central corneal thickness and age or sex. Data regarding the correlation between central corneal thickness and the duration of diabetes are inconsistent. Busted *et al.* [2] found no correlation while Lee *et al.* [4] showed a significant correlation between central corneal thickness and diabetes duration of over or under 10 years. Although the occurrence of multilaminar BM was more common in the diabetic eye than in the non-diabetic eye, the odds ratio was not statistically significant. The multilamination of BM, however, correlated more closely with the presence of the BM thickness than with the presence or absence of diabetes [5].

Abnormal Basement Membrane Formation

The corneas of diabetic patients are exposed to elevated glucose concentrations, and through the mechanism of non-enzymatic glycation, advanced glycation end products (AGEs) form and accumulate in the BM of the corneal epithelium. More specifically, the N-carboxymethyl lysine protein (CML), which is located in the laminin of epithelial BM, is the main AGEs antigen target.

In a study by Kaji *et al.*, age-matched diabetic and non-diabetic corneas were examined, and CML immunoreactivity was present in the epithelial BMs of most diabetic corneas, and absent in the corresponding areas of most non-diabetic corneas [6]. The presence of AGEs in the epithelial BM decreases adhesion and spread of the corneal epithelial cells. *In vitro* studies with glucose-6-phosphate (G-6-P) on glycation of laminin-coated matrix showed that glycation of laminin significantly diminished the number of attached corneal epithelial cells. When aminoguanidine, which inhibits CML formation with G-6-P, was added into the incubation mixture during glycation, both the number and the surface area of adherent corneal epithelial cells increased in a dose-dependent manner.

In addition to the presence of AGEs, another alteration that is specific to the diabetic cornea was the significant decrease in immunostaining of several major BM components and their binding epithelial integrins. The underlying mechanism is likely due to an increase in the degradation of these components by extracellular proteinases. Saghizadeh *et al.* studied various proteinases and noticed an increase in gene expression of matrix metalloproteinases (MMPs), which are a group of zinc enzymes responsible for degrading BM components [7]. This results in the weakening of the epithelial anchoring system, making the diabetic cornea more vulnerable to mechanical injuries and recurrent erosions.

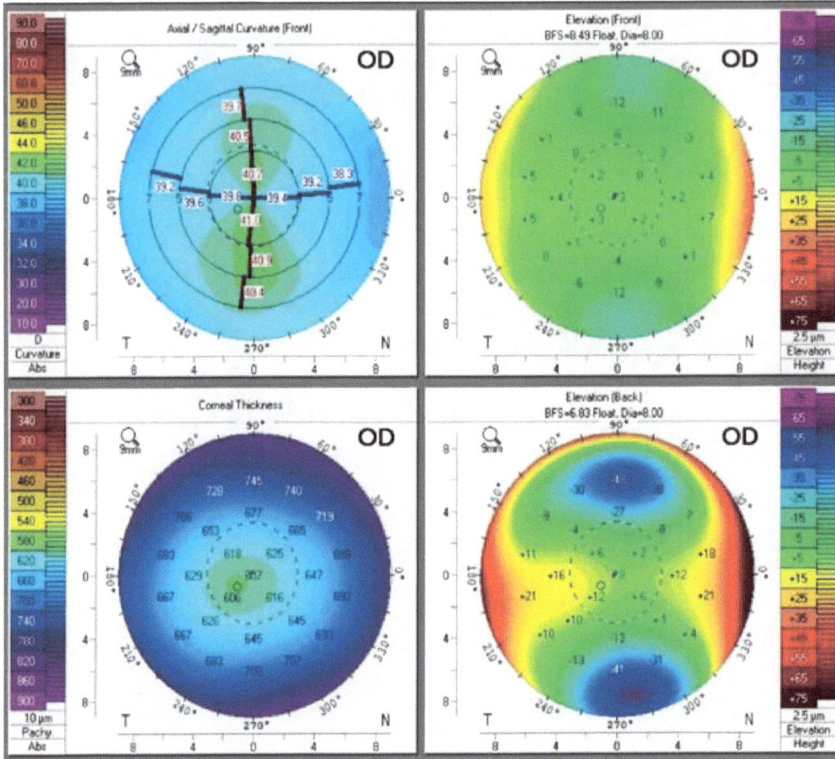

Fig. (2). Normal topography of cornea with mild central thinning.

Therefore, both the accumulation of AGEs on the BM and the proteolytic degradation of BM components due to the upregulation of MMPs are plausible causative culprits for the pathogenesis of corneal epithelial/Bowman's layer keratopathy.

Impaired Epithelial Barrier Function

As discussed above, the accumulation of AGEs on the epithelial BM alters the epithelial cell behavior, leading to a subsequent weakening of the epithelial barrier function in the diabetic cornea. Gekka *et al.* suggested a correlation between an increase in HbA1c level to an increase in the permeability of the epithelium [8]. Epithelial permeability to fluorescein was examined using a slit-lamp fluorophotometer, and a 5.4 fold increase in epithelial permeability to fluorescein was reported in patients with diabetes (average duration of disease was 11 years) compared to non-diabetic controls. Impaired corneal epithelial barrier function predisposes diabetic patients to corneal infections, such as infectious keratitis.

Increased Epithelial Fragility

In diabetic keratopathy, it has been well observed that the corneal epithelium often detaches easily from the stroma. This loosened epithelial adhesion and fragility is due to the thickened BM, the decreased penetration of the anchoring fibrils into the stroma [9], and the enhanced MMP activity in elevated glucose states.

Using the KKAy mouse model for type II diabetes, Watanabe *et al.* showed the characteristics of chronic epithelial detachment in these mice: thickened BM, fragile corneal epithelial cell attachment with poor adherence to the BM, widening of the intracellular spaces between corneal epithelial cells, and subepithelial opacities likely secondary to the continuous poor adhesion and the detachment of epithelial cells [10]. In response, activated keratocytes generate extracellular matrices and other molecules and signals to repair the wounded defects.

Poor Healing Capacity of Epithelial Defects

During corneal wound healing, epithelial cells migrate, proliferate, and undergo tissue remodeling. Proteinases, which include the MMP family, play an important role in the modulation of these processes. Under elevated glucose concentrations, Takahashi *et al.* reported not only a significant delay in the migration of human corneal epithelial cells but also an enhanced MMP activity [11]. This increased MMP activity further inhibits the migration phase by deteriorating cell attachments with BM components. In summary, corneal healing in the diabetic state is slowed by the combination of delays in the migration of epithelial cells and inhibitions in cell attachment with BM components.

CORNEAL INFECTIONS

Corneal ulcers can occur in diabetics more commonly than in non-diabetics. Due to poor healing and reduced sensitivity, diabetics can also take longer to heal when affected by ulcers. Unusual organisms should be considered in the differential diagnosis of microbial keratitis. Please see chapter 4 for reference and a more complete discussion.

CORNEAL STROMA

The corneal stroma is the thick transparent middle layer of the cornea (representing about 85-90% of the corneal thickness) composed of densely organized collagen fibers and proteoglycans. The collagen provides tensile strength and the proteoglycans allow for internal swelling pressure of about 60mmHg. The regular spacing of the collagen fibrils, uniform diameters of collagen and proteoglycans, and appropriate stromal hydration are essential for corneal transparency and optical function. The residing corneal keratocytes are fibroblasts responsible for general repair and maintenance.

Altered Collagen Synthesis

In diabetes, non-enzymatic glycosylation of collagen secondary to hyperglycemia affects many properties of the collage fibril, such as its ability to form supramolecular aggregates, its sensitivity to thermal degradation, its charge distribution, its crystalline structure, its molecular packing, and its turnover rate.

Increased glycosylation levels have been correlated with decreased diameter of stroma collagen fibers of mouse corneas, leading to corneal opacity and distortion of optical anisotropic properties. Additionally, collagen fibers in the diabetic mice cornea have been observed to be more crystalline and more densely packed than in the control, likely due to crosslinks mediated by nonenzymatic glycosylation of the collagens [12]. In diabetes, non-uniformed and irregular spacing of the collagen fibrils affect the biomechanics and transparency of cornea.

CORNEAL ENDOTHELIUM

The corneal endothelium lines the posterior surface of the cornea and faces the anterior chamber of the eye. It consists of a monolayer of specialized cells arrested in the G1 phase of the cell cycle with very low, if any, proliferation potential [13]. An age-related decrease in endothelial cell density has been well reported. The endothelial cells have incomplete zonula occludens, or leaky tight junctions, to allow for passage of nutrients and solutes from the aqueous humor through the posterior surface of the cornea to the stroma. At the same time, it actively pumps ions, and therefore water *via* the osmotic gradient, in the opposite direction from the stroma into the aqueous humor. The Na^+/K^+ ATPase and carbonic anhydrase play critical roles in controlling this energy-driven process. Actively regulating and maintaining corneal hydration is important for optical transparency [14].

Morphological Abnormalities

Structural changes in corneal endothelial cells secondary to the chronic metabolic stress in diabetes have been reported since the early 1980s, however, the results remain inconsistent. The four most commonly studied morphologies are coefficient of variation of cell area, percentage of hexagonal cells, endothelial cell density, and endothelium thickness. Different groups have reported various changes in either 1 or all 4 of these parameters, or no difference at all when comparing diabetic *versus* non-diabetic patients [15 - 19]. For example, Lee *et al.* reported an increase in polymegathism (coefficient of variation of cell area), decrease in pleomorphism (percentage of hexagonal cells), decrease in endothelial cell density and an increase in central corneal thickness [4]. On the contrary, Storr-Paulsen *et al.* showed a significant increase in central corneal thickness, but no significant difference in the other three parameters when comparing the diabetic patients to the non-diabetic patients [15].

At the present time, the morphology of the corneal endothelium in diabetes remains controversial. Nonetheless, it is important to carefully monitor the corneal endothelium for any abnormal changes in the diabetic patient.

Functional Abnormalities Leading to Increased Water Content in the Atroma and Folds in Descement's Membrane

In the diabetic state, hyperglycemia causes abnormal corneal hydration control and eventual stromal swelling. Elevated glucose level has been shown to reduce the activity of the Na^+/K^+ ATPase enzyme, which is a major component of the corneal endothelial fluid pump [20]. Inhibition of this endothelial pump causes increased water content in the stromal layer and eventually, increased corneal thickness. Herse *et al.* measured the activity of the Na^+/K^+ ATPase in normal *versus* rabbit endothelial homogenate. There was a 69% reduction in the Na^+/K^+ ATPase activity in the diabetic rabbit endothelial homogenate compared to the non-diabetic controls [21].

Since the cornea can only swell in the posterior direction, the presence of small folds in Descemet's membrane, which is the layer posterior to the stromal layer, has been used as an indicator for increased hydration of the cornea. Waite *et al.* and Henkind *et al.* have previously reported folds in Descemet's membrane in 26-33% of the diabetic patients under slit-lamp examination of the cornea. However, Keoleian *et al.* did not find any significant difference in corneal thickness or endothelial permeability to fluorescein in diabetic patients [22]. This inconsistency should be addressed and better defined with further research.

CORNEAL NERVES

The human cornea is one of the most densely innervated tissues of the body. The nerve bundles are either myelinated A-δ or unmeylinated C-nerve fibers. To maintain corneal transparency, the corneal nerves lose their perineurium and myelin sheaths as they enter the corneal surface, surrounded by only Schwann cell sheaths [23]. Anatomically, most of the corneal nerve fibers are sensory in origin, derived from the ophthalmic division of the trigeminal nerve. Nerve fibers *via* the anterior ciliary nerves enter the middle third of the stroma to form the subbasal epithelial plexus, with branches extending through Bowman's layer into the epithelium to innervate the basal and superficial epithelial cell layers. As nociceptors, they monitor mechanical, thermal, and chemical signals and perceptions. In addition to their sensory function, the corneal nerves serve a trophic role on the corneal epithelium for healthy maintenance and renewal of the ocular surface [24].

Reduced Corneal Sensation

Many factors, such as transforming growth factor-beta, fibroblast growth factor, and nerve growth factor, regulate nerve fiber integrity and repair. In the diabetic state, these factors are upregulated, which may contribute to damages in the corneal nerve fibers [25]. Other mechanisms that play a role in nerve damage include hyperglycemia-induced inflammation and oxidative stress and altered metabolic and signaling pathways [26]. Regardless, reductions in total nerve fiber and density have been related to the loss of both somatic and corneal sensations. With diminished sensation, the cornea is more vulnerable to trauma, erosion, and ulceration.

Morphologically, alterations with patches of thickening and thinning of Schwann cell basal lamina, axonal degeneration of the unmeylinated corneal nerves, increased tortuosity of corneal nerves, and irregularities in the periodicity of nerve beading have been demonstrated to be early pathological manifestations in the diabetic corneal innervation [25, 27].

Studies have shown decreased corneal sensitivity to be directly related to the degree of peripheral polyneuropathy and to the duration of diabetes in patients with keratopathy. These data suggest that keratopathy and corneal neuropathy may be manifestations of distal peripheral neuropathy of diabetes [28 - 30].

Loss of the Subbasal Nerve Plexus

In diabetic patients with no or mild/moderate neuropathy, corneal sensation remained normal, however the subbasal nerve plexus (SBNP) densities were decreased by an average of one nerve fiber bundle per confocal microscopic image. In diabetic patients with severe neuropathy, both the corneal sensitivity and SBNP densities were significantly reduced. Thus, it seems that the SBNP is affected earlier in the course of diabetic polyneuropathy than corneal mechanical sensitivity, and that confocal microscopy may be a useful tool to detect the beginning of diabetic neuropathy [31].

An explanation for this is that terminal epithelial nerves (TENs) are the ones responsible for relaying nociceptive sensory inputs. However, unlike the reduction in SBNP, which is influenced by hyperglycemia, the loss of terminal epithelial nerves (TENs) are due to normal maturation. Therefore, a greater degree of hyperglycemia impact on SBNP loss is required before substantial effects on the TENs would be seen. This would explain the above finding that SBNP loss is seen before corneal sensitivity is diminished [26].

Loss of Neurotrophic Support

Corneal nerves and endothelial cells support and influence one another trophically to maintain a healthy cornea and promote wound healing after injury. For example, corneal nerve fibers release neurotransmitters and neuropeptides to stimulate corneal epithelial cell growth, proliferation, differentiation, type VII collagen production, and corneal limbal stem cell maintenance. Corneal epithelial cells secrete soluble factors, such as nerve growth factors and glial cell-derived neurotrophic factor to promote neurite extension and survival. It has been well documented that dysfunction of the corneal innervation leads to neurotrophic keratitis [23].

It stands to reason that impaired corneal innervation leads to diminished release of endotheliotrophic substance, contributing to improper epithelial maintenance and problems in wound healing leading to recurrent erosions often seen in the diabetic eye. In diabetic patients with severe neuropathy, the corneal epithelium was significantly thinner than in diabetic patients with no neuropathy [31]. Notably, the subbasal nerve plexus (SBNP), which contains the highest number of nerve branches in the cornea, is reduced secondary to prolonged hyperglycemia. A reduction in basal epithelial cell density within the central and paracentral corneal epithelium has been observed, and it parallels the loss of the SBNP [26].

In addition to trophically supporting epithelial cells, the corneal nerves also influence limbal epithelial stem cell homeostasis. Located in the basal epithelial layer of the limbus, the limbal epithelial stem cells migrate centripetally to replace cells that desquamate during normal homeostasis and wound healing [32]. In mice model studies, depletion of sensory nerves by electrocoagulation of the ophthalmic branch of the trigeminal nerve significantly reduced the number of the limbal stem cells. When the diabetic mice were treated with insulin like growth factor-I (IGF-1), which accelerated recovery of the corneal subbasal nerve and epithelial branches, there was a significant increase in the number of the stem cells and corneal nerves.

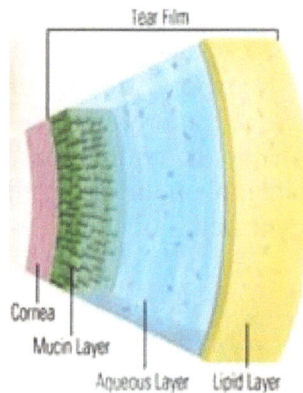

Fig. (3). Normal tear film.

In short, innervation plays a critical role in ocular surface health by influencing epithelial cells and maintaining limbal stem cells. Impairment in corneal innervation secondary to the diabetic state contributes to delayed wound healing, leading to persistent corneal neurotrophic ulcers. Administration of IGF-1 may be of therapeutic potential for these patients. The treatment of neurotrophic ulcers is beyond the scope of this chapter but can include frequent lubrication, serum plasma drops, tarsorraphy, nerve growth factor drops, and even nerve grafing.

TEAR DYNAMICS AND TEARING

The tear film is the outermost covering of the eye, functioning to keep the cornea moist to allow gas exchange, to deliver nutrients to the corneal epithelium and anterior stroma, to improve the quality of the image by lubricating and smoothing out the irregular corneal cellular surface, to prevent infection by bacteria and viruses, and to preserve the health and transparent nature of the cornea with vitamin A [33, 34]. It is composed of 3 layers, the outer surface lipid layer produced by meibomian glands, the middle aqueous layer produced by lacrimal glands, and the inner mucus layer produced by goblet cells in the conjunctiva [33] (Fig. **3**).

The aqueous tear is continuously produced at a basal level without stimulation by the accessory lacrimal glands and distributed over the ocular surface to form a constant tear film by blinking. Under physical or emotional stimulation, the main lacrimal glands produce reflex tears containing trophic substances such as vitamin A and epithelial growth factors important for epithelial wound healing [35].

Tear Film Dysfunction

Many diabetic patients often complain of dry eye symptoms such as eye fatigue, irritation, burning, and foreign body sensations. The prevalence of these symptoms is significantly higher with longer duration of diabetes, and not affected by sex and age [36].

Although controversial, tear film instability has been described in diabetic patients. An explanation for their poor tear film break up time compared to that of control groups could be due a reduction in corneal goblet cell numbers [29]. Since goblet cells produce mucin required for the mucus layer of the tear film, it stands to reason that a decrease in goblet cell numbers leads to tear film instability.

Additionally, concurrent squamous epithelial metaplasia of the cornea has been observed, and goblet cell loss which can contribute to a dysfunctional tear state is a well-known sign of squamous metaplasia [29]. Several mechanisms have been proposed. The loss of trigeminal sensory nerves and, in particular the subbasal nerve plexus with its subsequent decrease in trophic effects on the cornea, plays a role. Fluctuations in glycemic control affecting the aldose reductase and sorbital pathways have been implicated as well. Administration of aldose reductase inhibitors such as sorbinil, CT-112, and ONO-2235 has shown to be promising in improving nerve conduction, corneal sensitivity, corneal epithelial disease, and tear film dynamics significantly [29, 37, 38].

Decreased Reflex Tearing

The amount of provoked reflex tearing is significantly lower in diabetics than in non-diabetic patients when measured by the Schirmer testing, whereas the unstimulated basal tearing showed no differences [39]. The etiology is likely due to the diminished corneal sensitivity in diabetic patients. Additionally, damage of the microvasculature of the lacrimal glands and autonomic neuropathy in the diabetic state leading to impaired ability of the lacrimal glands to secrete is also responsible [40]. Since reflex tears contain trophic substances important in corneal epithelial wound healing, chronic dry eye can lead to recurrent scarring and perforation of the cornea, resulting in secondary bacterial infections and vision deficits. Therefore, diagnosing and treating dry eye with artificial lubricants and optimizing the ocular surface in the early stages is very important.

CORNEA CONSIDERATIONS IN OCULAR SURGERY

Chronic hyperglycemia places the cornea in a fragile state that is easily susceptible to stress-related injury. Common corneal complications in diabetes include persistent epithelial defects and instability, delayed wound healing, diminished corneal sensation secondary to denervation, and decreased tear production. Therefore, any ocular procedure that affects and distresses the diabetic cornea may result in increased corneal damage and complications compared to the non-diabetic cornea.

Cataract Surgery

Cataract surgery was considered high-risk for diabetic patients due to the risk of postoperative progression of retinopathy and development of macular edema that could compromise visual prognosis. With advancements of techniques such as small incision phacoemulsification, fewer postoperative complications with improved visual acuity have been reported after cataract surgery [41 - 43].

Somaiya *et al* [42] reported an 82% achievement of visual acuity of 20/40 in diabetic patients after small-incision phacoemulsification, compared to 95% in the nondiabetic patients. Postoperative visual acuity was worse in patients with diabetic retinopathy, but no significant difference was seen between patients with diabetes with no retinopathy *versus* patients without diabetes. Even though visual acuity did not improve to the same level as the nondiabetics, diabetic patients at all stages of preoperative retinopathy had significant improvements in visual acuity post surgery. No postoperative progression of retinopathy and maculopathy was observed in patients who were treated with photocoagulation before the cataract surgery [44].

Postoperative changes were higher in cataract patients who suffer from diabetes than in cataract patients without a systemic or local disease. Postoperative corneal edema recovery rate was slower in the diabetic group compared to the nondiabetic group [41]. Goebbels and Spitznas [45] performed fluorophotometry to evaluate endothelial permeability pre- and post-operatively. No difference in endothelial permeability was found before the operation, however, a 3-week delayed recovery of endothelial barrier function after surgery was seen in the diabetic group compared to the nondiabetic group.

A greater loss of endothelial cell density post cataract phacoemulsification was seen in diabetics compared to nondiabetics, 7% and 2% respectively [41]. This data is supported by several other studies [46 - 48], and can be attributed to the vulnerability of the corneal endothelium to mechanical stress in the diabetic state.

In summary, diabetic patients should not be excluded from cataract surgery. Significant improvements in visual acuity have been consistently achieved with modern surgical techniques and experienced surgeons [43]. Small-incision phacoemulsification is the better choice for diabetic patients because it minimizes ocular trauma and inflammation contributing to less breakdown of the blood-retina barrier. Good glycemic control is crucial both pre- and post-operatively. Since visual outcomes in eyes with advanced retinopathy is poorer compared to earlier stages of retinopathy, it may be advantageous to consider cataract surgery earlier in diabetic patients. For diabetic patients with vision threatening retinopathy, cataract surgery may aggravate the progression of retinopathy. Therefore, cataract surgery should be delayed if possible. When surgery is indicated, retinal photocoagulation is recommended preoperatively or immediately postoperatively when lens opacity precludes photocoagulation.

Refractive Surgery: PRK

Photorefractive keratotomy (PRK) uses a laser to refigure the curvature of the cornea by removing the surface of the corneal epithelium hence exposing the corneal stroma for a significant amount of time postoperatively until re-epithelialization is complete [49]. Diabetics are not ideal candidates for PRK due to their poor epithelial wound healing abilities that predisposes to complications such as scarring, making the procedure relatively although not absolutely contraindicated.

Refractive Surgery: LASIK

Laser *in situ* keratomileusis (LASIK) is a newer evolution of the photorefractory procedure with marked improvements in the healing process compared to PRK. In LASIK, a keratome or laser (intralase or femtosecond) is used to create a hinged flap of corneal epithelium and stroma, and then an excimer laser remodels the stroma by removing a precise amount of tissue from the corneal bed, and finally the flap is put back to its original position.

Even with major improvements in laser refractive surgery, the United States Food and Drug Administration still includes diabetes mellitus as a relative contraindication for LASIK. This generalized guideline is rather unclear, as it did not comment on the severity and duration of diabetes. Additionally, current literature, although limited, suggest that well-controlled diabetic patients may not be at increased risk for LASIK-related complications compared to poorly controlled diabetic patients [49, 50].

A study by Fraunfelder and Rich [51] concluded that diabetic patients treated with LASIK had significantly higher risk (47% *vs* 6.9% risk) in developing postoperative epithelial complications and poorer refractive outcomes than patients without diabetes. The common epithelial complications were non-healing or delayed healing epithelial defects and lingering punctate epithelial erosions. They attributed the high complication rates to preexisting diabetic keratopathy and LASIK-induced neuropathy.

During the passage of the microkeratome over the corneal surface in creating the LASIK flap, patients with epithelial basement membrane dystrophy such as diabetic keratopathy are at increased risk for epithelial sloughing due to the sliding trauma of the microkeratome [52]. This epithelial sloughing may cause distortions of the flap edges, creating a potential space for epithelial cells to migrate from the flap edge to grow beneath the flap forming a sheet of epithelium ingrowth, also known as interface epithelialization. Diabetic keratopathy is a risk factor for interface epithelialization after LASIK, which can lead to scarring, astigmatism, decreased best spectacle-corrected visual acuity, and blurry vision. Jabbur *et al*. [53] recommended limiting the number of anesthetic drops during lamellar procedures and using non-preserved carboxymethylcellulose sodium 0.5% solution before the microkeratome pass to decrease the incidence of epithelial defects. Additionally, in patients with uncontrolled diabetes, LASIK is not recommended.

During the creation of the LASIK flap, the corneal nerves are severed leading to diminished release of trophic factors for epithelial wound healing and decreased frequency of blinking. This explains the common complication of punctate epithelial erosions and rose Bengal staining on corneal flaps after LASIK [54]. Symptoms include dry eye discomfort and subjective complaints of decreased vision quality. LASIK-induced neutrotrophic epitheliopathy is a self-limited condition resolving after complete regeneration of the corneal nerves, which is approximately 6 months post-surgery. However, this complication is more common and severe in patients with pre-existing dry eye disease, such as in diabetic patients. Treatment is mainly palliative with non-preserved artificial tears and ointments.

Of note, Fraunfelder and Rich did not comment on the diabetic status of their patients in the study, such as the severity and duration of their disease and their glycemic control. Whether the increased LASIK complications occurred mostly in uncontrolled diabetics or at the same rate in all diabetics regardless of their glycemic control cannot be concluded.

In contrast, two studies on LASIK in well-controlled diabetic patients without keratopathy and neuropathy showed no significant risk for complications [49, 50]. The refractive outcomes in diabetic patients after LASIK were favorable, however 28% of the eyes still required enhancement surgery, compared to a 10% rate in the general population. Epithelial ingrowth rate was higher in the diabetic group than in the general population (4.3% vs 0.5%).

Lastly, patients with proliferative diabetic retinopathy should be cautioned against LASIK because of possible complications of transient retinal ischemia intraoperatively [55]. Patients with proliferative retinopathy have abnormally low ophthalmic arterial pressure due to increased vascular resistance and decreased ocular perfusion pressure. During LASIK, suctioning induces increased intraocular pressure, which disturbs choroidal blood flow and aggravates ischemia and diabetic retinopathy.

In general, the main considerations of LASIK for diabetic patients are the concern for wound healing complications, transient retinal ischemia due to increased intraoperative intraocular pressure during intraoperative suctioning, poorer refractive outcomes, and LASIK-induced neurotropic epitheliopathy. Diabetic patients with tight glycemic control and no corneal complications such as diabetic keratopathy or corneal neuropathy are at no greater risk for LASIK complications than the general population, and therefore are suitable candidates for LASIK. However, diabetic patients who are poorly controlled or with advanced systematic symptoms are not recommended for LASIK.

Penetrating Keratoplasty

As our understanding of corneal complications in diabetes increases, it is logical that ophthalmologists are reluctant to use diabetic donor corneas in penetrating keratoplasty to prevent graft complications. Chou *et al*. [56] revealed that the presence of diabetes in corneal graft donors is a significant risk factor for postoperative epithelial defects, whereas Lass *et al*. [57] and Sugar *et al*. [58] saw no significant adverse effect in graft failure or endothelial cell loss from diabetic graft donors. No formal clinical study has examined the effects of diabetic corneal donor on graft success and endothelial changes after penetrating keratoplasty.

Pterygium

Surgery for pterygium is generally a routine procedure with relatively good outcomes. Patients with diabetes can have postoperative healing issues due to aforementioned wound healing issues mentioned earlier in the chapter. (Fig. **4**) shows a postoperative diabetic patient whose epithelium did not heal and required additional surgery including amniotic membrane grafting.

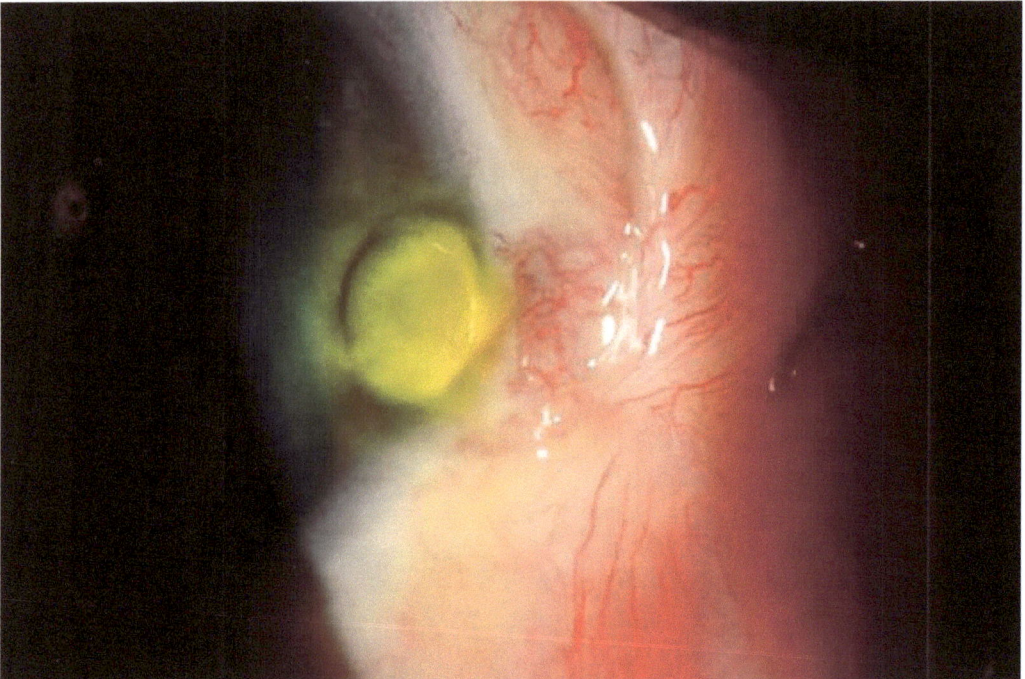

Fig. (4). Postoperative pterygium with persistent epithelial defect in a diabetic patient.

Closed Pars Plana Vitrectomy

Corneal epithelial defects following closed pars plana vitrectomy is a frequent complication mainly seen in diabetic patients. The pathophysiology is not entirely clear, but likely secondary to abnormal epithelium in the diabetic cornea.

Intraoperatively the epithelium of the diabetic cornea often becomes edematous and hazy, necessitating scraping of the cloudy parts of the epithelium for proper visualization of the vitreous. Due to the poor healing capacity of the diabetic cornea, these epithelial defects will have poor re-epithelialization and may occasionally develop into persistent epithelial defects requiring further surgery to prevent loss of visual acuity [59, 60].

In addition to diabetes, other risk factors for corneal complications after closed pars plana vitrectomy include decreased corneal sensitivity, intraoperative lensectomy, and history of vitreous surgery [59, 61]. Intraoperative lensectomy exposes the corneal endothelium to direct injury from the infusion stream and abrasion from the lens particles, leading to endothelial trauma. Foulks *et al.* reported that the combination of diabetes, decreased corneal touch sensitivity, and the need for intraoperative removal of the corneal epithelium or concurrent lensectomy are associated with postoperative corneal complication 80% of the time [59].

To reduce corneal complications, precautions should be taken for at risk patients to prevent direct trauma to the cornea [59 - 62]. Preoperative testing should be performed with soft contact lenses to avoid epithelial irritation. Intraoperatively, the eyelid speculum should be inserted carefully to avoid epithelial injury. Corneal contact lenses should be placed to prevent abrasion, and periodically removed to allow oxygen flow to the corneal epithelium to maintain corneal transparency. If lensectomy must be performed, techniques to avoid endothelial trauma should be followed. Ringer's solution or specifically prepared glutathione-containing solutions are superior and should be used for intraocular irrigation. Generous endothelial protecting viscoelastic substances should be used. If mechanical debridement of the corneal epithelium is required, topical corticosteroids should be avoided as steroids can further delay wound healing. Additionally, postoperative ointment use and pressure patching can be effective in promoting epithelial integrity. In cases of persistent epithelial defects, bandage soft contact lens therapy, amniotic membranes, plasma rich topical therapies can be utilized to promote healing. Most importantly, diabetic patients should be aggressively monitored for corneal complications to allow for early diagnosis and treatment before these complications become irreversible.

CONCLUSION

Diabetics have decreased corneal sensation and are at increased risk for corneal epithelial healing problems, and infections. Routine corneal abrasions may not be routine in the diabetic patient. These ocular surface issues can cause postoperative healing problems in the refractive surgery, pterygium and cataract patient among others. It is imperative to diagnose corneal infections promptly and treat them aggressively to avoid permanent vision changes. Likewise, one must remember that the corneal endothelium.

CONSENT FOR PUBLICATION

Not applicable.

CONFLICT OF INTEREST

The author declares no conflict of interest, financial or otherwise.

ACKNOWLEDGEMENTS

Declared none.

REFERENCES

[1]   Reinstein DZ, Archer TJ, Gobbe M, Silverman RH, Coleman DJ. Epithelial thickness in the normal cornea: three-dimensional display with Artemis very high-frequency digital ultrasound. J Refract Surg 2008; 24(6): 571-81.
[http://dx.doi.org/10.3928/1081597X-20080601-05] [PMID: 18581782]

[2]   Busted N, Olsen T, Schmitz O. Clinical observations on the corneal thickness and the corneal endothelium in diabetes mellitus. Br J Ophthalmol 1981; 65(10): 687-90.
[http://dx.doi.org/10.1136/bjo.65.10.687] [PMID: 7317320]

[3]   Claramonte PJ, Ruiz-Moreno JM, Sánchez-Pérez SI, *et al.* Variation of central corneal thickness in diabetic patients as detected by ultrasonic pachymetry. Arch Soc Esp Oftalmol 2006; 81(9): 523-6.
[PMID: 17016784]

[4]   Lee JS, Oum BS, Choi HY, Lee JE, Cho BM. Differences in corneal thickness and corneal endothelium related to duration in diabetes. Eye (Lond) 2006; 20(3): 315-8.
[http://dx.doi.org/10.1038/sj.eye.6701868] [PMID: 15832184]

[5]   Taylor HR, Kimsey RA. Corneal epithelial basement membrane changes in diabetes. Invest Ophthalmol Vis Sci 1981; 20(4): 548-53.
[PMID: 7216670]

[6]   Kaji Y, Usui T, Oshika T, *et al.* Advanced glycation end products in diabetic corneas. Invest Ophthalmol Vis Sci 2000; 41(2): 362-8.
[PMID: 10670463]

[7]   Saghizadeh M, Brown DJ, Castellon R, *et al.* Overexpression of matrix metalloproteinase-10 and matrix metalloproteinase-3 in human diabetic corneas: a possible mechanism of basement membrane and integrin alterations. Am J Pathol 2001; 158(2): 723-34.
[http://dx.doi.org/10.1016/S0002-9440(10)64015-1] [PMID: 11159210]

[8]   Gekka M, Miyata K, Nagai Y, *et al.* Corneal epithelial barrier function in diabetic patients. Cornea 2004; 23(1): 35-7.
[http://dx.doi.org/10.1097/00003226-200401000-00006] [PMID: 14701955]

[9]   Azar DT, Spurr-Michaud SJ, Tisdale AS, Gipson IK. Decreased penetration of anchoring fibrils into the diabetic stroma. A morphometric analysis. Arch Ophthalmol 1989; 107(10): 1520-3.
[http://dx.doi.org/10.1001/archopht.1989.01070020594047] [PMID: 2803103]

[10] Watanabe H, Katakami C, Miyata S, Negi A. Corneal disorders in KKAy mouse: a type 2 diabetes model. Jpn J Ophthalmol 2002; 46(2): 130-9.
[http://dx.doi.org/10.1016/S0021-5155(01)00487-7] [PMID: 12062217]

[11] Takahashi H, Akiba K, Noguchi T, *et al.* Matrix metalloproteinase activity is enhanced during corneal wound repair in high glucose condition. Curr Eye Res 2000; 21(2): 608-15.
[http://dx.doi.org/10.1076/0271-3683(200008)2121-VFT608] [PMID: 11148597]

[12]   Aldrovani M, Guaraldo AM, Vidal BC. Optical anisotropies in corneal stroma collagen fibers from diabetic spontaneous mice. Vision Res 2007; 47(26): 3229-37.
[http://dx.doi.org/10.1016/j.visres.2007.02.011] [PMID: 18028980]

[13]   Bourne WM. Biology of the corneal endothelium in health and disease. Eye (Lond) 2003; 17(8): 912-8.
[http://dx.doi.org/10.1038/sj.eye.6700559] [PMID: 14631396]

[14]   Joyce NC. Proliferative capacity of the corneal endothelium. Prog Retin Eye Res 2003; 22(3): 359-89.
[http://dx.doi.org/10.1016/S1350-9462(02)00065-4] [PMID: 12852491]

[15]   Storr-Paulsen A, Singh A, Jeppesen H, Norregaard JC, Thulesen J. Corneal endothelial morphology and central thickness in patients with type II diabetes mellitus. Acta Ophthalmol 2014; 92(2): 158-60.
[http://dx.doi.org/10.1111/aos.12064] [PMID: 23387877]

[16]   Inoue K, Kato S, Inoue Y, Amano S, Oshika T. The corneal endothelium and thickness in type II diabetes mellitus. Jpn J Ophthalmol 2002; 46(1): 65-9.
[http://dx.doi.org/10.1016/S0021-5155(01)00458-0] [PMID: 11853716]

[17]   Roszkowska AM, Tringali CG, Colosi P, Squeri CA, Ferreri G. Corneal endothelium evaluation in type I and type II diabetes mellitus. Ophthalmologica 1999; 213(4): 258-61.
[http://dx.doi.org/10.1159/000027431] [PMID: 10420110]

[18]   Larsson LI, Bourne WM, Pach JM, Brubaker RF. Structure and function of the corneal endothelium in diabetes mellitus type I and type II. Arch Ophthalmol 1996; 114(1): 9-14.
[http://dx.doi.org/10.1001/archopht.1996.01100130007001] [PMID: 8540858]

[19]   Schultz RO, Matsuda M, Yee RW, Edelhauser HF, Schultz KJ. Corneal endothelial changes in type I and type II diabetes mellitus. Am J Ophthalmol 1984; 98(4): 401-10.
[http://dx.doi.org/10.1016/0002-9394(84)90120-X] [PMID: 6486211]

[20]   McNamara NA, Brand RJ, Polse KA, Bourne WM. Corneal function during normal and high serum glucose levels in diabetes. Invest Ophthalmol Vis Sci 1998; 39(1): 3-17.
[PMID: 9430539]

[21]   Herse P, Adams L. Effect of hyperglycemia duration on rabbit corneal thickness and endothelial ATPase activity. Acta Ophthalmol Scand 1995; 73(2): 158-61.
[http://dx.doi.org/10.1111/j.1600-0420.1995.tb00659.x] [PMID: 7656146]

[22]   Keoleian GM, Pach JM, Hodge DO, Trocme SD, Bourne WM. Structural and functional studies of the corneal endothelium in diabetes mellitus. Am J Ophthalmol 1992; 113(1): 64-70.
[http://dx.doi.org/10.1016/S0002-9394(14)75755-1] [PMID: 1728148]

[23]   Müller LJ, Marfurt CF, Kruse F, Tervo TM. Corneal nerves: structure, contents and function. Exp Eye Res 2003; 76(5): 521-42.
[http://dx.doi.org/10.1016/S0014-4835(03)00050-2] [PMID: 12697417]

[24]   Müller LJ, Vrensen GF, Pels L, Cardozo BN, Willekens B. Architecture of human corneal nerves. Invest Ophthalmol Vis Sci 1997; 38(5): 985-94.
[PMID: 9112994]

[25]   Kallinikos P, Berhanu M, O'Donnell C, Boulton AJ, Efron N, Malik RA. Corneal nerve tortuosity in diabetic patients with neuropathy. Invest Ophthalmol Vis Sci 2004; 45(2): 418-22.
[http://dx.doi.org/10.1167/iovs.03-0637] [PMID: 14744880]

[26]   Cai D, Zhu M, Petroll WM, Koppaka V, Robertson DM. The impact of type 1 diabetes mellitus on corneal epithelial nerve morphology and the corneal epithelium. Am J Pathol 2014; 184(10): 2662-70.
[http://dx.doi.org/10.1016/j.ajpath.2014.06.016] [PMID: 25102563]

[27]   Ishida N, Rao GN, del Cerro M, Aquavella JV. Corneal nerve alterations in diabetes mellitus. Arch Ophthalmol 1984; 102(9): 1380-4.
[http://dx.doi.org/10.1001/archopht.1984.01040031122038] [PMID: 6236781]

[28] Tavakoli M, Kallinikos PA, Efron N, Boulton AJ, Malik RA. Corneal sensitivity is reduced and relates to the severity of neuropathy in patients with diabetes. Diabetes Care 2007; 30(7): 1895-7.
      [http://dx.doi.org/10.2337/dc07-0175] [PMID: 17372147]

[29] Dogru M, Katakami C, Inoue M. Tear function and ocular surface changes in noninsulin-dependent diabetes mellitus. Ophthalmology 2001; 108(3): 586-92.
      [http://dx.doi.org/10.1016/S0161-6420(00)00599-6] [PMID: 11237914]

[30] Schultz RO, Peters MA, Sobocinski K, Nassif K, Schultz KJ. Diabetic corneal neuropathy. Trans Am Ophthalmol Soc 1983; 81: 107-24.
      [PMID: 6676964]

[31] Rosenberg ME, Tervo TM, Immonen IJ, Müller LJ, Grönhagen-Riska C, Vesaluoma MH. Corneal structure and sensitivity in type 1 diabetes mellitus. Invest Ophthalmol Vis Sci 2000; 41(10): 2915-21.
      [PMID: 10967045]

[32] Ueno H, Hattori T, Kumagai Y, Suzuki N, Ueno S, Takagi H. Alterations in the corneal nerve and stem/progenitor cells in diabetes: preventive effects of insulin-like growth factor-1 treatment. Int J Endocrinol 2014; 2014312401
      [http://dx.doi.org/10.1155/2014/312401] [PMID: 24696681]

[33] Walcott B. The Lacrimal Gland and Its Veil of Tears. News Physiol Sci 1998; 13: 97-103.
      [http://dx.doi.org/10.1152/physiologyonline.1998.13.2.97] [PMID: 11390770]

[34] Tiffany JM. Tears in health and disease. Eye (Lond) 2003; 17(8): 923-6.
      [http://dx.doi.org/10.1038/sj.eye.6700566] [PMID: 14631398]

[35] Tsubota K. Tear dynamics and dry eye. Prog Retin Eye Res 1998; 17(4): 565-96.
      [http://dx.doi.org/10.1016/S1350-9462(98)00004-4] [PMID: 9777650]

[36] Manaviat MR, Rashidi M, Afkhami-Ardekani M, Shoja MR. Prevalence of dry eye syndrome and diabetic retinopathy in type 2 diabetic patients. BMC Ophthalmol 2008; 8: 10.
      [http://dx.doi.org/10.1186/1471-2415-8-10] [PMID: 18513455]

[37] Ramos-Remus C, Suarez-Almazor M, Russell AS. Low tear production in patients with diabetes mellitus is not due to Sjögren's syndrome. Clin Exp Rheumatol 1994; 12(4): 375-80.
      [PMID: 7955600]

[38] Fujishima H, Tsubota K. Improvement of corneal fluorescein staining in post cataract surgery of diabetic patients by an oral aldose reductase inhibitor, ONO-2235. Br J Ophthalmol 2002; 86(8): 860-3.
      [http://dx.doi.org/10.1136/bjo.86.8.860] [PMID: 12140204]

[39] Goebbels M. Tear secretion and tear film function in insulin dependent diabetics. Br J Ophthalmol 2000; 84(1): 19-21.
      [http://dx.doi.org/10.1136/bjo.84.1.19] [PMID: 10611093]

[40] Kaiserman I, Kaiserman N, Nakar S, Vinker S. Dry eye in diabetic patients. Am J Ophthalmol 2005; 139(3): 498-503.
      [http://dx.doi.org/10.1016/j.ajo.2004.10.022] [PMID: 15767060]

[41] Morikubo S, Takamura Y, Kubo E, Tsuzuki S, Akagi Y. Corneal changes after small-incision cataract surgery in patients with diabetes mellitus. Arch Ophthalmol 2004; 122(7): 966-9.
      [http://dx.doi.org/10.1001/archopht.122.7.966] [PMID: 15249359]

[42] Somaiya M, Burns JD, Mintz R, Warren RE, Uchida T, Godley BF. Factors affecting visual outcomes after small-incision phacoemulsification in diabetic patients. J Cataract Refract Surg 2002; 28(8): 1364-71.
      [http://dx.doi.org/10.1016/S0886-3350(02)01319-6] [PMID: 12160805]

[43] Flesner P, Sander B, Henning V, Parving HH, Dornonville de la Cour M, Lund-Andersen H. Cataract surgery on diabetic patients. A prospective evaluation of risk factors and complications. Acta

Ophthalmol Scand 2002; 80(1): 19-24.
[http://dx.doi.org/10.1034/j.1600-0420.2002.800105.x] [PMID: 11906299]

[44] Ivancić D, Mandić Z, Barać J, Kopić M. Cataract surgery and postoperative complications in diabetic patients. Coll Antropol 2005; 29 (Suppl. 1): 55-8.
[PMID: 16193678]

[45] Goebbels M, Spitznas M. Endothelial barrier function after phacoemulsification: a comparison between diabetic and non-diabetic patients. Graefes Arch Clin Exp Ophthalmol 1991; 229(3): 254-7.
[http://dx.doi.org/10.1007/BF00167879] [PMID: 1869062]

[46] Walkow T, Anders N, Klebe S. Endothelial cell loss after phacoemulsification: relation to preoperative and intraoperative parameters. J Cataract Refract Surg 2000; 26(5): 727-32.
[http://dx.doi.org/10.1016/S0886-3350(99)00462-9] [PMID: 10831904]

[47] Díaz-Valle D, Benítez del Castillo Sánchez JM, Castillo A, Sayagués O, Moriche M. Endothelial damage with cataract surgery techniques. J Cataract Refract Surg 1998; 24(7): 951-5.
[http://dx.doi.org/10.1016/S0886-3350(98)80049-7] [PMID: 9682116]

[48] Dick HB, Kohnen T, Jacobi FK, Jacobi KW. Long-term endothelial cell loss following phacoemulsification through a temporal clear corneal incision. J Cataract Refract Surg 1996; 22(1): 63-71.
[http://dx.doi.org/10.1016/S0886-3350(96)80272-0] [PMID: 8656366]

[49] Cobo-Soriano R, Beltran J, Baviera J. LASIK outcomes in patients with underlying systemic contraindications: a preliminary study. Ophthalmology 2006; 113(7): 1118.e1-8

[50] Simpson RG, Moshirfar M, Edmonds JN, Christiansen SM. Laser *in-situ* keratomileusis in patients with diabetes mellitus: a review of the literature. Clin Ophthalmol 2012; 6: 1665-74.
[PMID: 23109803]

[51] Fraunfelder FW, Rich LF. Laser-assisted *in situ* keratomileusis complications in diabetes mellitus. Cornea 2002; 21(3): 246-8.
[http://dx.doi.org/10.1097/00003226-200204000-00002] [PMID: 11917170]

[52] Dastgheib KA, Clinch TE, Manche EE, Hersh P, Ramsey J. Sloughing of corneal epithelium and wound healing complications associated with laser *in situ* keratomileusis in patients with epithelial basement membrane dystrophy. Am J Ophthalmol 2000; 130(3): 297-303.
[http://dx.doi.org/10.1016/S0002-9394(00)00504-3] [PMID: 11020408]

[53] Jabbur NS, Chicani CF, Kuo IC, O'Brien TP. Risk factors in interface epithelialization after laser *in situ* keratomileusis. J Refract Surg 2004; 20(4): 343-8.
[http://dx.doi.org/10.3928/1081-597X-20040701-07] [PMID: 15307396]

[54] Wilson SE. Laser *in situ* keratomileusis-induced (presumed) neurotrophic epitheliopathy. Ophthalmology 2001; 108(6): 1082-7.
[http://dx.doi.org/10.1016/S0161-6420(01)00587-5] [PMID: 11382633]

[55] Ghanbari H, Ahmadieh H. Aggravation of proliferative diabetic retinopathy after laser *in situ* keratomileusis. J Cataract Refract Surg 2003; 29(11): 2232-3.
[http://dx.doi.org/10.1016/S0886-3350(03)00355-9] [PMID: 14670438]

[56] Chou L, Cohen EJ, Laibson PR, Rapuano CJ. Factors associated with epithelial defects after penetrating keratoplasty. Ophthalmic Surg 1994; 25(10): 700-3.
[http://dx.doi.org/10.3928/1542-8877-19941101-09] [PMID: 7898864]

[57] Lass JH, Riddlesworth TD, Gal RL, *et al.* The effect of donor diabetes history on graft failure and endothelial cell density 10 years after penetrating keratoplasty. Ophthalmology 2015; 122(3): 448-56.
[http://dx.doi.org/10.1016/j.ophtha.2014.09.012] [PMID: 25439611]

[58] Sugar J, Montoya M, Dontchev M, *et al.* Donor risk factors for graft failure in the cornea donor study. Cornea 2009; 28(9): 981-5.
[http://dx.doi.org/10.1097/ICO.0b013e3181a0a3e6] [PMID: 19724216]

[59]   Foulks GN, Thoft RA, Perry HD, Tolentino FI. Factors related to corneal epithelial complications after closed vitrectomy in diabetics. Arch Ophthalmol 1979; 97(6): 1076-8.
[http://dx.doi.org/10.1001/archopht.1979.01020010530002] [PMID: 444136]

[60]   Perry HD, Foulks GN, Thoft RA, Tolentino FI. Corneal complications after closed vitrectomy through the pars plana. Arch Ophthalmol 1978; 96(8): 1401-3.
[http://dx.doi.org/10.1001/archopht.1978.03910060155011] [PMID: 678179]

[61]   Chung H, Tolentino FI, Cajita VN, Acosta J, Refojo MF. Reevaluation of corneal complications after closed vitrectomy. Arch Ophthalmol 1988; 106(7): 916-9.
[http://dx.doi.org/10.1001/archopht.1988.01060140062025] [PMID: 3390054]

[62]   Brightbill FS, Myers FL, Bresnick GH. Postvitrectomy keratopathy. Am J Ophthalmol 1978; 85(5 Pt 1): 651-5.
[http://dx.doi.org/10.1016/S0002-9394(14)77099-0] [PMID: 655244]

CHAPTER 8

Diabetes, Cataract, and Glaucoma

Frank Cao and **John Danias**[*]

SUNY Downstate College of Medicine, SUNY Downstate Medical Center, Brooklyn, NY, USA

Abstract: Diabetes Mellitus (DM) affects many parts of the eye. While we traditionally associate vision loss from DM with diabetic retinopathy, it can affect various structures of the eye other than the retina. In this chapter, we will focus on the disease's effects on the lens, and on the drainage apparatus of the eye. Specifically, we will look at cataract and glaucoma incidence in DM and its etiologic role, and then discuss treatment strategies.

Keywords: Cataract, Glaucoma, Glaucoma Implant, Intraocular pressure, Lens, Neovascular, Photocoagulation, Trabeculectomy, VEGF.

CATARACT

Anatomy

The crystalline lens occupies the space behind the iris anterior to the vitreous humor (Fig. **1**). It is formed in embryogenesis from surface ectoderm and serves to provide refractive power to help focus images on the retina, especially during accommodation. The lens sits within the capsular bag, which is held in place by zonules that attach to the ciliary body.

The crystalline lens is normally transparent. However, with age, or as a result of other causes, opacities to the lens often develop, which are collectively called cataracts. Anterior subcapsular cataracts are located just posterior to the anterior capsule, while posterior subcapsular cataracts are located anterior to the posterior capsule (Fig. **1**). The lens is anatomically categorized into an inner nucleus that occupies the center of the structure and is formed during embryogenesis, the surrounding cortex, and epi-nucleus that is the outermost layer. Nuclear sclerosis is defined by the opacification of the center(nucleus) of the lens (Fig. **2**), while cortical cataracts are characterized by the opacification of the cortical layer of the lens and may appear as spoking (Fig. **3**).

---

[*] **Corresponding author John Danias:** SUNY Downstate College of Medicine, SUNY Downstate Health Sciences University, Brooklyn, NY, USA; E-mail: John.Danias@downstate.edu

Douglas R. Lazzaro and Samy I. McFarlane (Eds.)

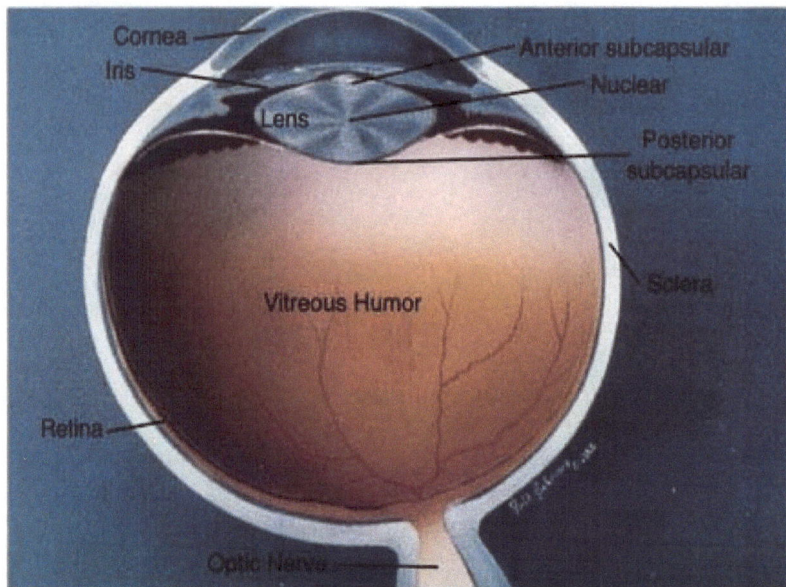

Fig. (1). Diagram of the eye and internal structures including lens. Based on "Normally Developing Eye". *National Eye Institute, National Institutes of Health.* https://www.flickr.com/photos/nationaleyeinstitute/7544655788/in/album-72157646829197286/. Accessed 4/10/2017.

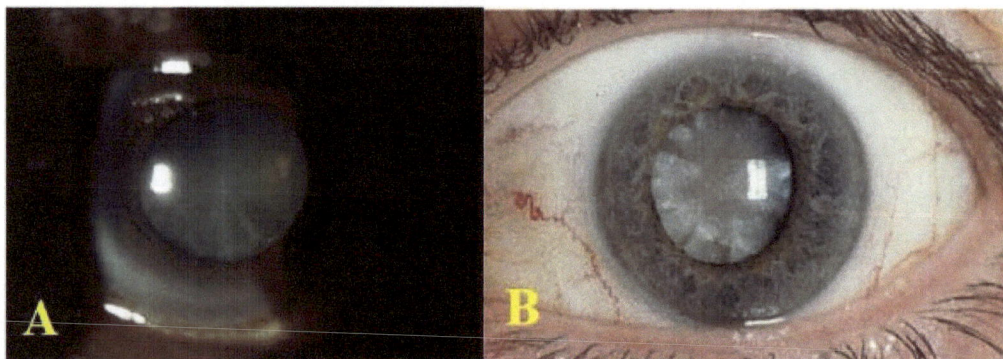

Fig. (2). Nuclear sclerotic cataracts. A. Moderate B. Severe. Image B is available at *National Eye Institute, National Institutes of Health.* https://www.flickr.com/photos/nationaleyeinstitute/7544344000/in/album-72157651546570359/. Accessed 6/8/2020.

Risk Factors

Cataract development is a multifactorial process that may involve ultraviolet light, smoking, medications, trauma, ocular inflammation, or a host of other factors. Cataracts have been shown to have associations with Diabetes Mellitus (DM). In individuals with diabetes, cataract develops at a younger age [1], and they have a 2-5 times higher risk of developing cataract than non-diabetic individuals [2, 3].

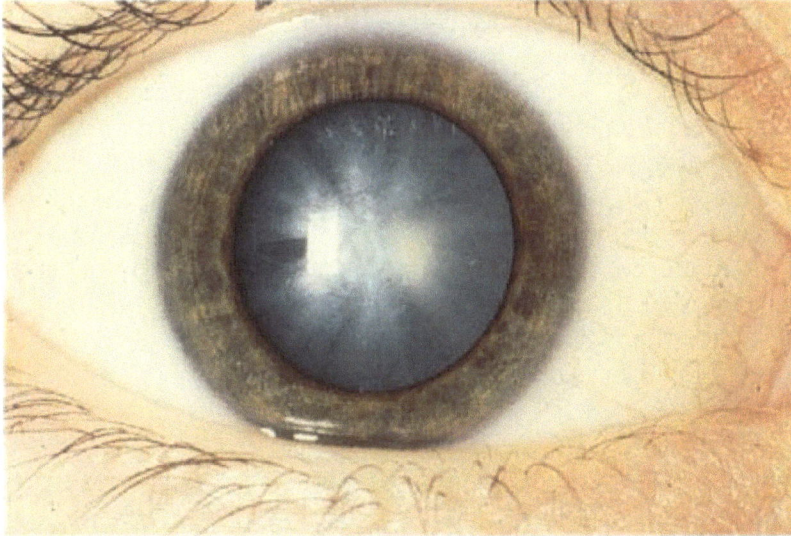

Fig. (3). Combined Cortical and Nuclear sclerotic cataract. Notice the "spoke" patterns of lens opacities. Image is available at *National Eye Institute, National Institutes of Health*. https://www.flickr.com/photos/ Accessed nationaleyeinstitute/7544344214/in/album-72157651546570359/. 6/8/2020.

The most common form of cataract among diabetic patients is a mixed cataract with a combination of posterior subcapsular and cortical cataract [4]. Among the non-mixed types, cortical cataract is reported as the most common [4], followed by the nuclear type [5]. The term *snowflake cataract* is used to describe bilateral, acute, widespread subcapsular lens changes, typically seen in younger patients. These cataracts are characterized by many gray-white subcapsular opacities with a snowflake appearance beginning in the lens cortex.

Pathophysiology

There have been multiple proposed mechanisms for the increased cataract formation in patients with DM. These include increased osmotic stress from activation of the polyol sorbitol-aldolase reductase pathway, increased oxidative stress, and non-enzymatic glycation of lens proteins [6 - 15]. The polyol pathway normally converts excess blood glucose to sorbitol. Sorbitol accumulates inside the lens because it can not easily cross cell membranes. Accumulation of sorbitol in the crystalline lens creates an osmotic gradient that causes fluid to accumulate inside the lens. High sorbitol concentrations also cause collapse and liquefaction of the lens fibers, resulting in loss of transparency and development of cataract [16, 17]. The increased osmotic stress also causes apoptosis of lens epithelial cells which contributes to cataract formation [16, 17].

Increased oxidative stress is caused by chronic hyperglycemia through direct increase of oxidative load and decreased ability in diabetic eyes to reduce free radical load [6, 10, 13]. These effects are mediated by increased glycation and defects in antioxidant enzyme activity. Non-enzymatic glycation also contributes to cataract formation by producing superoxide radicals and advanced glycation end (AGE) products. Accumulation of AGE products in the lens generates photosensitizers, which accelerates cataract formation [8, 9, 11, 12, 14, 18]. Control of blood glucose is important to prevent progression of diabetic cataracts. It has been suggested that other antioxidants may slow progression of cataracts, however definitive studies are lacking [19].

Clinical Evaluation

Clinical evaluation of cataracts in patients with DM should focus on a detailed history and visual complaints, visual acuity, slit-lamp examination, gonioscopy, measurement of IOP, and dilated fundus examination (DFE). History could include questionnaires such as the visual function index (VF-14) and the physician should focus the interview on difficulties with reading, driving, daily activities, such as watching TV, *etc.*, especially under conditions of limited lighting (*e.g.* at night) or when glare is present. Best corrected vision through refraction and glare testing are important to establish the level of visual impairment from cataract. Although central opacities can often be seen prior to dilation, the peripheral lens may only be fully appreciated when the pupil is dilated. In addition, visualization of the fundus may provide the clinician with a better idea of the level of lens opacity.

Treatment

Treatment of cataract is surgical and consists of removal of the cloudy lens and replacement with a small clear artificial intraocular lens (IOL). Cataract surgery is typically indicated when visual acuity is significantly decreased to interfere with daily activities. However, in patients with DM an additional indication is when, it interferes with the evaluation and treatment of the retina. Special considerations of cataract surgery in diabetics include difficulties with dilation due to iris ischemia, selection of intraocular lens, surgical technique, and exacerbation of diabetic retinal diseases, such as macular edema or diabetic retinopathy, after surgery. The iris of diabetic patients may not dilate well due to ischemia, necessitating special instrumentation such as pupillary expansion devices. Manual iris stretching may cause bleeding of the iris and may not be the best approach.

Intraocular multifocal lenses, which reduce contrast sensitivity in order to provide improved near vision, should be avoided in diabetic patients who have or will likely have compromised vision from their diabetic eye disease [20]. IOLs with larger diameter optics, the refractive part of the IOL, have been recommended to aid in visualization of the posterior segment [21]. Square edge designs may be preferred to decrease the incidence of posterior capsular opacification [22], as patients with DM seem to develop more severe PCO than non-diabetic patients [23]. Additionally, special consideration should be paid to the material of the intraocular lens. Silicone lenses should be avoided as silicone oil that may need to be placed in the eye to repair retinal detachment in the future can form droplets on silicone IOLs and degrade vision.

The femtosecond laser can perform some of the steps of cataract surgery, and reduces endothelial cell loss and achieves faster visual rehabilitation [24 - 26]. However, studies have not shown any difference in final vision with the laser [24 - 26]. Diabetic patients are at increased risk of persistent intraocular inflammation after cataract surgery [27], and may need to be treated with more peri- or postoperative steroids or non-steroidal medications. Diabetic patients also have an increased rate of progression of diabetic retinopathy after cataract surgery [28]. Foveal thickness and macular volume increase after cataract surgery in patients with diabetes, regardless of the presence of pre-existing diabetic retinopathy [29]. Similarly, the incidence of macular edema is higher in patients with moderate diabetic retinopathy compared to controls six weeks after cataract surgery [30]. Thus, close monitoring of the retina post operatively is indicated in order to timely diagnose and potentially treat diabetic retinopathy.

GLAUCOMA

Definition and Epidemiology

Glaucoma is an extremely common optic neuropathy in the US and worldwide [31, 32], and the first cause of non-reversible blindness is characterized by peripheral visual field loss and changes at the level of the optic disc. The incidence of glaucoma in the US in 2010 was 2.7 million patients, and this is expected to increase to 6.3 million in the year 2050 [31]. Worldwide, the prevalence was estimated to be over 60 million people in 2010 and was expected to increase to over 75 million people in 2020 [32]. Glaucoma is the second leading cause of blindness worldwide [32], and bilateral blindness from glaucoma was estimated to reach over 10 million people in 2020 [32]. While many forms of glaucoma are associated with increased intraocular pressure (IOP), glaucoma can also occur with IOPs within the normal range. Glaucoma is typically defined as an open or closed angle depending on the status of the anterior chamber angle of the eye (Fig. **4**). Aqueous humor is produced in the non-pigmented ciliary epithelium and travels via the pupil from the posterior segment of the eye to the anterior segment of the eye. The majority of aqueous humor is drained via the iridocorneal angle into the trabecular meshwork, and then into the canal of Schlemm. Eventually it passes into the episcleral veins which drain into the cavernous sinus via the superior ophthalmic vein. The status of the iridocorneal angle is evaluated by gonioscopy using a gonioprism, as the angle can not be viewed directly due to total internal reflection.

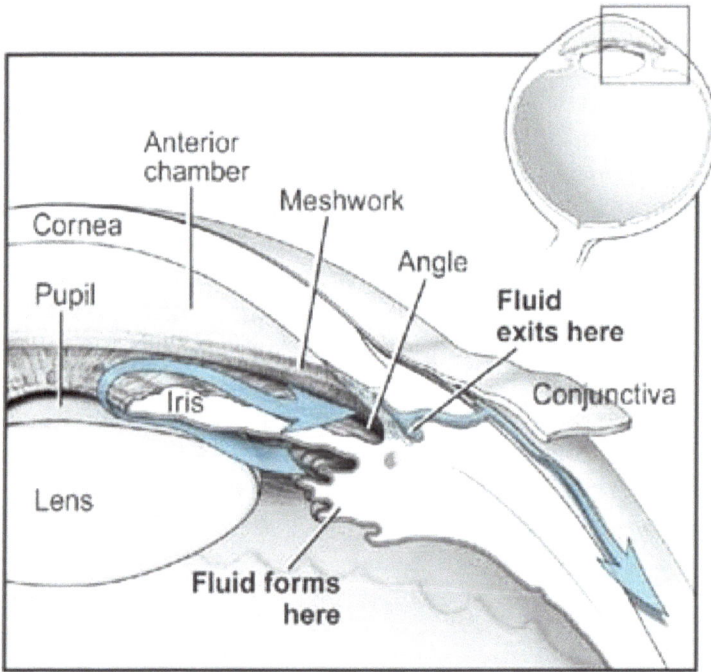

Fig. (4). Schematic diagram of aqueous humor flow. From *National Eye Institute, National Institutes of Health*.   https://www.flickr.com/photos/nationaleyeinstitute/7544457582/in/album-72157646829197286/. Accessed 6/8/2020.

Diabetes and Glaucoma Risk

The status of DM as a risk factor for primary open angle glaucoma (POAG), the most common type of glaucoma, has been somewhat controversial, with earlier large population based studies showing mixed results [2, 33]. However, a number of meta-analyses established that diabetic patients are at significantly increased risk of developing POAG and should be targeted for blindness prevention efforts [34 - 36]. A more recent systematic review of the available epidemiologic studies also concluded that diabetes, diabetes duration, and fasting glucose levels were associated with a significantly increased risk of glaucoma [36]. Longitudinal cohort studies which used billing codes to identify the development of OAG during a six year period have also detected an increased rate of incidence of glaucoma associated with the presence of DM [37, 38].

There are various plausible mechanisms by which DM may increase the risk of OAG. DM may affect retinal and optic nerve vascular perfusion, vascular autoregulation, glial reactivity with establishment of a pro-inflammatory environment or directly lead to RGC death. Indeed in animal models of DM accelerated apoptosis of retinal inner neurons and altered glial functions and vascular functions have been demonstrated [39 - 42]. These affects appear to be detectable in humans, as patients with DM have contrast sensitivity, color vision, and nerve fiber layer defects [43]. Since glaucoma also affects the RGCs in similar ways, DM may have an additive effect in the neurodegeneration. In animal models of the disease, it has been shown that DM increases apoptosis induced by glaucoma independent of IOP. Additionally, the loss of vascular autoregulation seen in DM may exacerbate hypoperfusion induced by increased IOP [44, 45]. Doppler flowmetry shows that OAG patients with diabetes fail to maintain retrobulbar blood flow and retinal microcirculation when ocular perfusion pressure decreases, either due to increased IOP or decreased mean arterial pressure [46].

Diabetes and Neovascular Glaucoma

Whether DM is associated with angle closure glaucoma is unsettled. However, neovascular glaucoma, a particular form of angle closure glaucoma has been clearly associated with DM. In neovascular glaucoma (NVG), ischemia to the retina and posterior segment leads to increased levels of angiogenic growth factors, such as vascular endothelial growth factor (VEGF), in the eye [47]. Many different cells from within the retina, such as Mueller cells, retinal pigment epithelial cells, retinal pericytes, endothelial cells, and ganglion cells, produce these growth factors [48]. In addition, the non pigmented epithelium of the ciliary body can also produce angiogenic factors. Additional inflammatory mediators that have been found to be elevated in eyes with NVG include cytokine IL-6, basic fibroblast growth factor, transforming growth factors, nitric oxide, and endothelin-1 [49 - 53]. These factors contribute to the growth and differentiation of new blood vessels, which are immature and thus fragile and bleed easily. These new blood vessels are able to grow onto the iris and iridocorneal angle and form fibrovascular membranes depending on their location, respectively, iris or angle neovascularization. Angle neovascularization can increase IOP causing decreased perfusion pressure to the retina and optic nerve head and leading to loss of vision. The presence of angle neovascularization typically precedes the rise in intraocular pressure [54]. While NVG may be caused by other ischemic retinal diseases, such as retinal vein occlusions or ocular ischemic syndrome, diabetes is among the most common etiologic factors for NVG [55]. Often, NVG is seen in patients who have coexisting proliferative diabetic retinopathy (PDR) [54].

Clinical Examination

A comprehensive eye exam with dilation is required in all patients suspected of having NVG. Rubeosis iridis, fine disorganized neovessels on the surface of the iris, which can be seen on slit lamp biomicroscopy, is diagnostic of the condition [56] (Fig. **5**). A mild anterior chamber inflammatory reaction characterized by flare is seen in almost all cases [54, 57]. In cases of acutely elevated IOP, the cornea may become edematous. The eye may be notably injected due to vascular changes and high IOP. Contraction of the fibrovascular membranes over the iris may result in ectropion uveae, a condition characterized by iris pigment epithelium visible on the anterior surface of the iris. Typically for DM, neovascularization will be visible on the iris before it is present in the angle [58]. Early NVI typically presents at the pupillary margin and is fine and delicate. In late stages of the disease, the angle may be closed due to contraction of the fibrovascular membranes that bridge the iris with the peripheral cornea forming extensive peripheral anterior synechiae (PAS). If the fragile neovessels bleed, there may be hyphema (layered blood in the anterior chamber). Gonioscopy to visualize the iridocorneal angle using a gonioprism, is necessary in order to detect NVA or PAS, and should be performed prior to dilation as a dilated iris may mask subtle NVA. Full dilated fundus examination is critical to diagnose diabetic retinopathy and examine the status of the optic nerve head, which may develop damage rapidly from high IOP. It is also critical to rule out other etiologies of retinal ischemia, such as central retinal vein occlusion that can cause NVG. It is also important to differentiate NVI from uveitis, which may present with dilated iris vessels and flare in the anterior chamber, normal iris vasculature in eyes with lightly pigmented irides, and carotid-cavernous fistulas, which may also have blood in Schlemm's canal and elevated IOP [54].

Adjunctive medical testing may aid in the clinical diagnosis of NVG. Fluorescein angiography (FA) of the retina may be useful to diagnose the causative retinal vascular disease and outline areas of retinal ischemia to guide prospective laser treatments. In contrast, fluorescein angiography of the iris is not routinely performed, although it may be used to demonstrate fluorescein leakage in borderline cases of NVG [54].

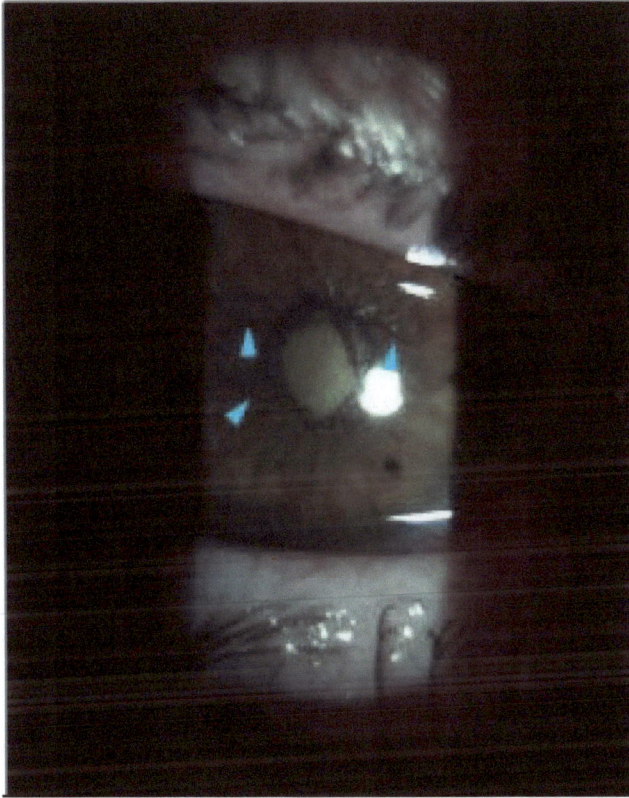

Fig. (5). Iris neovascularization. Notice the fine vessels on the surface of the iris (blue arrowheads). Courtesy of Dr Ilya Leskov.

The incidence is similar between genders, with a slightly higher prevalence in men [58]. NVG more commonly affects the elderly, and can be associated with significant health care costs due to medical and surgical care [58]. NVG has a particularly poor visual prognosis, with a large percentage of patients developing profound visual loss [59].

Treatment

Treatment of NVG is aimed at halting the neovascular drive of retinal ischemia and reducing IOP. To that end, ablation of the retina using laser with panretinal photocoagulation (PRP) has historically been performed. PRP inhibits and can even reverse the neovascularization in the anterior segment of the eye. The procedure is characterized by photocoagulating the peripheral ischemic retina with an argon laser [54]. PRP is typically performed for proliferative diabetic retinopathy in several sessions, but in cases of NVG should be performed as rapidly as it is safely possible. While typically performed in the clinic under topical anesthesia, patients may need to be taken to the operating room for PRP if deeper anesthesia is required. Clear ocular media are required for PRP. In cases where a cataract obstructs an adequate view to the retina, cataract surgery may need to be completed prior to successful PRP. Alternatively, in cases where a pars plana vitrectomy (PPV) is indicated, *e.g.* cases of tractional retinal detachment or non-clearing vitreous hemorrhage, PRP can be performed intraoperatively. PRP is successful in causing regression of retinal neovascularization in over two-thirds of cases, with IOP reduction achieved over 40% of the time and visual loss prevented in over half of the cases [60]. The amount of laser treatments can be titrated to achieve neovascularization regression.

In addition to PRP, anti-VEGF agents are used as adjunctive therapy for NVG [61]. These agents, such as bevacizumab and rainibizumab, which are antibodies, or aflibercept, which is an aptamer, either bind to the VEGF receptor or the VEGF molecule itself [62 - 64]. They are injected into the vitreous cavity using a 30 gauge needle and have been shown to decrease retinal neovascularization in various retinal vascular diseases. In NVG, these agents, when injected in the vitreous [61], have shown to cause regression of iris and angle neovascularization, and lower IOP if the angle has not been permanently occluded [65]. Typically, the effect of a single anti-VEGF agent administration lasts only 4-6 weeks [47] in cases of NVG, so additional definitive therapy with PRP or glaucoma surgery is still required. However, anti-VEGF therapy can delay the need for glaucoma surgery and, in some cases, obviate the need for such surgery [66]. Pre-operative use of anti-VEGF agents also provides the advantage of decreasing the incidence of [67, 68] postoperative hyphema and, in some studies, the number of glaucoma medications at the final visit [69]. Anti-VEGF agents result in rapid regression of iris and angle neovascularization in patients with early NVG and, more importantly, stabilize the endothelial barrier function of the immature blood vessels, thus decreasing the inflammatory extravasation of proteins that often contributes to IOP elevation [61, 70]. Similarly, intravitreal corticosteroids have also found to acutely decrease IOP via a similar mechanism [71].

Medical treatment should be initiated in cases of NVG with elevated IOP in order to prevent vision loss and relieve pain. Several classes of topical anti-glaucoma medications suppress aqueous humor formation, including α-2 agonists, β-adrenergic antagonists, and carbonic anhydrase inhibitors. Carbonic anhydrase inhibitors are also available in oral form, albeit with more systemic side effects, notably renal calculi, peripheral paresthesias, and renal compromise [72]. Care should be taken using beta blockers because of their bronchial constrictive effect and the possibility of inducing bradycardia. Prostaglandin-analogs, which are a popular class of topical anti-glaucoma medication used for many other forms of glaucoma, are not considered first line due to their tendency to breakdown the blood-aqueous barrier and worsen intraocular inflammation [58]. Direct cholinergic agonists such as pilocarpine may also incite inflammation and worsen synechiae angle closure by pulling the iris-lens diaphragm forward [58]. Topical atropine, an anticholinergic agent, is useful for its cycloplegic effects in paralyzing the ciliary body to prevent spasm and decrease pain, and reducing the incidence of hyphema [58]. Topical corticosteroids are also frequently used to reduce any intraocular inflammation, which frequently accompanies NVG.

While treating retinal ischemia with PRP and anti-VEGF agents is critical in reversing neovascularization, NVG often requires glaucoma surgery due to persistently elevated intraocular pressures because of complete obliteration of the angle. When this occurs, eyes become refractory to medical glaucoma therapy. Surgical options include trabeculectomy with antimetabolites, glaucoma drainage devices, cyclophotocoagulation, and other types of laser ablative procedures. Trabeculectomy, which involves creation of subconjunctival outflow for aqueous humor through a sclerostomy, has traditionally been used to treat many types of glaucoma refractory to medical therapy. NVG is associated with high rates of trabeculectomy failure [73, 74]. In fact, the presence of diabetes is a risk factor for trabeculectomy failure even in patients with open-angle glaucoma and no diabetic retinopathy or NVG [75]. Additionally, postoperative hyphema, which is a common complication in NVG patients, is also associated with higher failure rates [76]. Antimetabolites, such as mitomycin C, an alkylating agent, have been shown to increase success rates of trabeculectomy for all types of glaucoma, including NVG, however, even when MMC is used the success rate of trabeculectomy in cases of NVG is at best modest (~50% at 18 months) [77]. Glaucoma drainage devices (GDDs) are frequently used as first-line therapy for NVG. These devices shunt aqueous humor through a tube into a reservoir that is sutured onto the sclera 8-10 mm posterior to the limbus. The tube can be placed in the anterior chamber, ciliary sulcus behind the iris, or the vitreous cavity in vitrectomized eyes. Typically, the extraocular portion of the tube is covered with patch material to prevent exposure and erosion of the overlying conjunctiva. The device can be valved or non-valved. In the latter, the tube needs to be initially occluded to prevent early hypotony until a fibrous capsule has formed around the extraocular reservoir of the device. Although GDD use in NVG is currently preferred, its success is only slightly better than trabeculectomy and, in general, much worse than the success rate of GDDs in other forms of glaucoma [78 - 81]. In patients who have silicone oil placed in the eye, for example, as a result of surgical repair of a retinal detachment, GDDs are the only surgical option but should be placed in the inferior quadrants to prevent oil from occluding the tube. GDD combined with pars plana vitrectomy has been found to be safe and effective in patients with

PDR and NVG, although some patients experience decrease or even complete loss of vision [82, 83].

Cyclodestructive procedures involve the transscleral application of diode laser cyclophotocoagulation or cryotherapy to destroy the ciliary body epithelium and stroma in order to reduce the formation of aqueous humor. The non-pigmented ciliary epithelium of the ciliary body in the eye is an important source of VEGF in the anterior segment of the eye. Some studies suggest that treating the non-pigmented ciliary epithelium with cyclophotocoagulation or cyclocryotherapy may also be beneficial in cases where NVG is refractory to PRP [84]. Transscleral cyclophotocoagulation has been shown to be effective in lowering IOP and relieving pain in advanced cases of NVG, with or without adjunctive anti-VEGF therapy [85 - 87]. No difference in success rates has been found between diode cyclophotocoagulation and GDD implantation [88]. However, NVG is a risk factor for post-operative hypotony (IOP below 5mmHg), after transscleral cyclophotocoagulation [86, 87, 89]. Hypotony may lead to maculopathy and loss of vision and can be difficult to treat. As many as 1/4 of the eyes have been shown to develop severe long-term complications, including loss of vision, corneal decompensation, and phthisis bulbi in some series [90, 91]. To decrease the risk of hypotony, CPC can be performed in small increments and repeat treatments may be needed to maintain IOP control. Endo-cyclophotocoagulation, in which the ciliary body is treated through a probe inside the eye, was also found effective in treating NVG [92].

Because of the modest surgical success and high complication rate of NVG, novel surgical approaches such as attempting to remove fibrovascular membranes from the anterior chamber angle or GDDs made from different materials have been suggested [93]. However, to date, none of these efforts have resulted in increased efficacy or a significant reduction of adverse events and, thus, these procedures have not been widely adopted.

In cases of blind painful eyes with NVG, removal of the eye or intraocular contents via enucleation or evisceration can be considered. However, medical management with topical steroids, cycloplegic agents, and use of retrobulbar alcohol or chlorpromazine to permanently destroy pain nerve endings are typically attempted first [54].

CONSENT FOR PUBLICATION

Not applicable.

CONFLICT OF INTEREST

The author declares no conflict of interest, financial or otherwise.

ACKNOWLEDGEMENTS

We wish to acknowledge Dr. Ilya Leskov for providing one of the clinical photos above.

REFERENCES

[1]   Falck A, Laatikainen L. Diabetic cataract in children. Acta Ophthalmol Scand 1998; 76(2): 238-40.
        [http://dx.doi.org/10.1034/j.1600-0420.1998.760223.x] [PMID: 9591961]

[2]   Klein BE, Klein R, Jensen SC. Open-angle glaucoma and older-onset diabetes. The Beaver Dam Eye
        Study. Ophthalmology 1994; 101(7): 1173-7.
        [http://dx.doi.org/10.1016/S0161-6420(94)31191-2] [PMID: 8035979]

[3]   Klein BE, Klein R, Moss SE. Incidence of cataract surgery in the Wisconsin Epidemiologic Study of
        Diabetic Retinopathy. Am J Ophthalmol 1995; 119(3): 295-300.
        [http://dx.doi.org/10.1016/S0002-9394(14)71170-5] [PMID: 7872389]

[4]   Raman R, Pal SS, Adams JS, Rani PK, Vaitheeswaran K, Sharma T. Prevalence and risk factors for
        cataract in diabetes: Sankara Nethralaya Diabetic Retinopathy Epidemiology and Molecular Genetics
        Study, report no. 17. Invest Ophthalmol Vis Sci 2010; 51(12): 6253-61.
        [http://dx.doi.org/10.1167/iovs.10-5414] [PMID: 20610838]

[5]   Samanta A, Kumar P, Machhua S, Rao GN, Pal A. Incidence of cystoid macular oedema in diabetic
        patients after phacoemulsification and free radical link to its pathogenesis. Br J Ophthalmol 2014;
        98(9): 1266-72.
        [http://dx.doi.org/10.1136/bjophthalmol-2013-304438] [PMID: 24782476]

[6]   Agte VV, Tarwadi KV. Combination of diabetes and cataract worsens the oxidative stress and
        micronutrient status in Indians. Nutrition 2008; 24(7-8): 617-24.
        [http://dx.doi.org/10.1016/j.nut.2008.03.005] [PMID: 18472398]

[7]   Ahmed N. Advanced glycation endproducts--role in pathology of diabetic complications. Diabetes Res
        Clin Pract 2005; 67(1): 3-21.
        [http://dx.doi.org/10.1016/j.diabres.2004.09.004] [PMID: 15620429]

[8]   Araki N, Ueno N, Chakrabarti B, Morino Y, Horiuchi S. Immunochemical evidence for the presence
        of advanced glycation end products in human lens proteins and its positive correlation with aging. J
        Biol Chem 1992; 267(15): 10211-4.
        [PMID: 1587810]

[9]   Duhaiman AS. Glycation of human lens proteins from diabetic and (nondiabetic) senile cataract
        patients. Glycoconj J 1995; 12(5): 618-21.
        [http://dx.doi.org/10.1007/BF00731255] [PMID: 8595250]

[10]   Jeganathan VS, Wang JJ, Wong TY. Ocular associations of diabetes other than diabetic retinopathy.
        Diabetes Care 2008; 31(9): 1905-12.
        [http://dx.doi.org/10.2337/dc08-0342] [PMID: 18753669]

[11]   Lyons TJ, Silvestri G, Dunn JA, Dyer DG, Baynes JW. Role of glycation in modification of lens
        crystallins in diabetic and nondiabetic senile cataracts. Diabetes 1991; 40(8): 1010-5.
        [http://dx.doi.org/10.2337/diab.40.8.1010] [PMID: 1907246]

[12]   Nagaraj RH, Sell DR, Prabhakaram M, Ortwerth BJ, Monnier VM. High correlation between
        pentosidine protein crosslinks and pigmentation implicates ascorbate oxidation in human lens

senescence and cataractogenesis. Proc Natl Acad Sci USA 1991; 88(22): 10257-61.
[http://dx.doi.org/10.1073/pnas.88.22.10257] [PMID: 1946446]

[13]   Ookawara T, Kawamura N, Kitagawa Y, Taniguchi N. Site-specific and random fragmentation of Cu,Zn-superoxide dismutase by glycation reaction. Implication of reactive oxygen species. J Biol Chem 1992; 267(26): 18505-10.
[PMID: 1326527]

[14]   Shamsi FA, Sharkey E, Creighton D, Nagaraj RH. Maillard reactions in lens proteins: methylglyoxal-mediated modifications in the rat lens. Exp Eye Res 2000; 70(3): 369-80.
[http://dx.doi.org/10.1006/exer.1999.0800] [PMID: 10712823]

[15]   Srivastava SK, Ramana KV, Bhatnagar A. Role of aldose reductase and oxidative damage in diabetes and the consequent potential for therapeutic options. Endocr Rev 2005; 26(3): 380-92.
[http://dx.doi.org/10.1210/er.2004-0028] [PMID: 15814847]

[16]   Kinoshita JH. Cataracts in galactosemia. The Jonas S. Friedenwald Memorial Lecture. Invest Ophthalmol 1965; 4(5): 786-99.
[PMID: 5831988]

[17]   Kinoshita JH. Mechanisms initiating cataract formation. Proctor Lecture. Invest Ophthalmol 1974; 13(10): 713-24.
[PMID: 4278188]

[18]   Stitt AW. The maillard reaction in eye diseases. Ann N Y Acad Sci 2005; 1043: 582-97.
[http://dx.doi.org/10.1196/annals.1338.066] [PMID: 16037281]

[19]   Moïse MM, Benjamin LM, Doris TM, Dalida KN, Augustin NO. Role of Mediterranean diet, tropical vegetables rich in antioxidants, and sunlight exposure in blindness, cataract and glaucoma among African type 2 diabetics. Int J Ophthalmol 2012; 5(2): 231-7.
[PMID: 22762057]

[20]   Sokol S, Moskowitz A, Skarf B, Evans R, Molitch M, Senior B. Contrast sensitivity in diabetics with and without background retinopathy. Arch Ophthalmol 1985; 103(1): 51-4.
[http://dx.doi.org/10.1001/archopht.1985.01050010055018] [PMID: 3977675]

[21]   Javadi MA, Zarei-Ghanavati S. Cataracts in diabetic patients: a review article. J Ophthalmic Vis Res 2008; 3(1): 52-65.
[PMID: 23479523]

[22]   Nishi O, Nishi K, Wickström K. Preventing lens epithelial cell migration using intraocular lenses with sharp rectangular edges. J Cataract Refract Surg 2000; 26(10): 1543-9.
[http://dx.doi.org/10.1016/S0886-3350(00)00426-0] [PMID: 11033405]

[23]   Ebihara Y, Kato S, Oshika T, Yoshizaki M, Sugita G. Posterior capsule opacification after cataract surgery in patients with diabetes mellitus. J Cataract Refract Surg 2006; 32(7): 1184-7.
[http://dx.doi.org/10.1016/j.jcrs.2006.01.100] [PMID: 16857507]

[24]   Chee SP, Yang Y, Ti SE. Clinical outcomes in the first two years of femtosecond laser-assisted cataract surgery. Am J Ophthalmol 2015; 159(4): 714-9.
[http://dx.doi.org/10.1016/j.ajo.2015.01.016] [PMID: 25634531]

[25]   Lawless M, Bali SJ, Hodge C, Roberts TV, Chan C, Sutton G. Outcomes of femtosecond laser cataract surgery with a diffractive multifocal intraocular lens. J Refract Surg 2012; 28(12): 859-64.
[http://dx.doi.org/10.3928/1081597X-20121115-02] [PMID: 23231736]

[26]   Mastropasqua L, Toto L, Mastropasqua A, *et al.* Femtosecond laser *versus* manual clear corneal incision in cataract surgery. J Refract Surg 2014; 30(1): 27-33.
[http://dx.doi.org/10.3928/1081597X-20131217-03] [PMID: 24864325]

[27]   Krupsky S, Zalish M, Oliver M, Pollack A. Anterior segment complications in diabetic patients following extracapsular cataract extraction and posterior chamber intraocular lens implantation. Ophthalmic Surg 1991; 22(9): 526-30.

[PMID: 1945278]

[28]   Chung J, Kim MY, Kim HS, Yoo JS, Lee YC. Effect of cataract surgery on the progression of diabetic retinopathy. J Cataract Refract Surg 2002; 28(4): 626-30.
[http://dx.doi.org/10.1016/S0886-3350(01)01142-7] [PMID: 11955902]

[29]   Hayashi K, Igarashi C, Hirata A, Hayashi H. Changes in diabetic macular oedema after phacoemulsification surgery. Eye (Lond) 2009; 23(2): 389-96.
[http://dx.doi.org/10.1038/sj.eye.6703022] [PMID: 17962820]

[30]   Eriksson U, Alm A, Bjärnhall G, Granstam E, Matsson AW. Macular edema and visual outcome following cataract surgery in patients with diabetic retinopathy and controls. Graefes Arch Clin Exp Ophthalmol 2011; 249(3): 349-59.
[http://dx.doi.org/10.1007/s00417-010-1484-9] [PMID: 20827486]

[31]   https://nei.nih.gov/eyedata/glaucoma#5

[32]   Quigley HA. Number of people with glaucoma worldwide. Br J Ophthalmol 1996; 80(5): 389-93.
[http://dx.doi.org/10.1136/bjo.80.5.389] [PMID: 8695555]

[33]   Tielsch JM, Katz J, Quigley HA, Javitt JC, Sommer A. Diabetes, intraocular pressure, and primary open-angle glaucoma in the Baltimore Eye Survey. Ophthalmology 1995; 102(1): 48-53.
[http://dx.doi.org/10.1016/S0161-6420(95)31055-X] [PMID: 7831041]

[34]   Pasquale LR, Kang JH, Manson JE, Willett WC, Rosner BA, Hankinson SE. Prospective study of type 2 diabetes mellitus and risk of primary open-angle glaucoma in women. Ophthalmology 2006; 113(7): 1081-6.
[http://dx.doi.org/10.1016/j.ophtha.2006.01.066] [PMID: 16757028]

[35]   Wise LA, Rosenberg L, Radin RG, *et al.* A prospective study of diabetes, lifestyle factors, and glaucoma among African-American women. Ann Epidemiol 2011; 21(6): 430-9.
[http://dx.doi.org/10.1016/j.annepidem.2011.03.006] [PMID: 21549278]

[36]   Zhao D, Cho J, Kim MH, Friedman DS, Guallar E. Diabetes, fasting glucose, and the risk of glaucoma: a meta-analysis. Ophthalmology 2015; 122(1): 72-8.
[http://dx.doi.org/10.1016/j.ophtha.2014.07.051] [PMID: 25283061]

[37]   Newman-Casey PA, Talwar N, Nan B, Musch DC, Pasquale LR, Stein JD. The potential association between postmenopausal hormone use and primary open-angle glaucoma. JAMA Ophthalmol 2014; 132(3): 298-303.
[http://dx.doi.org/10.1001/jamaophthalmol.2013.7618] [PMID: 24481323]

[38]   Newman-Casey PA, Talwar N, Nan B, Musch DC, Stein JD. The relationship between components of metabolic syndrome and open-angle glaucoma. Ophthalmology 2011; 118(7): 1318-26.
[http://dx.doi.org/10.1016/j.ophtha.2010.11.022] [PMID: 21481477]

[39]   Galvao J, Elvas F, Martins T, Cordeiro MF, Ambrósio AF, Santiago AR. Adenosine A3 receptor activation is neuroprotective against retinal neurodegeneration. Exp Eye Res 2015; 140: 65-74.
[http://dx.doi.org/10.1016/j.exer.2015.08.009] [PMID: 26297614]

[40]   Lang GE. Mechanisms of retinal neurodegeneration as a result of diabetes mellitus. Klin Monatsbl Augenheilkd 2013; 230(9): 929-31.
[http://dx.doi.org/10.1055/s-0033-1350766] [PMID: 23986191]

[41]   Simó R, Hernández C, European R. Neurodegeneration in the diabetic eye: new insights and therapeutic perspectives. Trends Endocrinol Metab 2014; 25(1): 23-33.
[http://dx.doi.org/10.1016/j.tem.2013.09.005] [PMID: 24183659]

[42]   Wang L, Deng QQ, Wu XH, Yu J, Yang XL, Zhong YM. Upregulation of glutamate-aspartate transporter by glial cell line-derived neurotrophic factor ameliorates cell apoptosis in neural retina in streptozotocin-induced diabetic rats. CNS Neurosci Ther 2013; 19(12): 945-53.
[http://dx.doi.org/10.1111/cns.12150] [PMID: 23870489]

[43]   Nakamura M, Kanamori A, Negi A. Diabetes mellitus as a risk factor for glaucomatous optic neuropathy. Ophthalmologica 2005; 219(1): 1-10.
[http://dx.doi.org/10.1159/000081775] [PMID: 15627820]

[44]   Grunwald JE, Riva CE, Stone RA, Keates EU, Petrig BL. Retinal autoregulation in open-angle glaucoma. Ophthalmology 1984; 91(12): 1690-4.
[http://dx.doi.org/10.1016/S0161-6420(84)34091-X] [PMID: 6521997]

[45]   Sinclair SH, Grunwald JE, Riva CE, Braunstein SN, Nichols CW, Schwartz SS. Retinal vascular autoregulation in diabetes mellitus. Ophthalmology 1982; 89(7): 748-50.
[http://dx.doi.org/10.1016/S0161-6420(82)34720-X] [PMID: 7122050]

[46]   Shoshani YZ, Harris A, Shoja MM, *et al.* Endothelin and its suspected role in the pathogenesis and possible treatment of glaucoma. Curr Eye Res 2012; 37(1): 1-11.
[http://dx.doi.org/10.3109/02713683.2011.622849] [PMID: 22029631]

[47]   Wang JW, Zhou MW, Zhang X, *et al.* Short-term effect of intravitreal ranibizumab on intraocular concentrations of vascular endothelial growth factor-A and pigment epithelium-derived factor in neovascular glaucoma. Clin Exp Ophthalmol 2015; 43(5): 415-21.
[http://dx.doi.org/10.1111/ceo.12477] [PMID: 25488632]

[48]   Sall JW, Klisovic DD, O'Dorisio MS, Katz SE. Somatostatin inhibits IGF-1 mediated induction of VEGF in human retinal pigment epithelial cells. Exp Eye Res 2004; 79(4): 465-76.
[http://dx.doi.org/10.1016/j.exer.2004.06.007] [PMID: 15381031]

[49]   Chen KH, Wu CC, Roy S, Lee SM, Liu JH. Increased interleukin-6 in aqueous humor of neovascular glaucoma. Invest Ophthalmol Vis Sci 1999; 40(11): 2627-32.
[PMID: 10509659]

[50]   Chiou SH, Chang CJ, Chou CK, Hsu WM, Liu JH, Chiang CH. Increased nitric oxide levels in aqueous humor of diabetic patients with neovascular glaucoma. Diabetes Care 1999; 22(5): 861-2.
[http://dx.doi.org/10.2337/diacare.22.5.861a] [PMID: 10332703]

[51]   Iwabe S, Lamas M, Vásquez Pélaez CG, Carrasco FG. Aqueous humor endothelin-1 (Et-1), vascular endothelial growth factor (VEGF) and cyclooxygenase-2 (COX-2) levels in Mexican glaucomatous patients. Curr Eye Res 2010; 35(4): 287-94.
[http://dx.doi.org/10.3109/02713680903545315] [PMID: 20373895]

[52]   Tripathi RC, Borisuth NS, Tripathi BJ. Detection, quantification, and significance of basic fibroblast growth factor in the aqueous humor of man, cat, dog and pig. Exp Eye Res 1992; 54(3): 447-54.
[http://dx.doi.org/10.1016/0014-4835(92)90056-X] [PMID: 1521572]

[53]   Yu XB, Sun XH, Dahan E, *et al.* Increased levels of transforming growth factor-beta1 and -beta2 in the aqueous humor of patients with neovascular glaucoma. Ophthalmic Surg Lasers Imaging 2007; 38(1): 6-14.
[http://dx.doi.org/10.3928/15428877-20070101-01] [PMID: 17278530]

[54]   Hayreh SS. Neovascular glaucoma. Prog Retin Eye Res 2007; 26(5): 470-85.
[http://dx.doi.org/10.1016/j.preteyeres.2007.06.001] [PMID: 17690002]

[55]   Sayin N, Kara N, Pekel G. Ocular complications of diabetes mellitus. World J Diabetes 2015; 6(1): 92-108.
[http://dx.doi.org/10.4239/wjd.v6.i1.92] [PMID: 25685281]

[56]   Wilkinson-Berka JL, Miller AG. Update on the treatment of diabetic retinopathy. ScientificWorldJournal 2008; 8: 98-120.
[http://dx.doi.org/10.1100/tsw.2008.25] [PMID: 18264628]

[57]   Shazly TA, Latina MA. Neovascular glaucoma: etiology, diagnosis and prognosis. Semin Ophthalmol 2009; 24(2): 113-21.
[http://dx.doi.org/10.1080/08820530902800801] [PMID: 19373696]

[58] Rodrigues GB, Abe RY, Zangalli C, *et al.* Neovascular glaucoma: a review. Int J Retina Vitreous 2016; 2: 26.
[http://dx.doi.org/10.1186/s40942-016-0051-x] [PMID: 27895936]

[59] Albert DM, Jakobiec FA. Neovascular Glaucoma 1999.

[60] Lang GE. Laser treatment of diabetic retinopathy. Dev Ophthalmol 2007; 39: 48-68.
[http://dx.doi.org/10.1159/000098499] [PMID: 17245078]

[61] Olmos LC, Lee RK. Medical and surgical treatment of neovascular glaucoma. Int Ophthalmol Clin 2011; 51(3): 27-36.
[http://dx.doi.org/10.1097/IIO.0b013e31821e5960] [PMID: 21633236]

[62] Ferrara N, Hillan KJ, Novotny W. Bevacizumab (Avastin), a humanized anti-VEGF monoclonal antibody for cancer therapy. Biochem Biophys Res Commun 2005; 333(2): 328-35.
[http://dx.doi.org/10.1016/j.bbrc.2005.05.132] [PMID: 15961063]

[63] Lien S, Lowman HB. Therapeutic anti-VEGF antibodies. Handb Exp Pharmacol 2008; (181): 131-50.
[http://dx.doi.org/10.1007/978-3-540-73259-4_6] [PMID: 18071944]

[64] Stewart MW. Aflibercept (VEGF Trap-eye): the newest anti-VEGF drug. Br J Ophthalmol 2012; 96(9): 1157-8.
[http://dx.doi.org/10.1136/bjophthalmol-2011-300654] [PMID: 22446028]

[65] Horsley MB, Kahook MY. Anti-VEGF therapy for glaucoma. Curr Opin Ophthalmol 2010; 21(2): 112-7.
[http://dx.doi.org/10.1097/ICU.0b013e3283360aad] [PMID: 20040875]

[66] SooHoo JR, Seibold LK, Pantcheva MB, Kahook MY. Aflibercept for the treatment of neovascular glaucoma. Clin Exp Ophthalmol 2015; 43(9): 803-7.
[http://dx.doi.org/10.1111/ceo.12559] [PMID: 26016631]

[67] SooHoo JR, Seibold LK, Kahook MY. The link between intravitreal antivascular endothelial growth factor injections and glaucoma. Curr Opin Ophthalmol 2014; 25(2): 127-33.
[http://dx.doi.org/10.1097/ICU.0000000000000036] [PMID: 24406814]

[68] Zhou M, Xu X, Zhang X, Sun X. Clinical Outcomes of Ahmed Glaucoma Valve Implantation With or Without Intravitreal Bevacizumab Pretreatment for Neovascular Glaucoma: A Systematic Review and Meta-Analysis. J Glaucoma 2016; 25(7): 551-7.
[http://dx.doi.org/10.1097/IJG.0000000000000241] [PMID: 25719237]

[69] Arcieri ES, Paula JS, Jorge R, *et al.* Efficacy and safety of intravitreal bevacizumab in eyes with neovascular glaucoma undergoing Ahmed glaucoma valve implantation: 2-year follow-up. Acta Ophthalmol 2015; 93(1): e1-6.
[http://dx.doi.org/10.1111/aos.12493] [PMID: 24989855]

[70] Bates DO. Vascular endothelial growth factors and vascular permeability. Cardiovasc Res 2010; 87(2): 262-71.
[http://dx.doi.org/10.1093/cvr/cvq105] [PMID: 20400620]

[71] Jonas JB, Hayler JK, Söfker A, Panda-Jonas S. Regression of neovascular iris vessels by intravitreal injection of crystalline cortisone. J Glaucoma 2001; 10(4): 284-7.
[http://dx.doi.org/10.1097/00061198-200108000-00007] [PMID: 11558812]

[72] Centofanti M, Manni GL, Napoli D, Bucci MG. Comparative effects of intraocular pressure between systemic and topical carbonic anhydrase inhibitors: a clinical masked, cross-over study. Pharmacol Res 1997; 35(5): 481-5.
[http://dx.doi.org/10.1006/phrs.1997.0167] [PMID: 9299215]

[73] Allen RC, Bellows AR, Hutchinson BT, Murphy SD. Filtration surgery in the treatment of neovascular glaucoma. Ophthalmology 1982; 89(10): 1181-7.
[http://dx.doi.org/10.1016/S0161-6420(82)34672-2] [PMID: 6185899]

[74] Mietz H, Raschka B, Krieglstein GK. Risk factors for failures of trabeculectomies performed without antimetabolites. Br J Ophthalmol 1999; 83(7): 814-21.
[http://dx.doi.org/10.1136/bjo.83.7.814] [PMID: 10381669]

[75] Law SK, Hosseini H, Saidi E, *et al*. Long-term outcomes of primary trabeculectomy in diabetic patients with primary open angle glaucoma. Br J Ophthalmol 2013; 97(5): 561-6.
[http://dx.doi.org/10.1136/bjophthalmol-2012-302227] [PMID: 23355527]

[76] Nakatake S, Yoshida S, Nakao S, *et al*. Hyphema is a risk factor for failure of trabeculectomy in neovascular glaucoma: a retrospective analysis. BMC Ophthalmol 2014; 14: 55.
[http://dx.doi.org/10.1186/1471-2415-14-55] [PMID: 24766841]

[77] Sisto D, Vetrugno M, Trabucco T, Cantatore F, Ruggeri G, Sborgia C. The role of antimetabolites in filtration surgery for neovascular glaucoma: intermediate-term follow-up. Acta Ophthalmol Scand 2007; 85(3): 267-71.
[http://dx.doi.org/10.1111/j.1600-0420.2006.00810.x] [PMID: 17488455]

[78] Every SG, Molteno AC, Bevin TH, Herbison P. Long-term results of Molteno implant insertion in cases of neovascular glaucoma. Arch Ophthalmol 2006; 124(3): 355-60.
[http://dx.doi.org/10.1001/archopht.124.3.355] [PMID: 16534055]

[79] Krupin T, Kaufman P, Mandell AI, *et al*. Long-term results of valve implants in filtering surgery for eyes with neovascular glaucoma. Am J Ophthalmol 1983; 95(6): 775-82.
[http://dx.doi.org/10.1016/0002-9394(83)90064-8] [PMID: 6190402]

[80] Sidoti PA, Dunphy TR, Baerveldt G, *et al*. Experience with the Baerveldt glaucoma implant in treating neovascular glaucoma. Ophthalmology 1995; 102(7): 1107-18.
[http://dx.doi.org/10.1016/S0161-6420(95)30904-9] [PMID: 9121760]

[81] WuDunn D, Phan AD, Cantor LB, Lind JT, Cortes A, Wu B. Clinical experience with the Baerveldt 250-mm2 Glaucoma Implant. Ophthalmology 2006; 113(5): 766-72.
[http://dx.doi.org/10.1016/j.ophtha.2006.01.049] [PMID: 16650671]

[82] Faghihi H, Hajizadeh F, Mohammadi SF, Kadkhoda A, Peyman GA, Riazi-Esfahani M. Pars plana Ahmed valve implant and vitrectomy in the management of neovascular glaucoma. Ophthalmic Surg Lasers Imaging 2007; 38(4): 292-300.
[http://dx.doi.org/10.3928/15428877-20070701-04] [PMID: 17674919]

[83] Jeong HS, Nam DH, Paik HJ, Lee DY. Pars plana Ahmed implantation combined with 23-gauge vitrectomy for refractory neovascular glaucoma in diabetic retinopathy. Korean J Ophthalmol 2012; 26(2): 92-6.
[http://dx.doi.org/10.3341/kjo.2012.26.2.92] [PMID: 22511834]

[84] Tsai JC, Bloom PA, Franks WA, Khaw PT. Combined transscleral diode laser cyclophotocoagulation and transscleral retinal photocoagulation for refractory neovascular glaucoma. Retina 1996; 16(2): 164-6.
[http://dx.doi.org/10.1097/00006982-199616020-00016] [PMID: 8724965]

[85] Ghosh S, Singh D, Ruddle JB, Shiu M, Coote MA, Crowston JG. Combined diode laser cyclophotocoagulation and intravitreal bevacizumab (Avastin) in neovascular glaucoma. Clin Exp Ophthalmol 2010; 38(4): 353-7.
[http://dx.doi.org/10.1111/j.1442-9071.2010.02285.x] [PMID: 20665941]

[86] Iliev ME, Gerber S. Long-term outcome of trans-scleral diode laser cyclophotocoagulation in refractory glaucoma. Br J Ophthalmol 2007; 91(12): 1631-5.
[http://dx.doi.org/10.1136/bjo.2007.116533] [PMID: 17494956]

[87] Murphy CC, Burnett CA, Spry PG, Broadway DC, Diamond JP. A two centre study of the dose-response relation for transscleral diode laser cyclophotocoagulation in refractory glaucoma. Br J Ophthalmol 2003; 87(10): 1252-7.
[http://dx.doi.org/10.1136/bjo.87.10.1252] [PMID: 14507761]

[88]   Feldman RM, el-Harazi SM, LoRusso FJ, McCash C, Lloyd WC III, Warner PA. Histopathologic findings following contact transscleral semiconductor diode laser cyclophotocoagulation in a human eye. J Glaucoma 1997; 6(2): 139-40.
[http://dx.doi.org/10.1097/00061198-199704000-00011] [PMID: 9098823]

[89]   Yildirim N, Yalvac IS, Sahin A, Ozer A, Bozca T. A comparative study between diode laser cyclophotocoagulation and the Ahmed glaucoma valve implant in neovascular glaucoma: a long-term follow-up. J Glaucoma 2009; 18(3): 192-6.
[http://dx.doi.org/10.1097/IJG.0b013e31817d235c] [PMID: 19295370]

[90]   Delgado MF, Dickens CJ, Iwach AG, *et al.* Long-term results of noncontact neodymium:yttrium-aluminum-garnet cyclophotocoagulation in neovascular glaucoma. Ophthalmology 2003; 110(5): 895-9.
[http://dx.doi.org/10.1016/S0161-6420(03)00103-9] [PMID: 12750086]

[91]   Yap-Veloso MI, Simmons RB, Echelman DA, Gonzales TK, Veira WJ, Simmons RJ. Intraocular pressure control after contact transscleral diode cyclophotocoagulation in eyes with intractable glaucoma. J Glaucoma 1998; 7(5): 319-28.
[http://dx.doi.org/10.1097/00061198-199810000-00006] [PMID: 9786561]

[92]   Lima FE, Magacho L, Carvalho DM, Susanna R Jr, Avila MP. A prospective, comparative study between endoscopic cyclophotocoagulation and the Ahmed drainage implant in refractory glaucoma. J Glaucoma 2004; 13(3): 233-7.
[http://dx.doi.org/10.1097/00061198-200406000-00011] [PMID: 15118469]

[93]   Gil-Carrasco F, Jiménez-Román J, Turati-Acosta M, Bello-López Portillo H, Isida-Llerandi CG. Comparative study of the safety and efficacy of the Ahmed glaucoma valve model M4 (high density porous polyethylene) and the model S2 (polypropylene) in patients with neovascular glaucoma. Arch Soc Esp Oftalmol 2016; 91(9): 409-14.
[http://dx.doi.org/10.1016/j.oftal.2016.02.009] [PMID: 27068138]

CHAPTER 9

Optical Coherence Tomography and Fluorescein Angiography in Diabetic Retinopathy

Sruthi Arepalli, Justis P. Ehlers and **Peter K. Kaiser***

The Cole Eye Institute, Cleveland Clinic, Cleveland, OH, USA

Abstract: The assessment and monitoring of diabetic retinopathy are aided by multiple imaging techniques, including optical coherence tomography, optical coherence tomography angiography, and fluorescein angiography. We will discuss each modality in this chapter.

Keywords: Fluorescein angiography (FA), Optical coherence tomography (OCT), Optical coherence angiography (OCTA).

OPTICAL COHERENCE TOMOGRAPHY

Optical coherence tomography (OCT) has become an indispensable imaging technique in diabetic retinopathy and choroidopathy. OCT offers cross-sectional, detailed images of retinal tissue with high resolution on the level of microns [1 - 3]. This accuracy allows for the monitoring of disease progression and analysis of various characteristics associated with diabetic retinopathy.

Diabetic Macular Edema

Diabetic macular edema (DME), a major sequela of diabetes, presents at any stage of diabetic retinopathy and often results in a significant visual decline among working-aged individuals [4, 5]. In an epidemiological study reviewing the 10-year outcomes of patients with diabetes, DME occurred in 20.1% of the young-onset group and 25.4% in the older onset group taking insulin. This study estimates that DME will develop in over 800,000 patients, with clinically significant macular edema developing in over 550,000 people [6]. Therefore, the assessment and review of diabetic macular edema are integral to patient management and care.

---

* **Corresponding author Peter K. Kaiser:** From the Cole Eye Institute, Cleveland Clinic, Cleveland, OH;
E-mail: PKaiser@aol.com

The pathogenesis behind DME involves the alteration of endothelial cells and pericytes to create a hyperpermeable blood-retinal barrier, leading to the accumulation of plasma and lipid products in the macula [7]. This often leads to a detectable retinal elevation on fundoscopic examination. While the clinical examination was initially the standard for diagnosing macular edema, OCT can detect even minute amounts of edema invisible to the examiner [8]. This detailed view allows for the serial analysis and classification of various metrics in diabetes, including morphological retina edema patterns, evaluation of the vitreoretinal interface, measurement of retinal thickness and assessment of individual layers, and choroidal thickness [9]. This fact has also made the finding of clinically significant macular edema (CSME) as described in the Early Treatment Diabetic Retinopathy Study (ETDRS) replaced by the center-involved diabetic macular edema (CI-DME) based on OCT evaluation and not the clinical exam.

Morphological Patterns of Diabetic Macular Edema

Several morphological patterns of DME have been described in the literature [10 - 12]. The main classification system, set forth by Kim *et al.*, contains 5 categories: sponge-like, diffuse retinal thickening (DRT, defined as thickening greater than 200 um), cystoid macular edema (CME), serous retinal detachment (SRD), posterior hyaloid traction (PHT), and tractional retinal detachment (TRD) with PHT (Fig. **1**). These patterns of edema are not mutually exclusive and can present in conjunction with each other [10]. In this particular study, diffuse retinal thickening (present in 97% of scans) and cystoid macular edema (55% of scans) were the most common findings [10]. These results were compatible with previously published studies [11, 12]. DRT was the most commonly found sole presentation in eyes (39.5%), and DRT and CME were the most common combination (29% of scans) [10]. The same paper found that both CME and PHT without TRD were significantly associated with decreased vision. Additionally, cystic changes had the highest predisposition to decreased vision [10]. Kaiser *et al.* also described the unique form of DME associated with PHT, an entity that may be missed on clinical biomicroscopy alone. The recognition of this pattern is important as these patients may be more resistant to therapy and require surgical intervention earlier, although the exact mechanism of visual recovery is unknown [13].

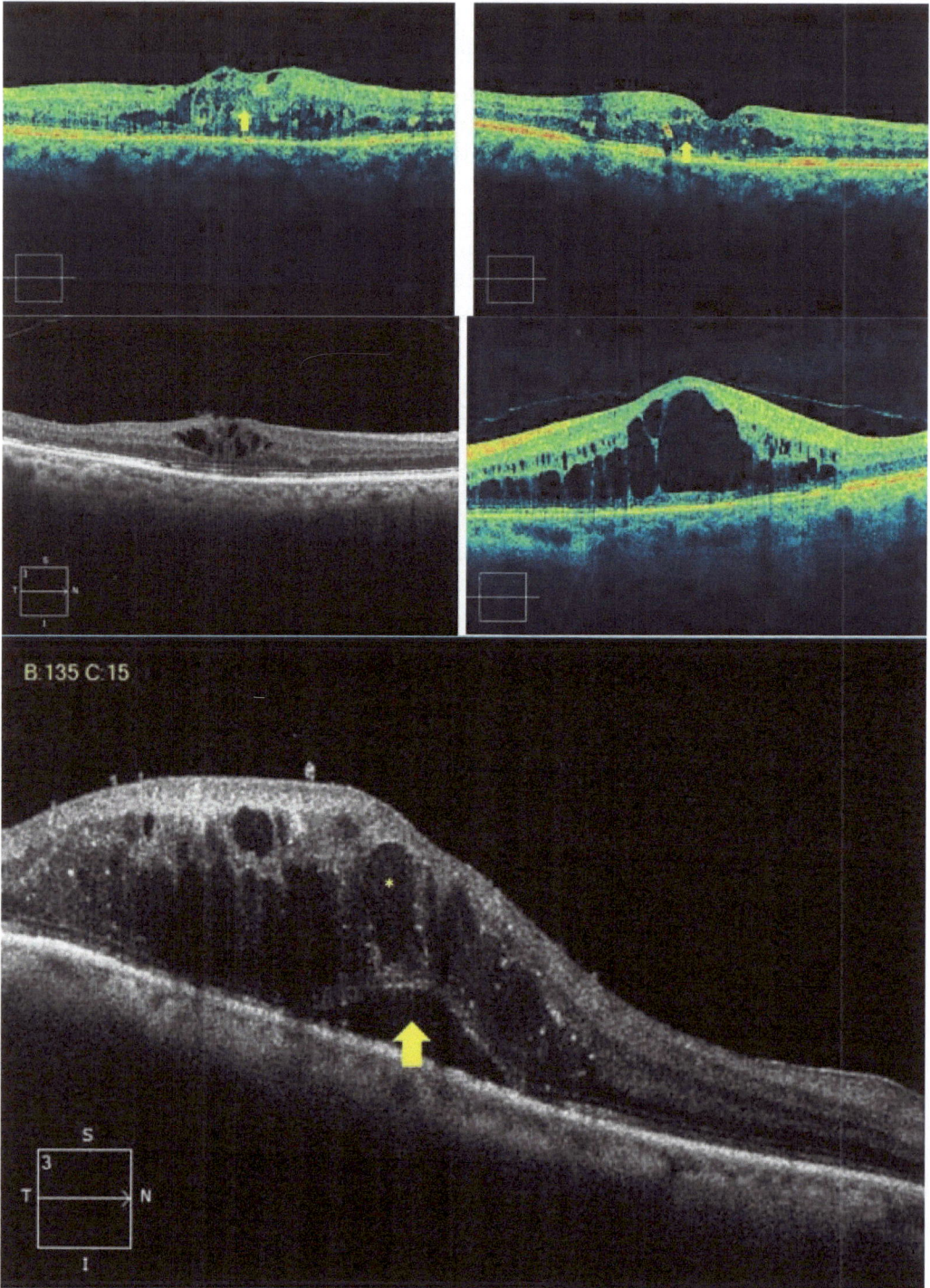

(Fig. 1) contd.....

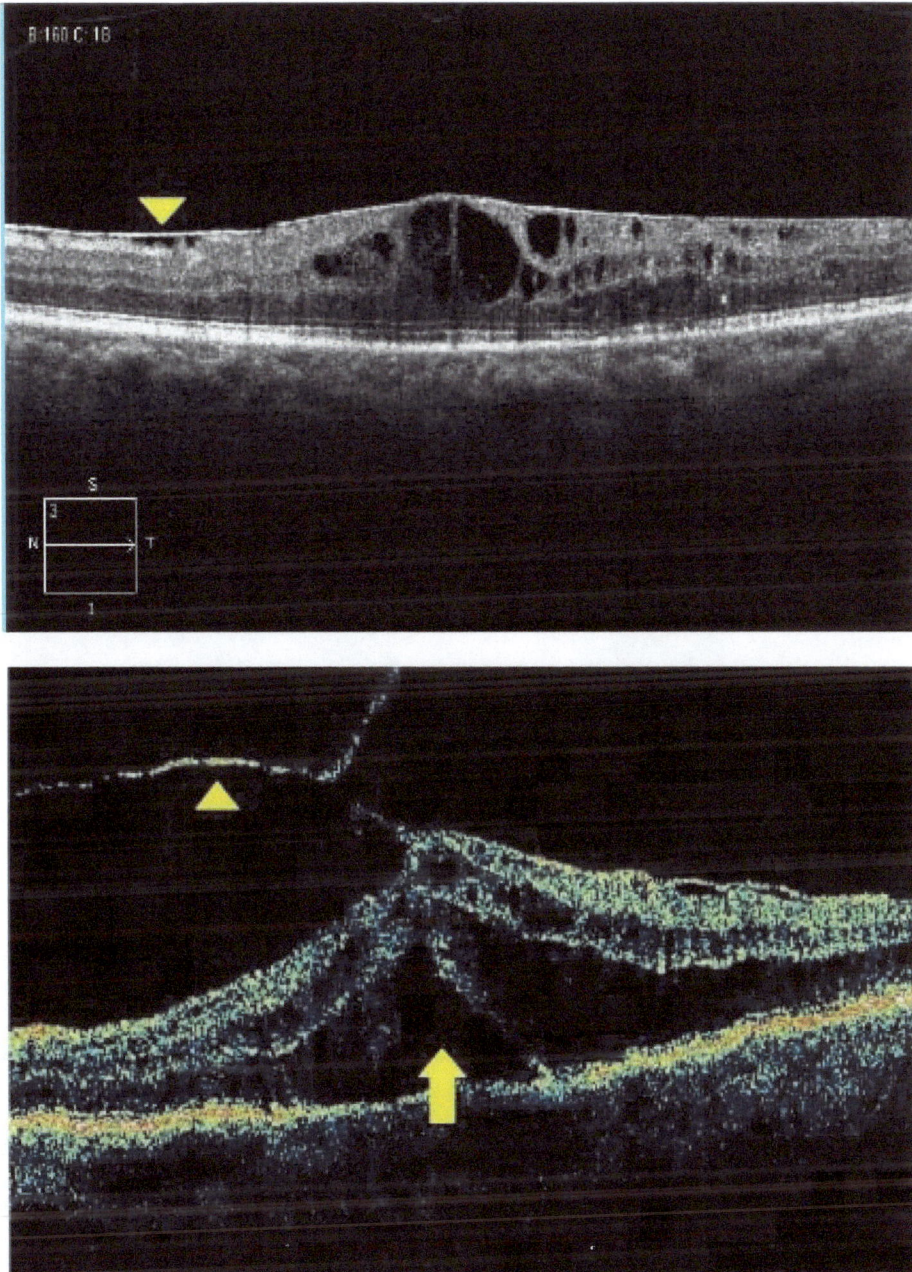

Fig. (1). Patterns of diabetic macular edema on OCT. **(A)** Sponge-like intraretinal swelling (yellow arrows); **(B)** early (left) and late (right) cystic changes; **(C)** subretinal fluid accumulation (arrow) associated with cystic changes (Asterisks); **(D)** posterior hyaloidal (arrowhead) traction without traction detachment; **(E)** posterior hyaloidal (arrowhead) traction with traction detachment (arrow).

Retinal Thickness and Individual Layer Integrity in Diabetic Macular Edema

Retinal Thickness

OCT enables the consistent measurement and comparison of retinal pathology, particularly retinal thickness and the integrity of the individual retinal layers. The increased retinal thickness on OCT is correlated with leakage on fluorescein angiography and tends to increase with diabetic progression [11, 14, 15]. While not a precise relationship, various studies have found a modest correlation between retinal thickness and visual acuity [10, 16]. This has led to the hypothesis that certain changes within the individual layers of the retina predispose to visual acuity changes more than others. Following the retinal thickness in patients being treated for diabetic macular edema gives feedback as to how well your therapy is working (Fig. **2**).

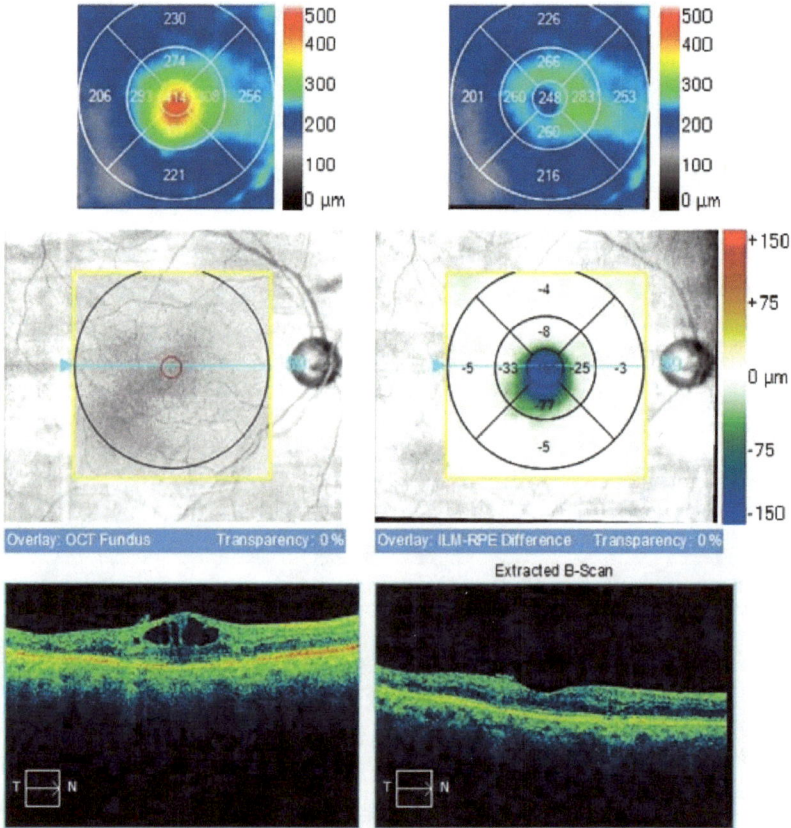

Fig. (2). Change analysis with treatment of DME. A patient with diabetic macular edema before (left) and after (right) treatment. The top panels show change in retinal thickness, while the bottom panels show a B-scan representation. The middle panels show the difference between the two visits.

Disorganization of the Retinal Inner Layers (DRIL)

Disorganization of the retinal inner layers (DRIL) in the presence of resolved or currently existing diabetic macular edema has been linked to worse visual acuity outcomes and worsening diabetic retinopathy [17, 18]. Longitudinal studies assessing the presence of foveal DRIL with central involving diabetic macular edema have found that it has a predictive effect on visual acuity [17]. The proposed mechanism of this includes a disruption of the connections between the inner retinal cells and the visual pathway [17]. DRIL has also been associated with increasing metamorphopsia [19]. Furthermore, the resolution of DRIL is linked to improving visual acuity [17].

Ellipsoid Zone

The importance of the ellipsoid zone (previously known as the IS/OS junction) in visual acuity is well established in various disease processes. In particular, a decline in photoreceptor outer segment thickness and volume is negatively correlated with visual acuity in DME [9, 20 - 22]. Moreover, retinal point sensitivity testing declines with the disruption and absence of the ellipsoid zone (Fig. **3**) [23]. Interestingly, in retinas with a thickness of over 300 *u*m, the ellipsoid disruption was strongly associated with declining retinal sensitivity. However, in atrophic retinas, either from long-standing edema or diabetic retinopathy, with thickness under 300 *u*ms, the destruction of the ellipsoid zone had less of an impact on visual acuity [22]. These findings support the movement towards resolving diabetic macular edema found on OCT sooner, rather than later, to preserve the functional ellipsoid zone [23].

Hard Exudates

Hard exudates are thought to be secondary to lipoprotein leakage from retinal capillaries [24]. The presence of these has been linked to decreasing vision; in one study, the severity of hard exudates was directly associated with the proportion of patients with worse than 20/40 vision, and the severity of hard exudates at initial presence was linked to a decrease from baseline by 3 or more lines at the fifth annual visit [24]. Hard exudates have also accumulated in the sub-retinal space in the presence of foveal serous retinal detachments [25].

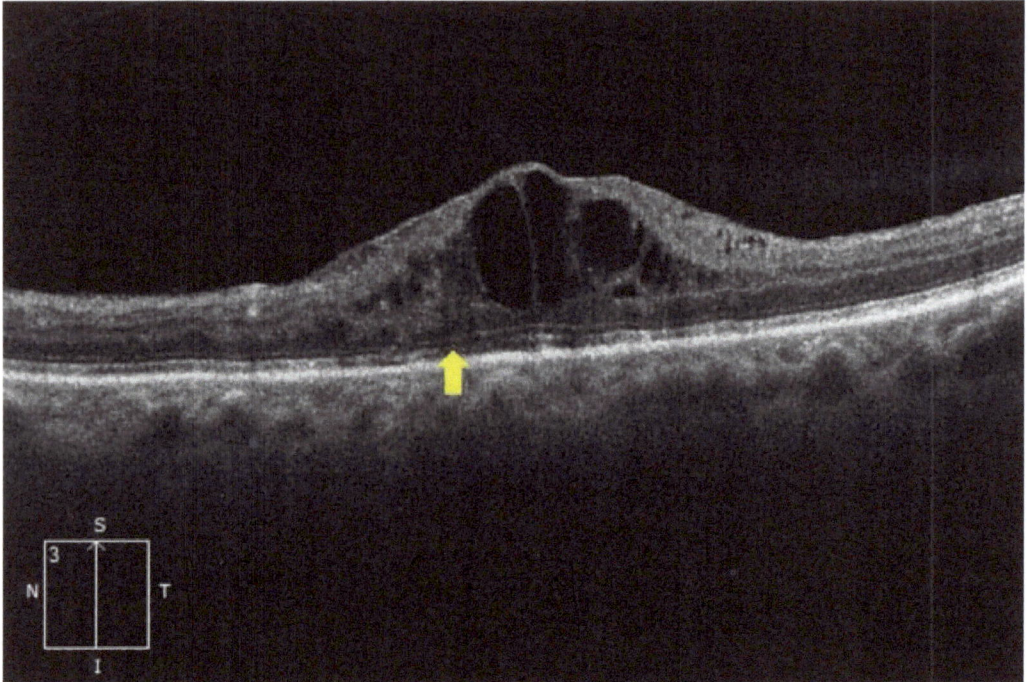

Fig. (3). Outer Retinal Changes in DME. The arrow points to an area of discontinuity of the ellipsoid zone indicating outer retinal changes.

Hyperreflective Foci and an External Limiting Membrane

The majority of eyes with DME have non-confluent hyperreflective foci within the retinal layers on OCT (Fig. **4**). These subclinical findings do not correspond to hemorrhage, exudates, or retinal thickening on biomicroscopy [26]. There are many theories on the origin of these foci.

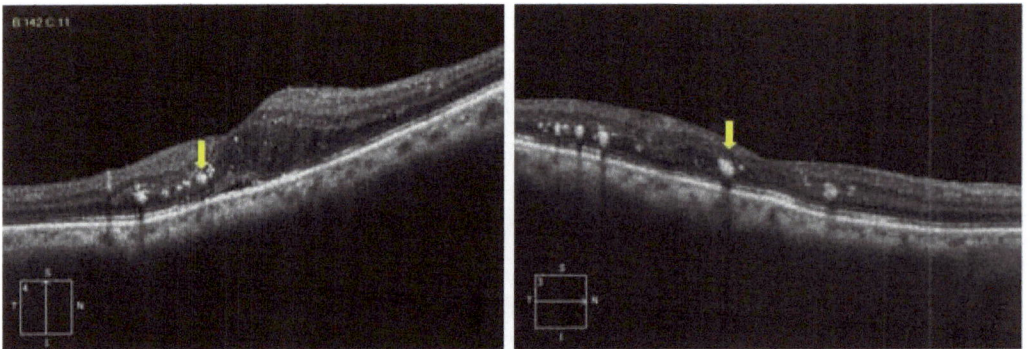

Fig. (4). Hard Exudates on OCT. Hard exudates appear as hyper-reflective foci within the retina (arrows).

Uji *et al.* hypothesize that these foci are excavated lipoprotein, which eventually progresses to hard exudates. They are more commonly found in the inner retinal layers, (99.1% of eyes), and less commonly in the outer retina (53.7% of eyes) [20]. The external limiting membrane (ELM) has been implicated in the migration of these foci from the inner retina to the outer retina, as it is a connection between Muller cells and photoreceptors, with previous studies revealing its barrier properties to macromolecules [27]. It has been hypothesized that the ELM also serves as a barrier to the progression of previously discussed hyperreflective foci into the outer retina, with the majority of patients with outer retinal foci having a disturbed ELM [20, 28].

Conversely, the presence of these changes in the outer retina may reflect a neurodegenerative process, involving the death of Muller cells, photoreceptors, or both. [26] Another theory, published by Vujosevic *et al.* and Midena *et al.*, attributes these foci to microglial activation. It is hypothesized that the later stages of activation involve the outer retina, while earlier stages remain in the inner retina [29, 30].

Regardless of their etiology, studies have linked photoreceptor and subsequent visual acuity decrease to the presence of hyperreflective foci in the outer retina and a disrupted ELM [20, 32]. Furthermore, studies have elucidated that an intact ELM and ellipsoid zone at the initial visit are more often associated with intact photoreceptors after DME absorption [21]. These findings emphasize the importance of an intact ELM in preventing photoreceptor damage in DME.

Macular Cube and Cystic Macular Edema

Segmentation algorithms allow for analysis of retinal thickness analysis and retinal topography, including cystic changes. These cystic changes typically occur in the inner nuclear and outer plexiform layers (Fig. **5**) [32, 33]. Cystoid changes have been found to correlate significantly with logMAR visual acuity, taken independently of retinal thickness changes or ellipsoid zone integrity [23, 32]. Novel imaging techniques have emerged to automatically quantify retinal fluid itself, rather than retinal thickness as a whole [34]. These algorithms can be used to track cystic volume changes as a response to treatment and disease progression. The visual aid also serves as a reinforcing educational device for patients to understand their disease process [35].

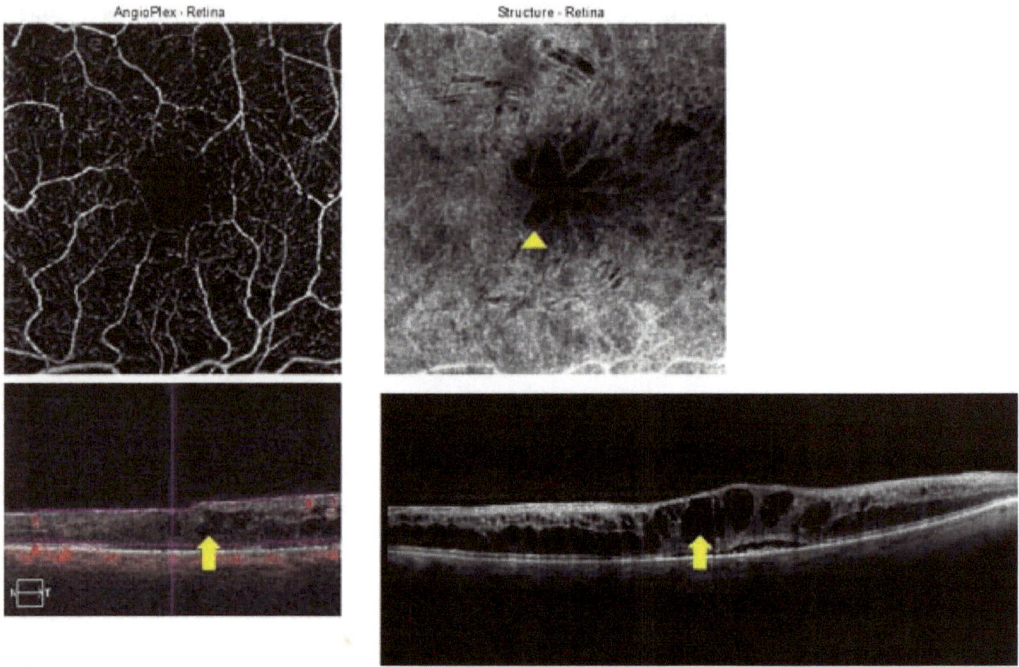

Fig. (5). Diabetic cystoid changes. The arrows point to cystic changes on the B-scan images of two different patients. The arrowhead points to a cystic change on the en-face image illustrating the petaloid pattern often seen with cystic changes.

Choroidal Thickness

While the retinal vascular changes have been well established and analyzed in diabetic retinopathy, choroidal pathology was previously poorly described. Advances in OCT technology have allowed for better visualization of the deeper structures, in some cases, up to the choroidoscleral interface. For example, swept-source OCT with a longer wavelength laser can image deep into the choroid. Standard spectral domain OCT can also focus on the choroid by moving the lens closer to the eye, or by using image averaging. These measurements focus on the chorioscleral interface, subfoveal choroidal thickness, and vessel thickness.

Adhi *et al.* found that in normal eyes, the choroidoscleral interface is normally a concave, "bowl shape." They contrasted this to patients with diabetic edema, as the contour changes of their choriodoscleral interface changes to an "S" shape with alternating concave-convex-concave areas. This irregular choroidoscleral interface occurred in 93% of diabetic edema eyes and in 0% of normal controls [36].

In general, investigators have found a reduction in the mean subfoveal choroidal thickness, as well as the combined thickness of the medium choroidal vessels and the choriocapillaris in eyes with DME [36, 37]. Adhi *et al.* found focal choroidal thinning in 86% of DME eyes, compared to 0% in controls [36]. Sheth and colleagues found a similar reduction in subfoveal choroidal thickness in eyes with diabetic retinopathy, noting a further significant decrease in eyes with macular ischemia as compared to eyes without macular ischemia (Fig. **6**) [38].

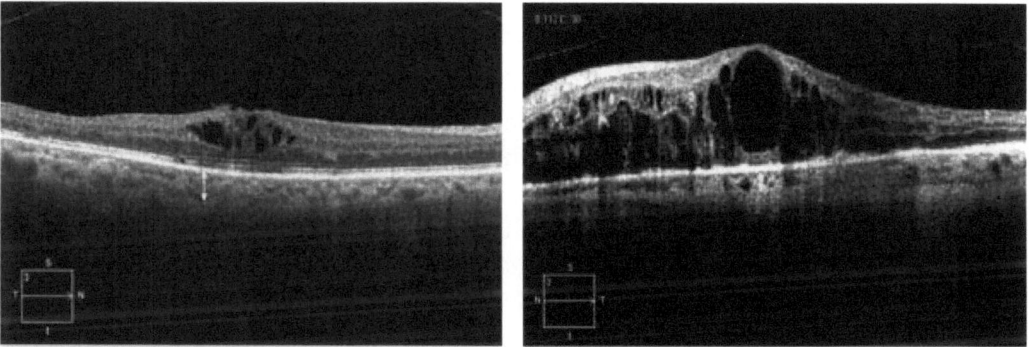

Fig. (6). Choroidal thickness. Two patients with different choroidal thickness (lines). Both are thinner than normal.

On the other hand, Kim *et al.* found an increase in choroidal thickness in eyes with diabetic macular edema [39]. The discrepancy in thickness measurements has been attributed to the different populations studied in each report. Patients with severe, proliferative diabetic retinopathy with an increased ischemic drive were included in the reports of the thicker choroid. Patients who had been previously treated were included in the study finding a thinner choroid, likely skewing results.

Summary

Optical coherence tomography is instrumental in monitoring structural changes from diabetic retinopathy, including macular edema, retinal thickness changes, disorganization and disturbance of retinal layers and extracellular accumulations. In terms of macular edema, diffuse retinal thickening and cystoid patterns are the most common. In addition to macular edema, the disorganization of the inner retinal layers, ellipsoid zone loss, and hard exudates portend a worse visual prognosis.

OPTICAL COHERENCE TOMOGRAPHY ANGIOGRAPHY

Optical coherence tomography angiography (OCTA) is a novel modification of OCT technology. It is a non-invasive, dye-free imaging technique that creates three-dimensional reconstructions of vascular flow within a tissue segment [35, 40, 41]. Put briefly, a segment of tissue is repeatedly scanned. The pixels in these

OCT scans from each segment are compared to each other, and the amount of variation between them calculated. These variations, if above a predetermined threshold, are attributed to the movement of blood cells within the vasculature [40]. Multiple algorithms exist to image tissue, including phase, amplitude, or a combination, and various statistical methods are used to interpret the data. Ultimately, they all aim to re-construct three-dimensional images of vascular flow.

As OCTA does not require dye, it cannot show leakage of vessels, an important pathology in diabetes. By the same token, it is able to visualize vascular layers more clearly than fluorescein angiography (FA) would, as these details would be missed from leakage. OCTA images are not without artifacts, which result from its complex data collection and require thoughtful interpretation [40, 41]. While it may be a powerful tool to image vascular pathology, further research is required to further the clinical applications of this imaging modality.

The ability for OCTA to image and differentiate multiple layers of vessels allows it to be an indispensable imaging method for the macula and the peripheral retina. The vasculature tree of the retina is composed of three main branches: the superficial capillary plexus (SCP), the deep capillary plexus (DCP), and the choriocapillaris. The SCP is responsible for supplying the retinal nerve fiber layer to the inner nuclear layer; the DCP is responsible for the outer border of the inner nuclear layer to the deep retina; and the choriocapillaris supplies the deep retina as well as the foveal avascular zone (FAZ) through diffusion [42, 43]. Variations in flow and vascular structure are present in the OCTA analyses of DME, central and peripheral ischemia, and neovascularization, all of which have been linked to decreased visual acuity. Interestingly, reports have contrasting findings on the specific pathology associated with each vascular level in the retina, likely secondary to the novel applications of this tool and the artifacts it produces [44 - 54].

Diabetic Macular Edema

Various studies have reported anomalies in the retinal vasculature of patients with DME, such as microaneurysms [44, 45]. Microaneurysmal changes in both the superficial and deep capillary plexus were significantly higher in eyes with DME as compared to control eyes [44]. Vascular flow density and area of avascular flow were also significantly decreased and increased, respectively, in the deep capillary plexus (DCP) between DME and control eyes [45]. This has led to the hypothesis that the DCP is involved in the pathogenesis of DME [44].

Macular Ischemia

OCTA can assess foveal ischemia (Fig. **7**). Studies focusing on foveal ischemia measure three main parameters: the foveal avascular zone (FAZ), perfusion and vessel density, and the presence of microaneurysms [44, 46].

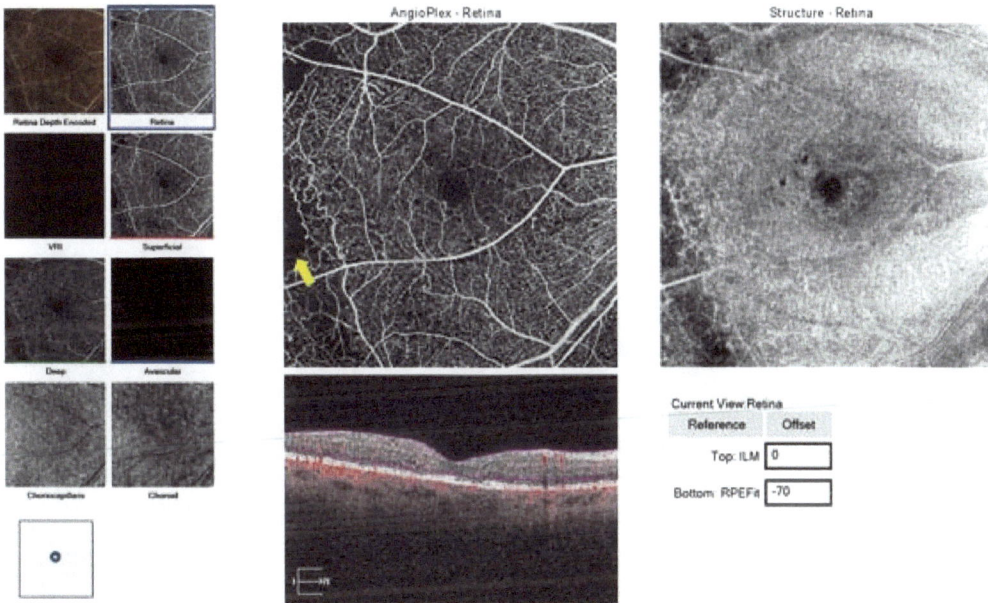

Fig. (7). OCT Angiography of macular ischemia. This patient has no diabetic macular edema but evidence of macular ischemia (arrow) on OCT angiography.

Increased FAZ

The FAZ in eyes without ocular pathology can vary [55]. Despite this, multiple reports document a significant increase in the FAZ diameter in diabetic patients in OCTA measurements [45]. In a comparison between eyes with diabetic retino-pathy and controls, there was a significant increase in the FAZ in both the SCP and DCP layers, with more of an increase noted in the DCP (Fig. **8**) [45, 47 - 51]. Tasake *et al.* showed an enlargement of the FAZ even in diabetes without any diabetic retinopathy [49].

Perfusion and Vessel Density

In DME, a loss of capillaries leads to non-perfusion and subsequent vascular remodeling throughout the retina [46]. These ischemic areas, which appear black on fluorescein angiography, can be imaged with OCTA, and have the vascular loss in these areas quantified [52]. In addition, OCTA images can be translated into perfusion maps, which further detailed loss of vascular supply. There have been conflicting reports on which retinal vascular layer (SCP *vs.* DCP) is more compromised in diabetic macular ischemia. This discrepancy could be in part due to the inherent artifacts associated with OCTA, as well as the different severity of diabetes included in each report.

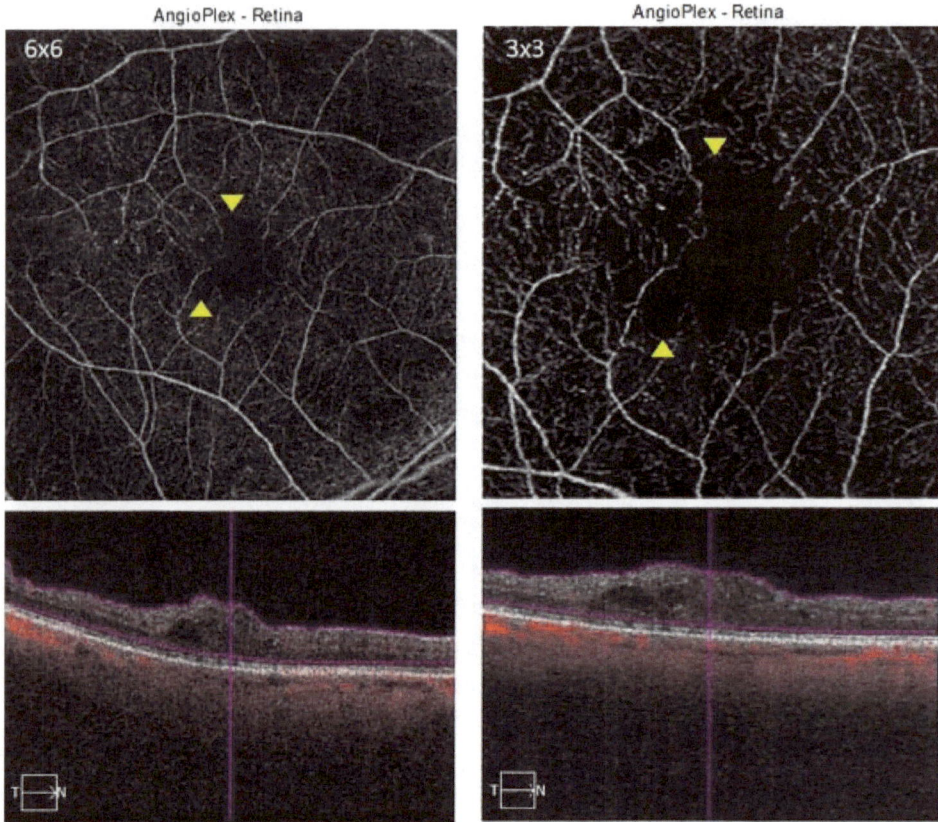

Fig. (8). OCT Angiography of enlarged FAZ. This is an OCT angiogram of the same patient using two different scan patterns: 6x6 mm (left) and 3x3mm (right). The enlargement of the foveal avascular zone (arrowheads) is easier to see on the 3x3 mm scan.

Agemy *et al.*, in a comparison between the perfusion maps of control eyes and eyes with diabetic retinopathy, reported a significant decrease in the perfusion density of the SCP, DCP, and choriocapillaris [46]. DCP and choriocapillaris showed the most decrease in perfusion. Samara *et al.* found a decrease in macular vessel density, measured by vessel area density and vessel length density in diabetic patients in both the SCP and DCP, also with the more pronounced changes located in the DCP [50]. These findings were correlated with worsening visual acuity [50]. The DCP has been termed a watershed zone of the retina, and its sensitivity to ischemia may predispose it to develop more ischemic findings on

OCTA. Furthermore, changes in the DCP are linked to early photoreceptor changes in diabetic retinopathy, leading to visual decline [45, 53]. Thus attention to and recognition of DCP pathology in OCTA can provide invaluable information regarding disease progression. In contrast, Al-Sheikh *et al.* found a decrease in vessel density seen in both the SCP and DCP, with the most drop-out seen in the SCP layer [45].

Microaneurysms

Microaneurysms serve as a surrogate marker for retinal ischemia, and their presence can be illustrated on OCTA, as fusiform, round or saccular outpunching of the vasculature [51, 54, 56]. Lee *et al.* found that these were increased in both the SCP and DCP [44]. In an OCTA image comparison between the DCP and SCP, Couturier *et al.* and Hasegawa *et al.* found significantly more microaneurysms in the DCP than the SCP in areas of diabetic macular edema [56, 57] Moreover, an increase in microaneurysms in the DCP was associated with the cystoid macular edema variant [57]. This also implicates the DCP in the pathogenesis of diabetic macular edema. However, it is important to note that microaneurysms may be missed, as the flow through these areas is too slow, and under the threshold set by the OCTA. It has also been hypothesized that the flow through these microaneurysms may be plasma only, without blood cells, thus limiting OCTA's ability to detect vasculature [56]. These caveats do limit the application of OCTA findings but do serve as interesting points for further investigation [56].

Peripheral Ischemia

In addition to highlighting ischemic changes in the fovea of diabetic patients, OCTA provides a peripheral view of capillary nonperfusion in patients with diabetic retinopathy [58]. In a study evaluating proliferative diabetic retinopathy, 92% of eyes were noted to have PDR into the vitreous above an area of retinal ischemia, portrayed as capillary drop-out on OCTA [58]. This highlights the relationship between ischemia and diabetic retinopathy and can serve as a potential area to monitor serial OCTA scans. Hwang *et al.* were able to identify areas of capillary drop out in all eyes beyond the FAZ and found that OCTA was more reliable that fluorescein angiography in depicting ischemia, as there was no loss of detail from leakage [48].

Proliferative Diabetic Retinopathy

In proliferative diabetic retinopathy (PDR), ischemia is an instigating force behind the growth of pathological retinal blood vessels extending through the internal limiting membrane and into the vitreous space [59]. While fluorescein angiography can highlight neovascular changes in diabetes, the details and level of vascular pathology can be obscured by leakage [52]. OCTA enables *en face* imaging of different levels of the vitreoretinal interface, including preretinal neovascularization, retinal neovascularization, and intraretinal microvascular abnormalities [58, 60].

De Carlo *et al.* provided the first OCTA imaging of neovascularization into the vitreous cavity, highlighting the presence of capillary drop-out and ischemia surrounding the areas, and associated IRMA in 50% of the cases [58]. Hwang *et al.* highlighted the ability for OCTA to depict early retinal neovascularization, which was initially interpreted as microaneurysms on fluorescein angiography. This may elucidate why some diabetic patients with vitreous hemorrhage do not have clearly delineated neovascularization on FA [48]. Ishibazawa *et al.* argue that OCTA can be used to track neovascular growths and to categorize the proliferative growths as active or inactive, based on the pattern of small caliber vessels associated with them [54]. Given the results of these studies, the potential application of OCTA in assessing and monitoring proliferative diabetic retinopathy is immense.

Summary

Optical coherence tomography angiography allows for dye-less, non-invasive imaging of multiple retinal layers. In particular, it is able to highlight a higher number of microaneurysmal changes in the superficial and deep capillary plexus in patients with diabetic macular edema. It can also be utilized to monitor an increasing foveal avascular zone throughout both the capillary layers, especially in the deep capillary plexus. OCTA also shows a decrease in perfusion of the superficial, deep capillary plexus and the choriocapillaris. It is also instrumental in documenting the number of microaneurysms, and an increase is correlated to worsening diabetic macular edema. Moreover, it can monitor for the development of neovascular fronds, especially in cases missed with fluorescein angiography.

FLUORESCEIN ANGIOGRAPHY

Novotny and Alvis first described fluorescein angiography (FA) as an imaging method in 1960 to visualize both the retinal and choroidal vasculature. FA is currently the gold standard in documenting areas of retinal ischemia, leakage, neovascularization, and microaneurysms, making it integral to the assessment of diabetic retinopathy. There are drawbacks to its administration, including time requirements, dye injection with rare side effects, and obscuration of vascular details from leakage [55]. The fluorescein angiography images produce a composite of all retinal vascular layers, which complicates delineating what level of retinal vasculature is involved.

Diabetic Ischemia

Like OCTA, FA allows for the measurement of ischemia in the fovea and periphery. Ischemia causes capillary loss, portrayed as a black area without vasculature perfusion, with a concurrent enlargement of the FAZ if the ischemia is macular (Fig. **9**) [61]. Analysis of the FAZ with FA shows an increase in size in diabetic patients compared to normal controls [62]. Bresnick *et al.* and Sim *et al.* elucidated a correlation between the increase in FAZ and worsening diabetic retinopathy [61, 63]. Conrath and colleagues also reported an increase in FAZ, even in the earliest stages [62]. Contrastingly, Sander *et al.* and Hilmantel found that the FAZ dimensions only significantly increase with later stage diabetic retinopathy [64, 65]. These variable findings may be due to the large range of FAZ dimensions in normal subjects [61].

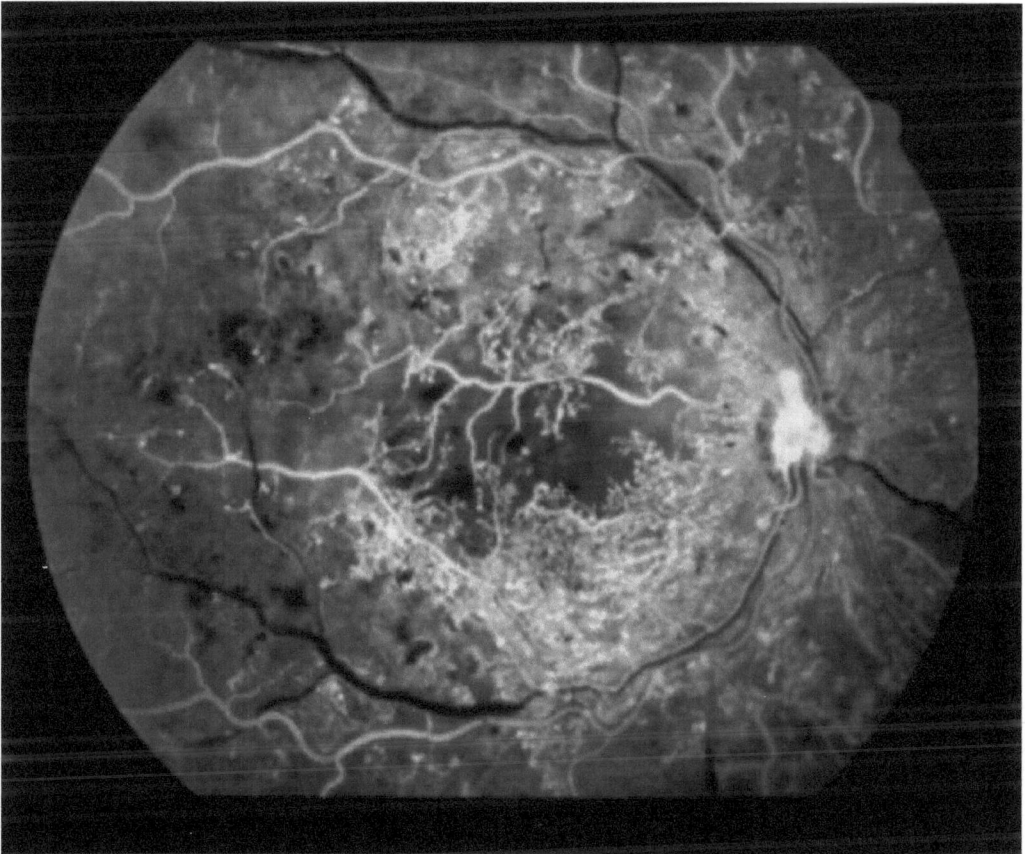

Fig. (9). Fluorescein angiogram of macular ischemia. This patient has extensive macular ischemia and neovascularization of the disc.

Diabetic Leakage

FA is integral in imaging leakage, either from microaneurysms, neovascularization, or from macular edema. Microaneurysms tend to produce focal, pinpoint areas of leakage, while neovascularization creates a broader, widespread leakage pattern that is elevated over the retinal surface. Two main leakage patterns are associated with cystoid macular edema – petaloid and honeycomb (Fig. **10**). There is some variation in the association of these patterns with structural changes found on OCT. In general, petaloid is more commonly associated with cystic changes in the outer nuclear layer and outer plexiform layer, while honeycomb appearance is more linked to cystic swelling in the inner nuclear layer [66 - 68].

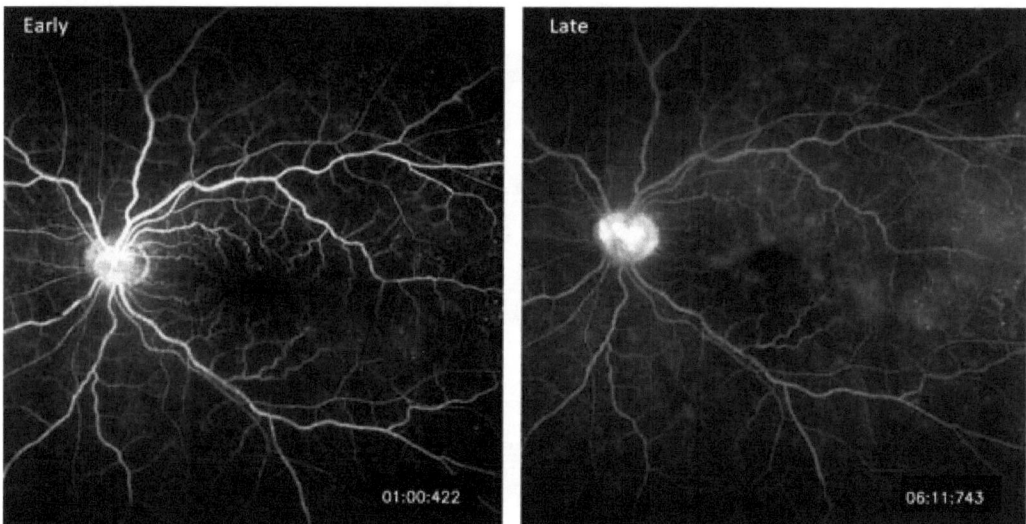

Fig. (10). Fluorescein angiogram of CME. The early views (left) show minimal leakage but in late views (right) the petaloid leakage characteristic of CME is evident.

Interestingly, diffuse leakage noted on FA was not linked to a specific OCT edema morphology, and in some cases, no morphological changes were found on OCT at all. This further consolidates the importance of FA in documenting leakage in diabetic retinopathy, even without morphology present on OCT imaging [66]. These findings would have been missed if the patients were imaged with solely OCT or OCTA.

Leakage patterns of FA are also integral to treatment planning. In cases of diffuse, widespread leakage, or large amounts of macular edema, intravitreal injection of an anti-vascular endothelial growth factor may be beneficial [35]. However, in the case of focal, extrafoveal leakage, a targeted focal laser may allow for resolution.

WIDE FIELD FLUORESCEIN ANGIOGRAPHY

Wide field fluorescein angiography (WF-FA) allows for an increased field of view and better characterization of disease that may be missed with standard imaging practices, while maintaining its depiction of pathology in the posterior pole [3, 35]. Talks *et al.* found a 30% increase in the number of peripheral neovascular changes on WF-FA as compared to standard imaging [69].

The documentation of far peripheral ischemia may alert clinicians to monitor a patient more closely for possible macular edema changes in the future (Fig. **11**). Wessel *et al.* highlighted the relationship between an increased likelihood of developing macular edema when peripheral retinal ischemia was present [70]. Furthermore, areas of diabetic macular edema that are difficult to treat have been associated with larger areas of peripheral non-perfusion [71]. Interestingly, WF-FA also allows for the monitoring of retinal non-perfusion, and studies have shown that more frequent dosing of aflibercept was correlated with decreasing amounts of non-perfusion [72]. Moreover, wide-field FA allows for the depiction of microanyeurms in the periphery of patients who were previously thought to have no diabetic retinopathy or highlights neovascular peripheral changes that may have otherwise been missed [3]. Silva *et al.* argue that peripheral changes in the retina can predispose to a more accelerated course of diabetic retinopathy as well [73].

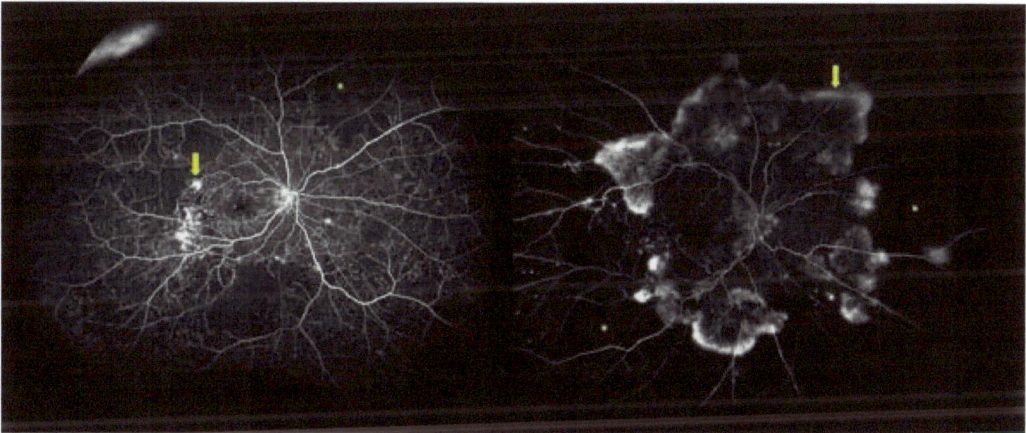

Fig. (11). Wide field fluorescein angiogram. Wide-field fluorescein angiography of two patients illustrating neovascularization elsewhere (arrows) and peripheral ischemia (asterisks) due to proliferative diabetic retinopathy.

Summary

Fluorescein angiography can be used to monitor the size of the FAZ, which is commonly increased in diabetics. Additionally, it provides valuable information regarding microaneurysms number, the presence of neovascularization, peripheral leakage and can confirm the presence macular edema. Fluorescein angiography can also document widespread leakage and atypical vasculature, which may occur without the presence of OCT changes.

CONCLUSION

The pathology of diabetic retinopathy is extensive and varied. It includes macular edema, ischemia and neovascularization. Optical coherence tomography allows visualization of individual retinal layers as well as fluid accumulation patterns and architectural disorganization. Optical coherence tomography angiography allows for the visualization of vasculature in separate layers and may provide a more detailed view of the vasculature as compared to fluorescein angiography. Fluorescein angiography is able to depict vascular changes, ischemia, and vascular leakage, and ultrawide field imaging provides information previously missed with traditional imaging. The available imaging modalities each augment our understanding of diabetes and allow for more careful monitoring of disease progression and response to treatment.

CONSENT FOR PUBLICATION

Not applicable.

CONFLICT OF INTEREST

The author declares no conflict of interest, financial or otherwise.

ACKNOWLEDGEMENTS

Declared none.

REFERENCES

[1]   Huang D, Swanson EA, Lin CP, *et al.* Optical coherence tomography. Science 1991; 254(5035): 1178-81.
[http://dx.doi.org/10.1126/science.1957169] [PMID: 1957169]

[2]   Hee MR, Izatt JA, Swanson EA, Huang D, Schuman JS, Lin CP, *et al.* Optical coherence tomography of the human retina 1995.
[http://dx.doi.org/10.1001/archopht.1995.01100030081025]

[3]   Kong M, Lee MY, Ham DI. Ultrawide-field fluorescein angiography for evaluation of diabetic retinopathy. Korean J Ophthalmol 2012; 26(6): 428-31.
[http://dx.doi.org/10.3341/kjo.2012.26.6.428] [PMID: 23204797]

[4]   Patz A, Schatz H, Berkow JW, Gittelsohn AM, Ticho U. Macular edema--an overlooked complication of diabetic retinopathy. Transactions - American Academy of Ophthalmology and Otolaryngology American Academy of Ophthalmology and Ophthalmol 1973; 77(1): Op34-42.

[5]   Ding J, Wong TY. Current epidemiology of diabetic retinopathy and diabetic macular edema. Curr

Diab Rep 2012; 12(4): 346-54.
[http://dx.doi.org/10.1007/s11892-012-0283-6] [PMID: 22585044]

[6]   Klein R, Klein BEK, Moss SE, Cruickshanks KJ. The wisconsin epidemiologic study of diabetic retinopathy. XV. The long-term incidence of macular edema. Ophthalmol 1995; 102(1): 7-16.
[http://dx.doi.org/10.1016/S0161-6420(95)31052-4] [PMID: 7831044]

[7]   Das A, McGuire PG, Rangasamy S. Diabetic macular edema: pathophysiology and novel therapeutic targets. Ophthalmol 2015; 122(7): 1375-94.
[http://dx.doi.org/10.1016/j.ophtha.2015.03.024] [PMID: 25935789]

[8]   BuAbbud JC. Al-latayfeh MM, Sun JK. Optical coherence tomography imaging for diabetic retinopathy and macular edem. Curr Diab Rep 2010; 10(4): 264-9.
[http://dx.doi.org/10.1007/s11892-010-0129-z] [PMID: 20556548]

[9]   Alasil T, Keane PA, Updike JF, *et al.* Relationship between optical coherence tomography retinal parameters and visual acuity in diabetic macular edema. Ophthalmol 2010; 117(12): 2379-86.
[http://dx.doi.org/10.1016/j.ophtha.2010.03.051] [PMID: 20561684]

[10]   Kim BY, Smith SD, Kaiser PK. Optical coherence tomographic patterns of diabetic macular edema. Am J Ophthalmol 2006; 142(3): 405-12.
[http://dx.doi.org/10.1016/j.ajo.2006.04.023] [PMID: 16935584]

[11]   Otani T, Kishi S, Maruyama Y. Patterns of diabetic macular edema with optical coherence tomography. Am J Ophthalmol 1999; 127(6): 688-93.
[http://dx.doi.org/10.1016/S0002-9394(99)00033-1] [PMID: 10372879]

[12]   Yamamoto S, Yamamoto T, Hayashi M, Takeuchi S. Morphological and functional analyses of diabetic macular edema by optical coherence tomography and multifocal electroretinograms. Graefes Arch Clin Exp Ophthalmol 2001; 239(2): 96-101.
[http://dx.doi.org/10.1007/s004170000238] [PMID: 11372551]

[13]   Kaiser PK, Riemann CD, Sears JE, Lewis H. Macular traction detachment and diabetic macular edema associated with posterior hyaloidal traction. Am J Ophthalmol 2001; 131(1): 44-9.
[http://dx.doi.org/10.1016/S0002-9394(00)00872-2] [PMID: 11162978]

[14]   Kang SW, Park CY, Ham DI. The correlation between fluorescein angiographic and optical coherence tomographic features in clinically significant diabetic macular edema. Am J Ophthalmol 2004; 137(2): 313-22.
[http://dx.doi.org/10.1016/j.ajo.2003.09.016] [PMID: 14962423]

[15]   Lattanzio R, Brancato R, Pierro L, *et al.* Macular thickness measured by optical coherence tomography (OCT) in diabetic patients. Eur J Ophthalmol 2002; 12(6): 482-7.
[http://dx.doi.org/10.1177/112067210201200606] [PMID: 12510717]

[16]   Browning DJ, Glassman AR, Aiello LP, *et al.* Relationship between optical coherence tomography-measured central retinal thickness and visual acuity in diabetic macular edema. Ophthalmol 2007; 114(3): 525-36.
[http://dx.doi.org/10.1016/j.ophtha.2006.06.052] [PMID: 17123615]

[17]   Sun JK, Lin MM, Lammer J, *et al.* Disorganization of the retinal inner layers as a predictor of visual acuity in eyes with center-involved diabetic macular edema. JAMA Ophthalmol 2014; 132(11): 1309-16.
[http://dx.doi.org/10.1001/jamaophthalmol.2014.2350] [PMID: 25058813]

[18]   Das R, Spence G, Hogg RE, Stevenson M, Chakravarthy U. Disorganization of Inner Retina and Outer Retinal Morphology in Diabetic Macular Edema. JAMA Ophthalmol 2018; 136(2): 202-8.
[http://dx.doi.org/10.1001/jamaophthalmol.2017.6256] [PMID: 29327033]

[19]   Nakano E, Ota T, Jingami Y, Nakata I, Hayashi H, Yamashiro K. Correlation between metamorphopsia and disorganization of the retinal inner layers in eyes with diabetic macular edema. Graefe's archive for clinical and experimental ophthalmology. Albrecht Von Graefes Arch Klin Exp

Ophthalmol 2019; 257(9): 1873-8.
[http://dx.doi.org/10.1007/s00417-019-04393-0]

[20]   Uji A, Murakami T, Nishijima K, Akagi T, Horii T, Arakawa N, *et al*. Association between hyperreflective foci in the outer retina, status of photoreceptor layer, and visual acuity in diabetic macular edema 2012.
[http://dx.doi.org/10.1016/j.ajo.2011.08.041]

[21]   Shin HJ, Lee SH, Chung H, Kim HC. Association between photoreceptor integrity and visual outcome in diabetic macular edema. Graefe's archive for clinical and experimental ophthalmology =. Albrecht Von Graefes Arch Klin Exp Ophthalmol 2012; 250(1): 61-70.
[http://dx.doi.org/10.1007/s00417-011-1774-x]

[22]   Seo KH, Yu SY, Kim M, Kwak HW. Visual and morphologic outcomes of intravitreal ranibizuman for diabetic macular edema based on optical coherence tomography patterns. Retina 2016; 36(3): 588-95.
[http://dx.doi.org/10.1097/IAE.0000000000000770] [PMID: 26398695]

[23]   Yohannan J, Bittencourt M, Sepah YJ, *et al*. Association of retinal sensitivity to integrity of photoreceptor inner/outer segment junction in patients with diabetic macular edema. Ophthalmol 2013; 120(6): 1254-61.
[http://dx.doi.org/10.1016/j.ophtha.2012.12.003] [PMID: 23499060]

[24]   Chew EY, Klein ML, Ferris FL 3rd, Remaley NA, Murphy RP, Chantry K, *et al*. Association of elevated serum lipid levels with retinal hard exudate in diabetic retinopathy. 1996.
[http://dx.doi.org/10.1001/archopht.1996.01100140281004]

[25]   Ota M, Nishijima K, Sakamoto A, *et al*. Optical coherence tomographic evaluation of foveal hard exudates in patients with diabetic maculopathy accompanying macular detachment. Ophthalmol 2010; 117(10): 1996-2002.
[http://dx.doi.org/10.1016/j.ophtha.2010.06.019] [PMID: 20723993]

[26]   Bolz M, Schmidt-Erfurth U, Deak G, Mylonas G, Kriechbaum K, Scholda C. Optical coherence tomographic hyperreflective foci: a morphologic sign of lipid extravasation in diabetic macular edema. Ophthalmol 2009; 116(5): 914-20.
[http://dx.doi.org/10.1016/j.ophtha.2008.12.039] [PMID: 19410950]

[27]   Bunt-Milam AH, Saari JC, Klock IB, Garwin GG. Zonulae adherentes pore size in the external limiting membrane of the rabbit retina. Invest Ophthalmol Vis Sci 1985; 26(10): 1377-80.
[PMID: 4044165]

[28]   Murakami T, Yoshimura N. Structural changes in individual retinal layers in diabetic macular edema. J Diabetes Res 2013; 2013920713
[http://dx.doi.org/10.1155/2013/920713] [PMID: 24073417]

[29]   Vujosevic S, Bini S, Midena G, Berton M, Pilotto E, Midena E. Hyperreflective intraretinal spots in diabetics without and with nonproliferative diabetic retinopathy: an *in vivo* study using spectral domain OCT. J Diabetes Res 2013; 2013491835
[http://dx.doi.org/10.1155/2013/491835] [PMID: 24386645]

[30]   Midena E, Bini S. Multimodal retinal imaging of diabetic macular edema: toward new paradigms of pathophysiology. Graefe's archive for clinical and experimental ophthalmology =. Albrecht Von Graefes Arch Klin Exp Ophthalmol 2016; 254(9): 1661-8.
[http://dx.doi.org/10.1007/s00417-016-3361-7]

[31]   Chung H, Park B, Shin HJ, Kim HC. Correlation of fundus autofluorescence with spectral-domain optical coherence tomography and vision in diabetic macular edema. Ophthalmology 2012; 119(5): 1056-65.
[http://dx.doi.org/10.1016/j.ophtha.2011.11.018] [PMID: 22342014]

[32]   Tso MO. Pathology of cystoid macular edema. Ophthalmology 1982; 89(8): 902-15.
[http://dx.doi.org/10.1016/S0161-6420(82)34698-9] [PMID: 7133637]

[33]   Cunha-Vaz J, Santos T, Ribeiro L, Alves D, Marques I, Goldberg M. M G. OCT- Leakage: a new method to identify and locate abnormal fluid accumulation in diabetic retinal edema. Invest Ophthalmol Vis Sci 2016; 57(15): 6776-83.
[http://dx.doi.org/10.1167/iovs.16-19999] [PMID: 27978559]

[34]   Wang J, Zhang M, Pechauer AD, *et al.* Automated volumetric segmentation of retinal fluid on optical coherence tomography. Biomed Opt Express 2016; 7(4): 1577-89.
[http://dx.doi.org/10.1364/BOE.7.001577] [PMID: 27446676]

[35]   Modi Y, Ehlers JP. Imaging modalities for the management of diabetic macular edema. 2015.

[36]   Adhi M, Brewer E, Waheed NK, Duker JS. Analysis of morphological features and vascular layers of choroid in diabetic retinopathy using spectral-domain optical coherence tomography. JAMA Ophthalmol 2013; 131(10): 1267-74.
[http://dx.doi.org/10.1001/jamaophthalmol.2013.4321] [PMID: 23907153]

[37]   de Freytas A, Gallego Pinazo R, Cisneros Lanuza Á. Subfoveal choroidal thickness in eyes with diabetic macular oedema using swept source optical coherence tomography. Arch Soc Esp Oftalmol 2016; 91(5): 228-31.
[http://dx.doi.org/10.1016/j.oftal.2015.12.015] [PMID: 26832156]

[38]   Sheth JU, Giridhar A, Rajesh B, Gopalakrishnan M. Characterization of macular choroidal thickness in ischemic and nonischemic diabetic maculopathy. Retina 2017; 37(3): 522-8.
[http://dx.doi.org/10.1097/IAE.0000000000001172] [PMID: 28225723]

[39]   Kim JT, Lee DH, Joe SG, Kim JG, Yoon YH. Changes in choroidal thickness in relation to the severity of retinopathy and macular edema in type 2 diabetic patients. Invest Ophthalmol Vis Sci 2013; 54(5): 3378-84.
[http://dx.doi.org/10.1167/iovs.12-11503] [PMID: 23611988]

[40]   Spaide RF, Fujimoto JG, Waheed NK. Optical Coherence Tomography Angiography. Retina 2015; 35(11): 2161-2.
[http://dx.doi.org/10.1097/IAE.0000000000000881] [PMID: 26502006]

[41]   Chalam KV, Sambhav K. Optical Coherence Tomography Angiography in Retinal Diseases. J Ophthalmic Vis Res 2016; 11(1): 84-92.
[http://dx.doi.org/10.4103/2008-322X.180709] [PMID: 27195091]

[42]   Snodderly DM, Weinhaus RS. Retinal vasculature of the fovea of the squirrel monkey, Saimiri sciureus: three-dimensional architecture, visual screening, and relationships to the neuronal layers. J Comp Neurol 1990; 297(1): 145-63.
[http://dx.doi.org/10.1002/cne.902970111] [PMID: 2376631]

[43]   Linsenmeier RA, Braun RD. Oxygen distribution and consumption in the cat retina during normoxia and hypoxemia. J Gen Physiol 1992; 99(2): 177-97.
[http://dx.doi.org/10.1085/jgp.99.2.177] [PMID: 1613482]

[44]   Lee J, Moon BG, Cho AR, Yoon YH. Optical Coherence Tomography Angiography of DME and Its Association with Anti-VEGF Treatment Response. Ophthalmology 2016; 123(11): 2368-75.
[http://dx.doi.org/10.1016/j.ophtha.2016.07.010] [PMID: 27613201]

[45]   Al-Sheikh M, Akil H, Pfau M, Sadda SR. Swept-Source OCT Angiography Imaging of the Foveal Avascular Zone and Macular Capillary Network Density in Diabetic Retinopathy. Invest Ophthalmol Vis Sci 2016; 57(8): 3907-13.
[http://dx.doi.org/10.1167/iovs.16-19570] [PMID: 27472076]

[46]   Agemy SA, Scripsema NK, Shah CM, *et al.* Retinal vascular perfusion density mapping using optical coherence tomography angiography in normals and diabetic retinopathy patients. Retina 2015; 35(11): 2353-63.
[http://dx.doi.org/10.1097/IAE.0000000000000862] [PMID: 26465617]

[47]   Freiberg FJ, Pfau M, Wons J, Wirth MA, Becker MD, Michels S. Optical coherence tomography

angiography of the foveal avascular zone in diabetic retinopathy. Graefe's archive for clinical and experimental ophthalmology =. Albrecht Von Graefes Arch Klin Exp Ophthalmol 2016; 254(6): 1051-8.
[http://dx.doi.org/10.1007/s00417-015-3148-2]

[48]   Hwang TS, Jia Y, Gao SS, *et al.* Optical coherence tomography angiography features of diabetic retinopathy. Retina 2015; 35(11): 2371-6.
[http://dx.doi.org/10.1097/IAE.0000000000000716] [PMID: 26308529]

[49]   Takase N, Nozaki M, Kato A, Ozeki H, Yoshida M, Ogura Y. Enlargement of foveal avascular zone in diabetic eyes evauated by en face optical coherence tomography angiography. Retina 2015; 35(11): 2377-83.
[http://dx.doi.org/10.1097/IAE.0000000000000849] [PMID: 26457396]

[50]   Samara WA, Shahlaee A, Adam MK, *et al.* Quantification of Diabetic Macular Ischemia Using Optical Coherence Tomography Angiography and Its Relationship with Visual Acuity. Ophthalmology 2017; 124(2): 235-44.
[http://dx.doi.org/10.1016/j.ophtha.2016.10.008] [PMID: 27887743]

[51]   Salz DA, de Carlo TE, Adhi M, *et al.* Select Features of Diabetic Retinopathy on Swept-Source Optical Coherence Tomographic Angiography Compared With Fluorescein Angiography and Normal Eyes. JAMA Ophthalmol 2016; 134(6): 644-50.
[http://dx.doi.org/10.1001/jamaophthalmol.2016.0600] [PMID: 27055248]

[52]   Lee J, Rosen R. Optical Coherence Tomography Angiography in Diabetes. Curr Diab Rep 2016; 16(12): 123.
[http://dx.doi.org/10.1007/s11892-016-0811-x] [PMID: 27766583]

[53]   Yu S, Pang CE, Gong Y, Freund KB, Yannuzzi LA, Rahimy E, *et al.* The spectrum of superficial and deep capillary ischemia in retinal artery occlusion 2015.
[http://dx.doi.org/10.1016/j.ajo.2014.09.027]

[54]   Ishibazawa A, Nagaoka T, Yokota H, *et al.* Characteristics of Retinal Neovascularization in Proliferative Diabetic Retinopathy Imaged by Optical Coherence Tomography Angiography. Invest Ophthalmol Vis Sci 2016; 57(14): 6247-55.
[http://dx.doi.org/10.1167/iovs.16-20210] [PMID: 27849310]

[55]   Yannuzzi LA, Rohrer KT, Tindel LJ, *et al.* Fluorescein angiography complication survey. Ophthalmology 1986; 93(5): 611-7.
[http://dx.doi.org/10.1016/S0161-6420(86)33697-2] [PMID: 3523356]

[56]   Couturier A, Mané V, Bonnin S, *et al.* Capillary plexus anomalies in diabetic retinopathy on optical coherence tomography angiography. Retina 2015; 35(11): 2384-91.
[http://dx.doi.org/10.1097/IAE.0000000000000859] [PMID: 26469531]

[57]   Hasegawa N, Nozaki M, Takase N, Yoshida M, Ogura Y. New Insights Into Microaneurysms in the Deep Capillary Plexus Detected by Optical Coherence Tomography Angiography in Diabetic Macular Edema. Invest Ophthalmol Vis Sci 2016; 57(9): OCT348-55.
[http://dx.doi.org/10.1167/iovs.15-18782] [PMID: 27409492]

[58]   de Carlo TE, Bonini Filho MA, Baumal CR, *et al.* Evaluation of Preretinal Neovascularization in Proliferative Diabetic Retinopathy Using Optical Coherence Tomography Angiography. Ophthalmic Surg Lasers Imaging Retina 2016; 47(2): 115-9.
[http://dx.doi.org/10.3928/23258160-20160126-03] [PMID: 26878443]

[59]   Lee CS, Lee AY, Sim DA, *et al.* Reevaluating the definition of intraretinal microvascular abnormalities and neovascularization elsewhere in diabetic retinopathy using optical coherence tomography and fluorescein angiography. Am J Ophthalmol 2015; 159(1): 101-10.e1.
[http://dx.doi.org/10.1016/j.ajo.2014.09.041] [PMID: 25284762]

[60]   Jia Y, Bailey ST, Hwang TS, *et al.* Quantitative optical coherence tomography angiography of vascular abnormalities in the living human eye. Proc Natl Acad Sci USA 2015; 112(18): E2395-402.

[http://dx.doi.org/10.1073/pnas.1500185112] [PMID: 25897021]

[61]   Sim DA, Keane PA, Zarranz-Ventura J, *et al.* The effects of macular ischemia on visual acuity in diabetic retinopathy. Invest Ophthalmol Vis Sci 2013; 54(3): 2353-60.
[http://dx.doi.org/10.1167/iovs.12-11103] [PMID: 23449720]

[62]   Conrath J, Giorgi R, Raccah D, Ridings B. Foveal avascular zone in diabetic retinopathy: quantitative *vs* qualitative assessment. Eye (Lond) 2005; 19(3): 322-6.
[http://dx.doi.org/10.1038/sj.eye.6701456] [PMID: 15258601]

[63]   Bresnick GH, Condit R, Syrjala S, Palta M, Groo A, Korth K. Abnormalities of the foveal avascular zone in diabetic retinopathy 1984.
[http://dx.doi.org/10.1001/archopht.1984.01040031036019]

[64]   Sander B, Larsen M, Engler C, Lund-Andersen H, Parving HH. Early changes in diabetic retinopathy: capillary loss and blood-retina barrier permeability in relation to metabolic control. Acta Ophthalmol (Copenh) 1994; 72(5): 553-9.
[http://dx.doi.org/10.1111/j.1755-3768.1994.tb07179.x] [PMID: 7887152]

[65]   Hilmantel G, Applegate RA, van Heuven WA, Stowers SP, Bradley A, Lee BL. Entoptic foveal avascular zone measurement and diabetic retinopathy 1999.
[http://dx.doi.org/10.1097/00006324-199912000-00017]

[66]   Bolz M, Ritter M, Schneider M, Simader C, Scholda C, Schmidt-Erfurth U. A systematic correlation of angiography and high-resolution optical coherence tomography in diabetic macular edema. Ophthalmology 2009; 116(1): 66-72.
[http://dx.doi.org/10.1016/j.ophtha.2008.09.042] [PMID: 19118697]

[67]   Soliman W, Sander B, Hasler PW, Larsen M. Correlation between intraretinal changes in diabetic macular oedema seen in fluorescein angiography and optical coherence tomography. Acta Ophthalmol 2008; 86(1): 34-9.
[http://dx.doi.org/10.1111/j.1600-0420.2007.00989.x] [PMID: 17651471]

[68]   Otani T, Kishi S. Correlation between optical coherence tomography and fluorescein angiography findings in diabetic macular edema. Ophthalmology 2007; 114(1): 104-7.
[http://dx.doi.org/10.1016/j.ophtha.2006.06.044] [PMID: 17070586]

[69]   Talks SJ, Manjunath V, Steel DH, Peto T, Taylor R. New vessels detected on wide-field imaging compared to two-field and seven-field imaging: implications for diabetic retinopathy screening image analysis. Br J Ophthalmol 2015; 99(12): 1606-9.
[http://dx.doi.org/10.1136/bjophthalmol-2015-306719] [PMID: 26271269]

[70]   Wessel MM, Aaker GD, Parlitsis G, Cho M, D'Amico DJ, Kiss S. Ultra-wide-field angiography improves the detection and classification of diabetic retinopathy. Retina 2012; 32(4): 785-91.
[http://dx.doi.org/10.1097/IAE.0b013e3182278b64] [PMID: 22080911]

[71]   Patel RD, Messner LV, Teitelbaum B, Michel KA, Hariprasad SM. Characterization of ischemic index using ultra-widefield fluorescein angiography in patients with focal and diffuse recalcitrant diabetic macular edema. Am J Ophthalmol 2013; 155(6): 1038-1044.e2.
[http://dx.doi.org/10.1016/j.ajo.2013.01.007] [PMID: 23453693]

[72]   Wykoff CC, Nittala MG, Zhou B, *et al.* Intravitreal Aflibercept for Retinal Nonperfusion in Proliferative Diabetic Retinopathy: Outcomes from the Randomized RECOVERY Trial. Ophthalmol Retina 2019; 3(12): 1076-86.
[http://dx.doi.org/10.1016/j.oret.2019.07.011] [PMID: 31542339]

[73]   Silva PS, Dela Cruz AJ, Ledesma MG, *et al.* Diabetic Retinopathy Severity and Peripheral Lesions Are Associated with Nonperfusion on Ultrawide Field Angiography. Ophthalmology 2015; 122(12): 2465-72.
[http://dx.doi.org/10.1016/j.ophtha.2015.07.034] [PMID: 26350546]

Diabetes: Current and Future Developments, 2021, *Vol. 2*, 171-184

Classification of Proliferative and Non-Proliferative Diabetic Retinopathy and its Implications

Ferhina S. Ali and Sunir J. Garg*

The Retina Service of Wills Eye Hospital, Professor of Ophthalmology Thomas Jefferson University 840 Walnut Street, Suite 1020 Philadelphia, PA 19107, USA

Abstract: An understanding of the classification scheme of nonproliferative and proliferative diabetic retinopathy is essential for the proper management of diabetic eye disease. The level of retinopathy is based on clinical findings seen on fundus examination.

Keywords: Anti-VEGF, Diabetic Retinopathy Study (DRS), Diabetic retinopathy, Early Treatment of Diabetic Retinopathy Study, Mild, Moderate, Nonproliferative, Neovascularization, Proliferative, Severe.

BACKGROUND

The global prevalence of diabetes has been increasing rapidly, with a projected estimate of over 360 million people worldwide affected by the year 2030. As such, the need to identify and to treat diabetic retinopathy is critical to prevent vision loss. Central to this is an understanding of the classification and severity stages of diabetic retinopathy [1].

In 1968, an expert panel developed the Airlie House classification scheme for diabetic retinopathy that was subsequently modified and used in the landmark Diabetic Retinopathy Study (DRS) and the Early Treatment Diabetic Retinopathy Study (ETDRS) [2, 3]. The classification is based on grading seven-field 30-degree standard stereo-photographs [4]. While this has been the gold standard for clinical trials, it remains challenging to use in daily clinical practice. Simplification of this classification occurred through the International Clinical

---

* **Corresponding authors Sunir J. Garg:** The Retina Service of Wills Eye Hospital Professor of Ophthalmology Thomas Jefferson University 840 Walnut Street, Suite 1020 Philadelphia, PA 19107, USA; Tel: (800) 331-6634; Fax: (610) 667-1328; E-mail: SunirGarg@yahoo.com

Douglas R. Lazzaro and Samy I. McFarlane (Eds.)

Disease Severity Scale for Diabetic Retinopathy that consists of five scales with increasing degrees of retinopathy observed on dilated ophthalmoscopy (Table **1**) [2].

Table 1. International Clinical Diabetic Retinopathy Disease Severity Scale (adapted from the American Academy of Ophthalmology Diabetic Retinopathy Preferred Practice Patterns 2019).

Proposed Disease Severity Level	Findings Observable upon Dilated Ophthalmoscopy
No Apparent Retinopathy	No abnormalities
Mild Non-Proliferative Diabetic Retinopathy	Microaneurysms only
Moderate Non-Proliferative Diabetic Retinopathy	More than just microaneurysms but less than Severe NPDR
Severe Non-Proliferative Diabetic Retinopathy	Any of the following: More than 20 intraretinal hemorrhages in each of 4 quadrants Definite venous beading in 2+ quadrants Prominent IRMA in 1+ quadrant and no signs of proliferative retinopathy
Proliferative Diabetic Retinopathy	One or more of the following: Neovascularization Vitreous/preretinal hemorrhage

CLINICAL MANIFESTATIONS OF NONPROLIFERATIVE DIABETIC RETINOPATHY

Diabetic retinopathy is a microvascular disease that has a characteristic clinical appearance that results from damage to the retinal capillaries and smaller retinal vessels. A brief description of the common clinical findings follows below.

Intraretinal hemorrhages have a diverse appearance in diabetic retinopathy. Eyes can develop focal, round, well-defined hemorrhages called dot-blot hemorrhages (Fig. **1**, arrow). These occur in the outer retina and/or inner plexiform layers, which are vertically oriented. This results in the round focal appearance of these hemorrhages. Flame-shaped hemorrhages are larger with less distinct margins with morphology that corresponds to the orientation of the retinal nerve fiber layer (Fig. **1**, asterisk). As a result, they are horizontal and linear. In contrast to microaneurysms, intraretinal hemorrhages are hypofluorescent on fluorescein angiography because blood blocks the normal choroidal fluorescence (Fig. **2**, asterisk).

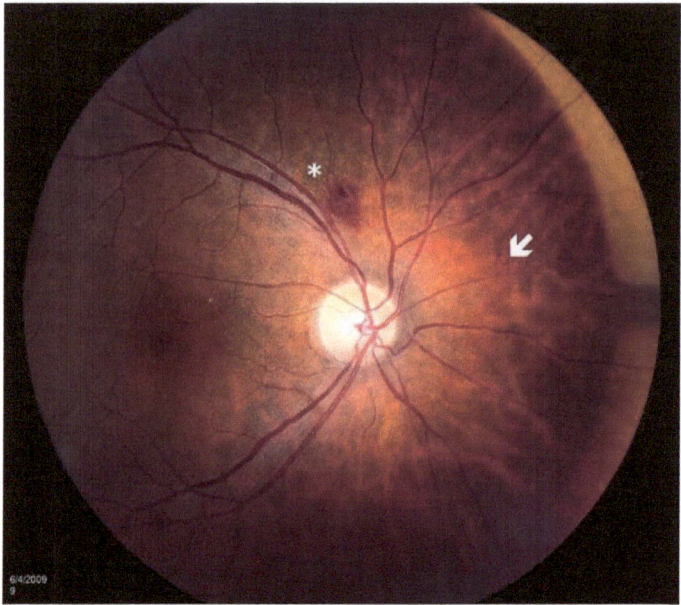

Fig. (1). Dot blot hemorrhage (arrow) and flame hemorrhage (asterisk).

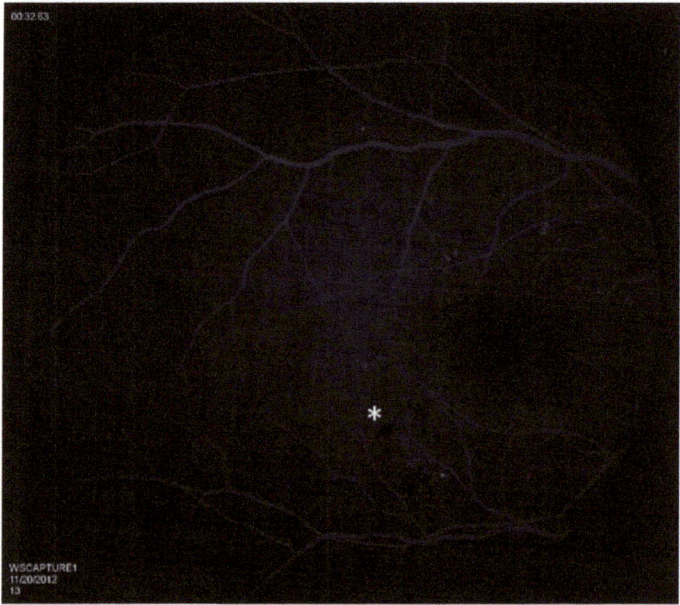

Fig. (2). Hypofluorescence of retinal hemorrhage (asterisk).

Hard exudates are discrete yellow-white deposits in the retina, usually at the border of edematous and nonedematous retina. These occur from incompetent vessels that allow fluid exudation. Over time, the associated edema may get absorbed, but the lipid remains. Leaking microaneurysms may create a ring of exudate surrounding the microaneurysm called a circinate exudate (Fig. **3**, arrow).

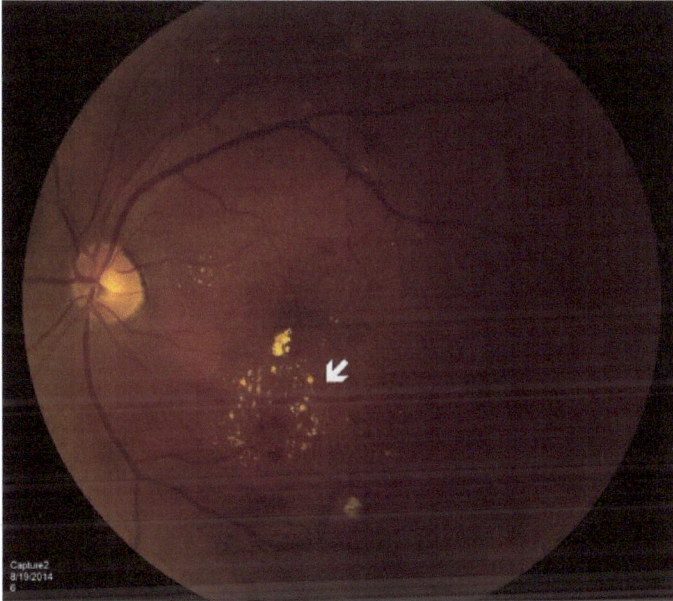

Fig. (3). Circinate exudate (arrow).

Nerve fiber layer infarcts (more commonly called cotton wool spots) are another common manifestation of diabetic eye disease. They represent areas of relative ischemia affecting the retinal nerve fiber layer (Fig. **4**, arrow). Another type of infarct that can occur in diabetic eye disease is an infarct of the optic nerve, also referred to as diabetic optic neuropathy, which is a form of ischemic optic neuropathy that occurs secondary to the underlying diabetic vasculopathy. This typically resolves over several weeks, leaving an atrophic optic disc.

Moderate and severe diabetic retinopathy may exhibit additional changes, including attenuation of the arterioles (Fig. **5**) as well as dilation and tortuosity of the venules (Fig. **6**). Venous beading occurs when there is relative dilation and constriction of the venules (Fig. **7**, arrow). Intraretinal microvascular abnormal-ities (IRMA), one of the defining attributes of severe nonproliferative diabetic retinopathy, represent tortuous retinal microvasculature within retinal vessels (Fig. **4**, asterisk). On fluorescein angiography, these changes hyperfluoresce during arteriovenous transit and usually occur at the borders of capillary nonperfusion (Fig. **8**, asterisk) [5].

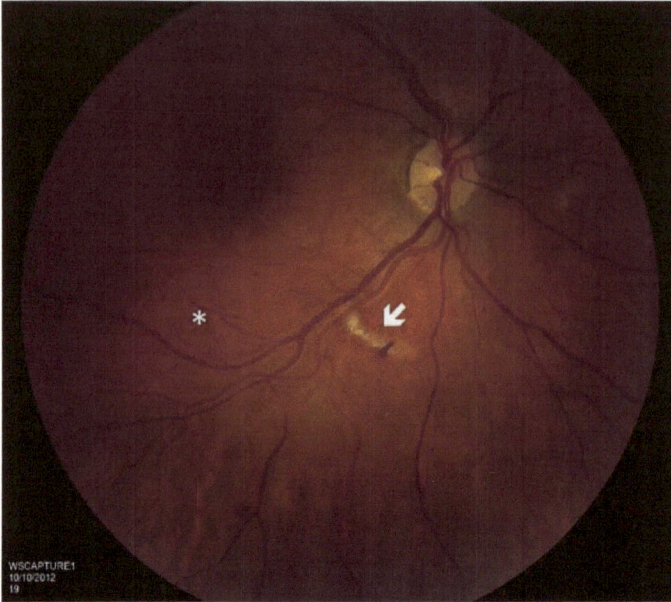

Fig. (4). Cotton wool spot (arrow) and IRMA (asterisk).

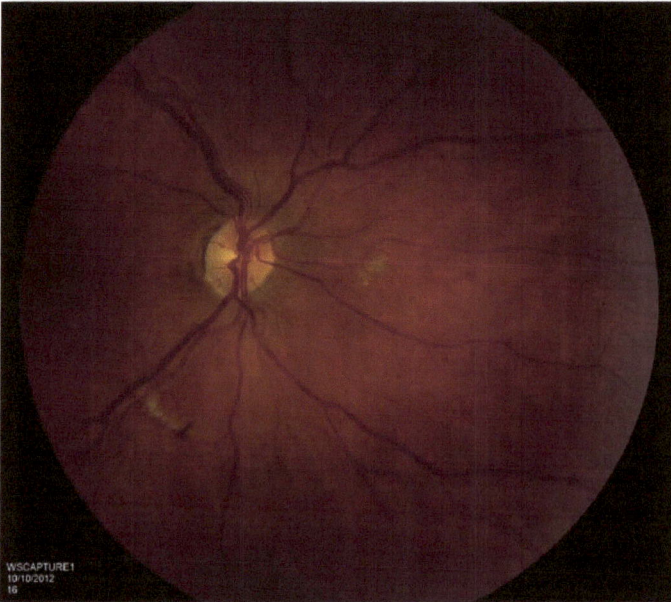

Fig. (5). Attenuation of arterioles.

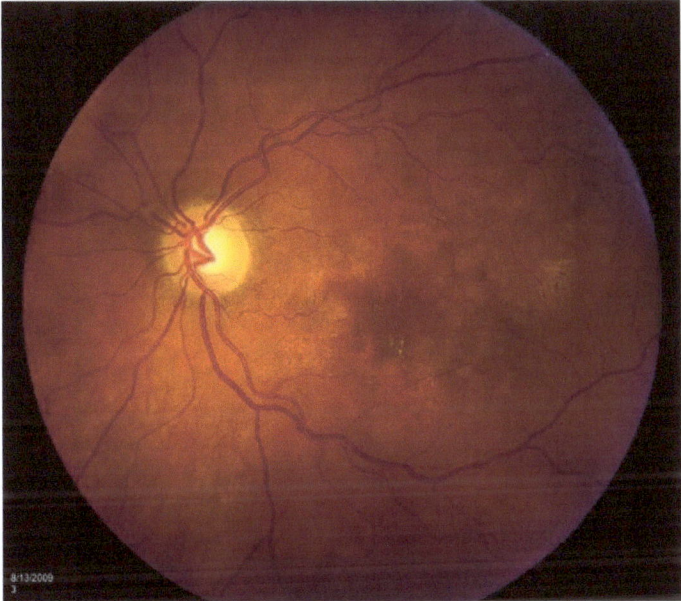

Fig. (6). Dilation and tortuosity of venules.

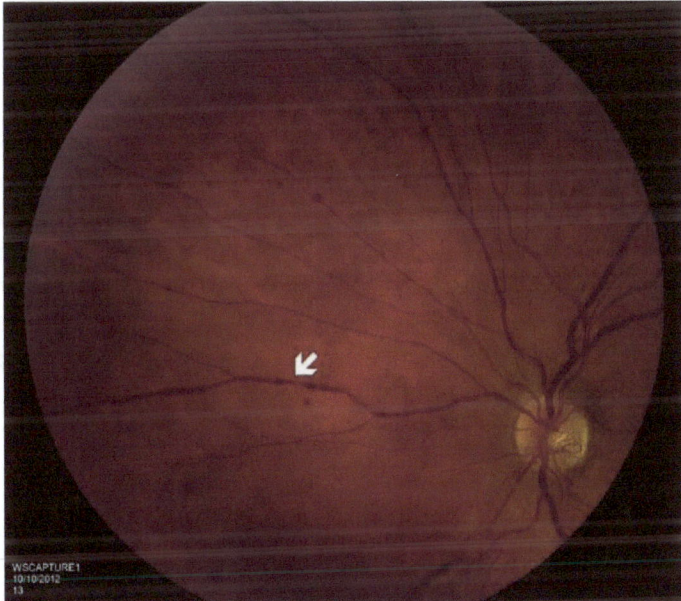

Fig. (7). Venous beading (arrow).

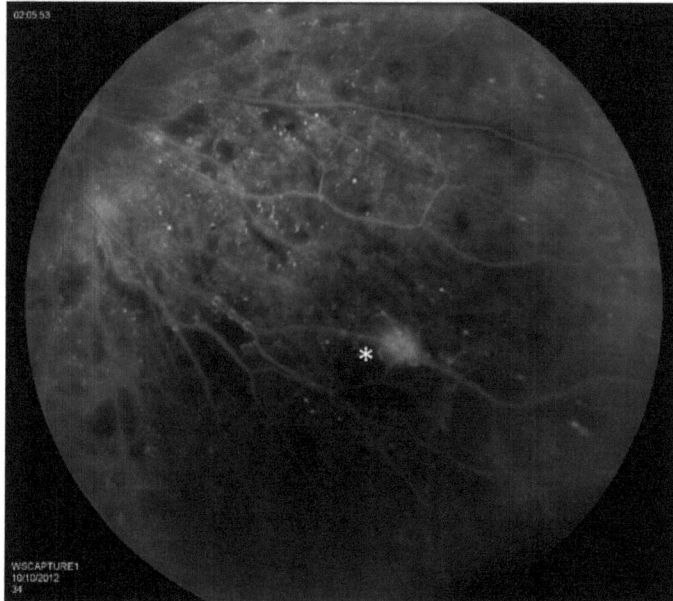

Fig. (8). Capillary nonperfusion (asterisk).

NONPROLIFERATIVE DIABETIC RETINOPATHY

Mild Nonproliferative Diabetic Retinopathy

Mild nonproliferative diabetic retinopathy (NPDR) is characterized by the presence of microaneurysms only. Microaneurysms are the first sign of diabetic retinopathy and histopathologically are outpouchings of the capillary wall. Although microaneurysms are visible on clinical exam, fluorescein angiography is more sensitive for detecting microaneurysms. These first appear during the arteriovenous transit phase and may or may not reveal evidence of leakage in later frames (Fig. **9**, asterisk). Microaneurysms most commonly arise in the posterior pole but may also be present in the periphery. They can appear and disappear over time and, in the absence of exudation, do not affect vision and do not warrant ophthalmic treatment [5].

Moderate and Severe Nonproliferative Diabetic Retinopathy

Moderate nonproliferative diabetic retinopathy is defined by microaneurysms, intraretinal hemorrhages and/or venous beading, but by definition (Fig. **10**), less than the changes that occur in severe nonproliferative diabetic retinopathy (Fig. **11**) [2].

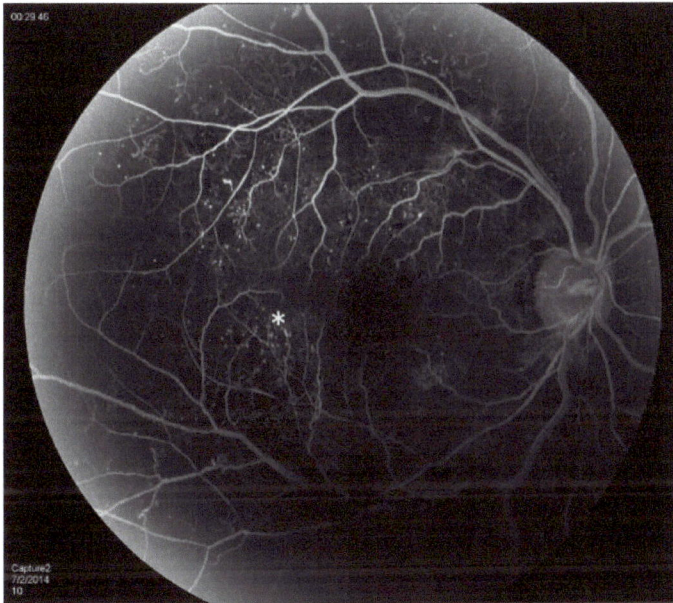

Fig. (9). Fluorescein angiography of microaneurysms (asterisk).

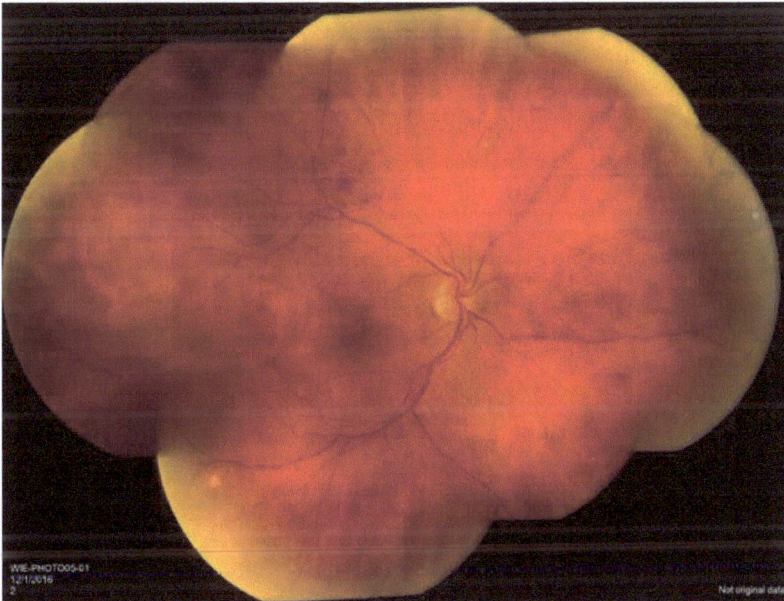

Fig. (10). Moderate nonproliferative diabetic retinopathy.

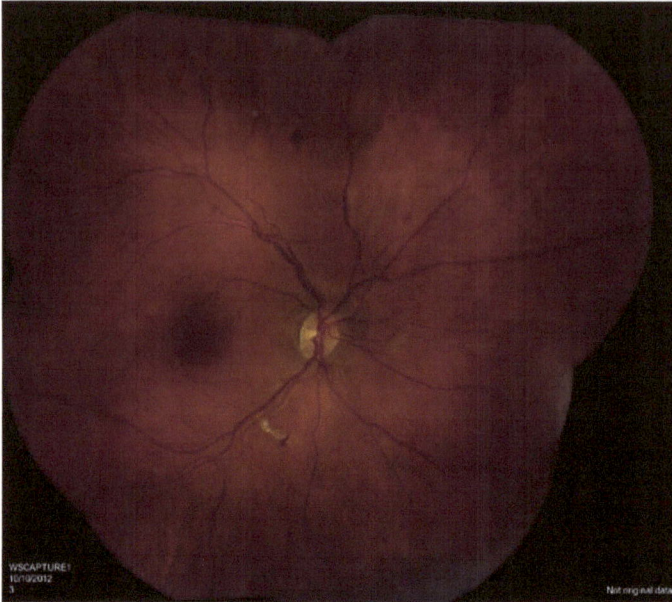

Fig. (11). Severe nonproliferative diabetic retinopathy.

Both the Early Treatment of Diabetic Retinopathy Study and the International Clinical Disease Severity for Diabetic Retinopathy Scale defined severe NPDR based on the *4:2:1 rule.* Specifically, the presence of any 1 of the following defines severe NPDR: diffuse intraretinal hemorrhages and microaneurysms in 4 quadrants, venous beading in 2 quadrants, or intraretinal microvascular abnormality (IRMA) in 1 quadrant. The ETDRS revealed that eyes with severe NPDR had a 15% risk of progression to high-risk PDR (as defined below) within 1 year. Very severe NPDR, as defined by the presence of 2 features from the 4:2:1 rule, had a 45% chance of progression to high-risk PDR within 1 year [2, 5].

PROLIFERATIVE DIABETIC RETINOPATHY

Proliferative diabetic retinopathy (PDR) is defined as the presence of retinal neovascularization that may also have vitreous/preretinal hemorrhage [2]. Retinal ischemia creates an angiogenic stimulus that results in PDR. Although vascular endothelial growth factor (VEGF) is the most common cytokine discussed, others including angiopoietin, erythropoietin, platelet derived growth factor, tumor growth factor, insulin-like growth factor, and basic fibroblast growth factor also contribute to angiogenesis [5].

The risk of progression from NPDR to PDR primarily depends on the duration of diabetes as well as the degree of systemic control. In the Wisconsin Epidemiologic Study of Diabetic Retinopathy, nearly 50% of patients who had

Type 1 diabetes for 20 years or more developed PDR [6] In patients with Type 2 diabetes, PDR develops in 2% of patients with disease duration of less than 5 years, but in 25% of patients who have had diabetes for 25 years or more [7]. In both types of disease, landmark studies have underscored the role of glycemic control in slowing the progression of retinopathy [8, 9].

Proliferative diabetic retinopathy is characterized by new vessels growing along the surface of the optic disc, the retina, and/or less commonly on the iris or trabecular meshwork. The neovascularization often grows within a fibrous scaffold and contraction of this tissue can lead to vitreous hemorrhage (Fig. **12**) and tractional retinal detachment (Fig. **13**) [5].

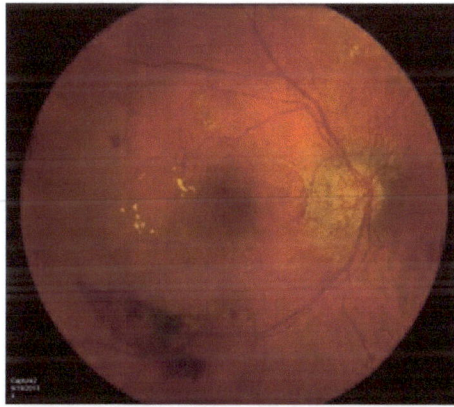

Fig. (12). Vitreous hemorrhage.

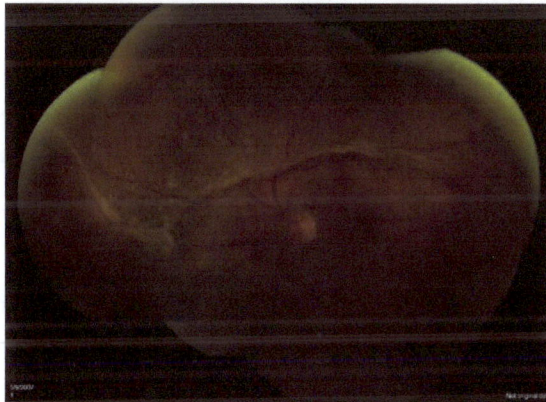

Fig. (13). Diabetic tractional retinal detachment.

The Diabetic Retinopathy Study found that panretinal laser photocoagulation was beneficial for patients who had what was defined as high-risk characteristics for severe vision loss. High-risk characteristics include: 1) new vessels within one disc diameter of the optic nerve head (neovascularization of the disk, NVD) that are larger than one-third disc area (Fig. **14**); 2) any NVD with vitreous or preretinal hemorrhage or; 3) neovascularization elsewhere on the retina (NVE) one-half disc area or more in size with vitreous hemorrhage (Fig. **15**, asterisk).

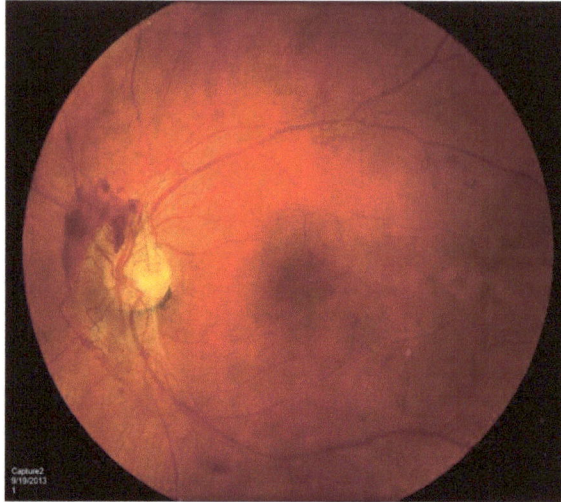

Fig. (14). Neovascularization of the disc.

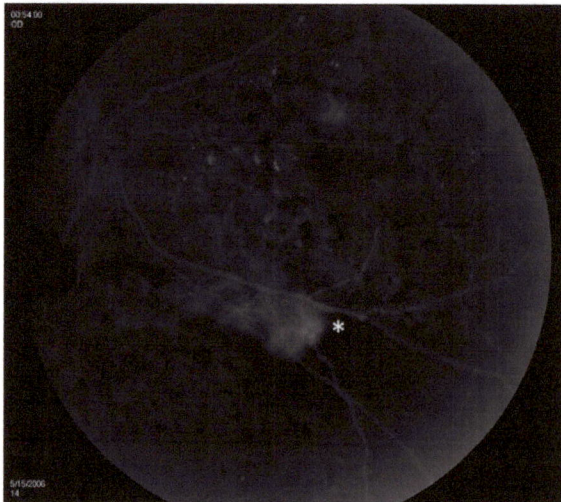

Fig. (15). Neovascularization elsewhere at the border of perfused and nonperfused retina (asterisk).

Panretinal Laser Photocoagulation

As established by the Diabetic Retinopathy Study in 1978, panretinal laser photocoagulation (PRP) has been the primary treatment for proliferative diabetic retinopathy [10]. The application of ablative laser to the peripheral ischemic retina decreases proangiogenic growth factors. The DRS provided strong evidence that prompt PRP decreased the incidence of severe vision loss related to high-risk PDR by 50%. Per the DRS protocol, PRP was defined as argon laser or xenon arc laser scatter treatment with burns spaced one-half to one burn width apart extending from the posterior pole to the equator in approximately 800-1600 laser burns, 500 um shots, often in one sitting (Fig. **16**). For eyes with severe NPDR or PDR without high-risk characteristics, the DRS concluded that prompt treatment *versus* close observation is acceptable, considering patient-specific factors. The ETDRS found that for patients who adhere to scheduled follow up appointments, there was no benefit to PRP prior to development of high-risk characteristics in patients with Type 2 diabetes [11]. Although effective in preventing severe vision loss, patients can experience side effects, including peripheral vision loss and worsening of macular edema.

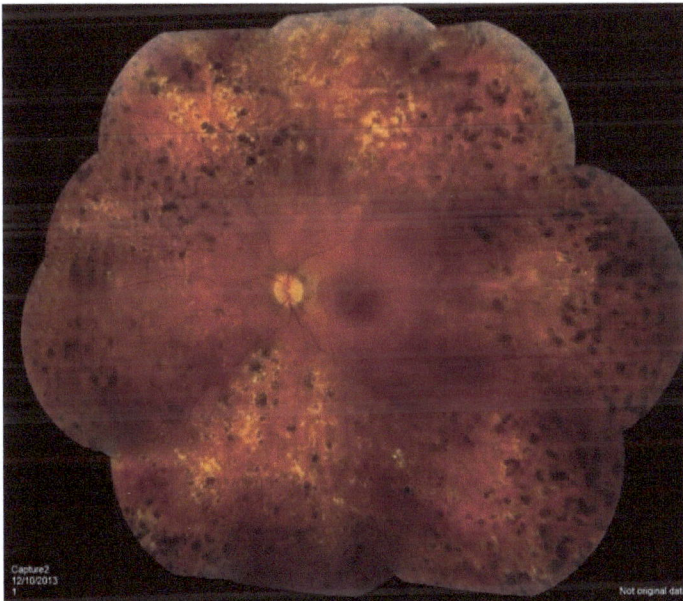

Fig. (16). Panretinal photocoagulation.

Anti-Vascular Endothelial Growth Factor (anti-VEGF) Therapy

Currently, the most common treatment for center-involving diabetic macula edema is anti-VEGF therapy [12 - 14]. The data from the anti-VEGF for diabetic edema treatment trials found that for patients receiving anti-VEGF therapy for macular edema, not only did the edema resolve, but the diabetic retinopathy reversed in some eyes, while other eyes demonstrated capillary reperfusion [15].

A recent non-inferiority trial by the Diabetic Retinopathy Clinic Research Network (DRCR.net) treated eyes with proliferative diabetic retinopathy (however not exclusively with high-risk characteristics). Protocol S compared PRP to serial intravitreal anti-VEGF injection with ranibizumab. The trial found that ranibizumab treatment, when compared to PRP, was non-inferior to PRP laser treatment for 2 years. Furthermore, patients in the ranibizumab arm had slightly better visual acuity outcomes, and significantly better preservation of peripheral visual field compared to eyes that received PRP. However, patients in a clinical trial may be more likely to adhere to recommended follow up intervals, and in patients who are less likely to adhere to scheduled visits, PRP is still useful [16].

CONCLUSION

We have discussed the way in which diabetic retinopathy is classified in this chapter. We also have presented how the classification drives the treatments. The ophthalmologist should be aware that the American Academy of Ophthalmology has outlined in their preferred practice patterns recommendations for follow up frequency according to the severity of retinopathy. Follow up recommendations differ significantly if macular edema or traction retinal detachment is present, and this is discussed elsewhere in this book.

CONSENT FOR PUBLICATION

Not applicable.

CONFLICT OF INTEREST

The author declares no conflict of interest, financial or otherwise.

ACKNOWLEDGEMENTS

The authors would like to thank photographer Elaine Gonzales of MidAtlantic Retina for the photographs in this chapter.

REFERENCES

[1]   Sabanayagam C, Yip W, Ting DS, Tan G, Wong TY. Ten emerging trends in the epidemiology of diabetic retinopathy. Ophthalmic Epidemiol 2016; 23(4): 209-22.
[http://dx.doi.org/10.1080/09286586.2016.1193618] [PMID: 27355693]

[2]   Wilkinson CP, Ferris FL III, Klein RE, *et al.* Proposed international clinical diabetic retinopathy and diabetic macular edema disease severity scales. Ophthalmology 2003; 110(9): 1677-82.
[http://dx.doi.org/10.1016/S0161-6420(03)00475-5] [PMID: 13129861]

[3]   Fine SL, Goldberg MF, Tasman W. Historical Perspectives on the Management of Macular Degeneration, Diabetic Retinopathy, and Retinal Detachment: Personal Reminiscences. Ophthalmology 2016; 123(10S): S64-77.
[http://dx.doi.org/10.1016/j.ophtha.2016.04.058] [PMID: 27664288]

[4]   Wu L, Fernandez-Loaiza P, Sauma J, Hernandez-Bogantes E, Masis M. Classification of diabetic retinopathy and diabetic macular edema. World J Diabetes 2013; 4(6): 290-4.
[http://dx.doi.org/10.4239/wjd.v4.i6.290] [PMID: 24379919]

[5]   Ryan SJ. Retina. 5th ed., Philadelphia, PA, USA: Elsevier, Inc 2013.

[6]   Hirai FE, Knudtson MD, Klein BE, Klein R. Clinically significant macular edema and survival in type 1 and type 2 diabetes. Am J Ophthalmol 2008; 145(4): 700-6.
[http://dx.doi.org/10.1016/j.ajo.2007.11.019] [PMID: 18226797]

[7]   Klein R, Klein BE, Moss SE, Davis MD, DeMets DL. The Wisconsin epidemiologic study of diabetic retinopathy. III. Prevalence and risk of diabetic retinopathy when age at diagnosis is 30 or more years. Arch Ophthalmol 1984; 102(4): 527-32.
[http://dx.doi.org/10.1001/archopht.1984.01040030405011] [PMID: 6367725]

[8]   Nathan DM, Genuth S, Lachin J, *et al.* The effect of intensive treatment of diabetes on the development and progression of long-term complications in insulin-dependent diabetes mellitus. N Engl J Med 1993; 329(14): 977-86.
[http://dx.doi.org/10.1056/NEJM199309303291401] [PMID: 8366922]

[9]   Nasr CE, Hoogwerf BJ, Faiman C, Reddy SS. United Kingdom Prospective Diabetes Study (UKPDS). Effects of glucose and blood pressure control on complications of type 2 diabetes mellitus. Cleve Clin J Med 1999; 66(4): 247-53.
[http://dx.doi.org/10.3949/ccjm.66.4.247] [PMID: 10199061]

[10]   Photocoagulation treatment of proliferative diabetic retinopathy: the second report of diabetic retinopathy study findings. Ophthalmology 1978; 85(1): 82-106.
[http://dx.doi.org/10.1016/S0161-6420(78)35693-1] [PMID: 345173]

[11]   Early photocoagulation for diabetic retinopathy. ETDRS report number 9. Ophthalmology 1991; 98(5) (Suppl.): 766-85.
[http://dx.doi.org/10.1016/S0161-6420(13)38011-7] [PMID: 2062512]

[12]   Wells JA, Glassman AR, Ayala AR, *et al.* Aflibercept, Bevacizumab, or Ranibizumab for Diabetic Macular Edema: Two-Year Results from a Comparative Effectiveness Randomized Clinical Trial. Ophthalmology 2016; 123(6): 1351-9.
[http://dx.doi.org/10.1016/j.ophtha.2016.02.022] [PMID: 26935357]

[13]   Heier JS, Korobelnik JF, Brown DM, *et al.* Intravitreal Aflibercept for Diabetic Macular Edema: 148-Week Results from the VISTA and VIVID Studies. Ophthalmology 2016; 123(11): 2376-85.
[http://dx.doi.org/10.1016/j.ophtha.2016.07.032] [PMID: 27651226]

[14]   Boyer DS, Nguyen QD, Brown DM, Basu K, Ehrlich JS. Outcomes with As-Needed Ranibizumab after Initial Monthly Therapy: Long-Term Outcomes of the Phase III RIDE and RISE Trials. Ophthalmology 2015; 122(12): 2504-13.e1.
[http://dx.doi.org/10.1016/j.ophtha.2015.08.006] [PMID: 26452713]

[15]   Spaide RF, Fisher YL. Intravitreal bevacizumab (Avastin) treatment of proliferative diabetic retinopathy complicated by vitreous hemorrhage. Retina 2006; 26(3): 275-8.
[http://dx.doi.org/10.1097/00006982-200603000-00004] [PMID: 16508426]

[16]   Gross JG, Glassman AR, Jampol LM, *et al.* Writing committee for the diabetic retinopathy clinical research network. Panretinal photocoagulation *vs* intravitreous ranibizumab for proliferative diabetic retinopathy: a randomized clinical trial. JAMA 2015; 314(20): 2137-46.
[http://dx.doi.org/10.1001/jama.2015.15217] [PMID: 26565927]

CHAPTER 11

Current Treatment for Diabetic Retinopathy

Joseph Bogaard and **Judy E. Kim**[*]

Department of Ophthalmology and Visual Sciences, Medical College of Wisconsin, Milwaukee, USA

Abstract: This chapter will review most common therapies currently used for diabetic retinopathy. Specifically, the treatments being used for diabetic macular edema (DME) and proliferative diabetic retinopathy will be discussed.

Keywords: Anti-VEGF, Diabetes, DME, Edema, Laser, Laser, Macula, Retinopathy, Steroids, Treatment, Vitrectomy.

INTRODUCTION

Diabetic retinopathy is the most common microvascular complication of diabetes. Ten percent of people with diabetes have vision-threatening diabetic retinopathy (DR). It is also a major public health threat and is the leading cause of blindness in working-aged individuals in industrialized nations [1]. Diabetic macular edema (DME) accounts for the majority of diabetic retinopathy-related vision loss, followed by complications resulting from proliferative diabetic retinopathy (PDR). Tremendous advances have been made in the treatment of DME and PDR in recent years, particularly with the discovery of the role that vascular endothelial growth factor (VEGF) plays in diabetic retinopathy and the advent of intravitreal anti-vascular endothelial growth factor (anti-VEGF) therapy.

The VEGF family is the master regulator of angiogenesis, vasculogenesis and lymphangiogenesis. It consists of six members VEGF-A, VEGF-B, VEGF-C, VEGF-D, viral VEGF-E, and placental growth factor (PIGF). Of these, VEGF-A is the most important member and is what most of our anti-VEGF therapies currently target. VEGF is an anti-parallel homodimeric peptide with numerous cysteine residues that form intramolecular disulphide bonds, making it a member of the "cys-loop" superfamily of proteins.

[*] **Corresponding author Judy E. Kim**: Department of Ophthalmology and Visual Sciences, Medical College of Wisconsin, Milwaukee, Milwaukee, USA; E-mail:jekim@mcw.edu

Douglas R. Lazzaro and Samy I. McFarlane (Eds.)
All rights reserved-© 2021 Bentham Science Publishers

The human VEGF-A gene located on chromosome 6 consists of 8 exons with alternate splice sites in exons 6, 7 and 8 leading to 16 currently known different isoforms of the VEGF-A protein, each with different biological properties and activities. These isoforms are most commonly from six transcripts: $VEGF_{111}$, $VEGF_{121}$, $VEGF_{145}$, $VEGF_{165}$, $VEGF_{189}$, and $VEGF_{206}$. Exon 8 contains a major site of alternative splicing resulting in either the prototypical $VEGF_{xxxa}$ form or the "anti-angiogenic" $VEGF_{xxxb}$ isoform. The shorter isoforms $VEGF_{111}$ and $VEGF_{121}$ are freely diffusible due to their excluded exons 6 and 7 which contain heparin and Neuropilin-1 binding sites. Longer isoforms $VEGF_{145}$, $VEGF_{189}$, and $VEGF_{206}$ have high affinity binding to heparin sulfate glycoproteins which tightly tether them to the extracellular matrix. Finally, $VEGF_{165}$ represents an intermediate between freely diffusible and tightly bound isoforms [2, 3].

VEGF plays an important role in the development of both PDR and DME. VEGF production is induced in response to ischemia or hypoxia through a DNA binding protein called hypoxia-inducible factor 1 (HIF-1) which leads to increased transcription of VEGF mRNA [4]. VEGF molecules bind to tyrosine kinase receptors on the endothelial cell surface causing them to dimerize and activate *via* transphosphorylation. This transphosphorylation induces a cascade of intracellular signaling pathways shown in Fig. (**1**). This complex signal cascade causes an increase in vascular permeability, cell proliferation, cell migration, and cell survival. This cascade also causes the release of matrix metalloproteinases and urokinase-type plasminogen resulting in the destruction of basement membranes allowing for migration, proliferation, and creation of new basement membranes [5].

Anti-VEGF agents currently Food and Drug Administration (FDA) approved for the treatment of DME include aflibercept (Eylea, Regeneron, Eastview, New York, United States) and ranibizumab (Lucentis, Genentech, South San Francisco, California, United States). Bevacizumab (Avastin, Genentech, South San Francisco, California, United States) is also used off-label. These anti-VEGF agents have been shown to prevent progression of PDR, reverse diabetic retinopathy severity scores, and improve visual acuity (VA) and retinal thickness in eyes with center-involved DME. Despite these advances, many challenges remain in the treatment of diabetic retinopathy, including patient access to health care services, early screening, and increasing costs related to drug therapy. Future therapeutic agents may help by decreasing the socioeconomic treatment burden and durability of treatment effect.

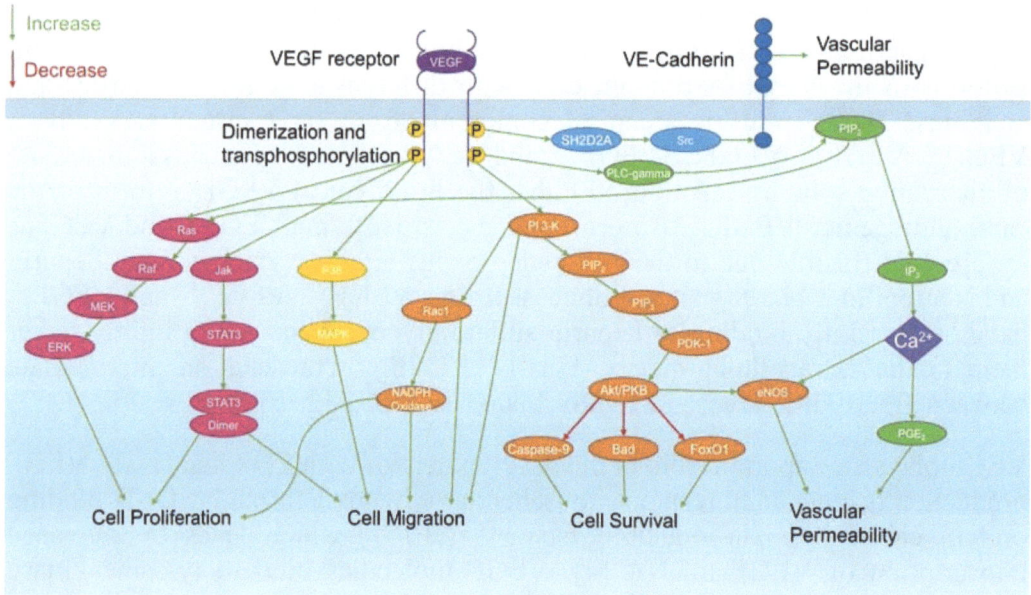

Fig. (1). MEK – Mitogen-activated protein kinase kinases ERK – Extracellular signal-regulated kinases Jak – Janus kinases STAT3 – Signal transducer and activator of transcription 3 MAPK- Mitogen-activated protein kinases Rac1 – Ras-related C3 botulinum toxin substrate 1 NADPH Oxidase - Nicotinamide adenine dinucleotide phosphate oxidase PI 3-K – Phosphoinositide 3-kinases PIP_2 – Phosphatidylinositol 4,5-bisphosphate PIP_3 – Phosphatidylinositol (3,4,5)-trisphosphate PDK-1 – Pyruvate dehydrogenase lipoamide kinase isozyme 1 AKT/PKB – Protein Kinase B BAD – B cell lymphoma 2 associated death promoter FoxO1 – Forkhead box protein O1 eNOS – Endothelial nitric oxide synthase SH2D2A – SH2 domain-containing protein 2A PLC-gamma – Phospholipase C gamma IP_3 – inositol 1,4,5-trisphosphate Ca^{2+} – Ionic Calcium 2+ PGE2 – Prostaglandin E2.

Diabetic Retinopathy

Management of DR requires timely diagnosis and and access to treatments when needed. Perhaps the most effective form of treatment for DR is prevention and early diagnosis. This is often a collaborative effort with primary care providers and endocrinologists and involves appropriate diabetes screening and blood sugar control, followed by routine eye examinations to detect DR in the earliest stages. Despite well-established screening guidelines [6 - 8] and education programs directed at both physicians and patients [9], only 50% of patients with diabetes undergo screening eye examinations within a given year, and only 16% receive exams in two consecutive years [10]. Non-adherence to screening guidelines has been attributed to socioeconomic, cultural, and geographic reasons [11]. In developing countries, screening examinations may be limited by an insufficient number of physicians [12]. Telemedicine may help ease the burden of screening exams by allowing patients to be examined in locations that are more convenient or accessible to them. The fundus images obtained from a camera can be sent through an established telemedicine program to an ophthalmologist's office or a reading center for interpretation. Based on the reading of the photographic images, appropriate and timely referral is made if indicated. Smartphone-based imaging systems have also been developed, which can further increase patient access to screening in a cost-effective manner [13]. As telemedicine grows with the development of more portable, affordable, and reliably gradable fundus imaging systems, the influx of patient data may outstrip the ability of qualified eye care providers to read these images [14]. Therefore, automated image reading software utilizing artificial intelligence algorithms have been developed and have been FDA approved.

Treatment of Diabetic Macular Edema

Anti-VEGF Therapy for DME

According to the Early Treatment of Diabetic Retinopathy Study (ETDRS), focal/grid laser photocoagulation of eyes with clinically-significant DME decreased the risk of moderate vision loss (15 letters) by 50% over three years [15]. As a result, focal/grid laser photocoagulation remained the gold standard for treatment of clinically significant DME for over three decades. Recently, however, a paradigm shift has occurred, and anti-VEGF agents are the first-line therapy for center-involved DME (ci-DME) with vision loss, based on results from several multi-center randomized clinical trials. It should be noted that most of the initial clinical trials for DME therapy with an anti-VEGF agent were performed with ranibizumab, since the drug was designed specifically for intraocular use, was available prior to aflibercept, and bevacizumab was not approved by the U.S. FDA for intraocular use. Nevertheless, many clinicians have used and continue to use bevacizumab in an off-label fashion for DME treatment, as they do for neovascular AMD treatment. In addition to the off-label nature of bevacizumab, another key difference among currently available anti-VEGF agents for DME (aflibercept, bevacizumab, and ranibizumab) is the cost of the drugs. Bevacizumab is significantly less expensive. From one bottle of bevacizumab, which is intended for intravenous cancer treatment, multiple syringes of the drug can be aliquoted for individual use in the eye. This preparation is usually performed by compounding or hospital pharmacies. On the other hand, aflibercept and ranibizumab are drawn from individual bottles in the office using aseptic technique prior to use. Recently, pre-filled syringes of ranibizumab and aflibercept have become available.

Intravitreal injections with anti-VEGF agents have been shown to not only prevent vision loss, but to significantly improve VA in patients with vision loss due to center-involved DME in pivotal phase III clinical trials. In the RESTORE study, ranibizumab groups with and without laser were compared to laser alone.

Intravitreal ranibizumab was given monthly for 3 months, then pro re nata (PRN). Both ranibizumab groups were found to be superior to laser monotherapy at one year [16]. Patients switched to individualized treatment regimens maintained the VA improvement over a three-year period even with progressively decreasing number of injections each year [17]. The Diabetic Retinopathy Clinical Research network (DRCR.net) protocol I study evaluated the efficacy of intravitreal ranibizumab injections with prompt or deferred laser treatment for at least six months and triamcinolone with prompt laser treatment. These three groups were compared to prompt laser with sham injection as the control group. Both ranibizumab groups were found to be superior to triamcinolone with prompt laser treatment and laser alone at one- and two-year follow-up [18, 19]. Evidence for superiority of anti-VEGF therapy was strengthened with the RISE and RIDE trials, which showed that monthly injections of ranibizumab significantly reduced central subfield thickness on optical coherence tomography (OCT) and improved VA with both 0.3 and 0.5 mg doses [20]. The open label extension to these studies demonstrated that VA gains could be maintained with less-than-monthly ranibizumab injections [21].

Comparison of Anti-VEGF Agents for DME

Aflibercept is a recombinant fusion protein that binds to and inhibits VEGF-A. Aflibercept administered at either four- or eight-week intervals has been shown to be significantly superior to focal/grid laser photocoagulation at improving VA [22]. Aflibercept has been shown in DRCR.net protocol T to be more effective than ranibizumab and bevacizumab for improving VA in center-involved DME, when baseline visual acuity is approximately 20/50 or worse [23]. When the baseline VA was 20/32 to 20/40, all three VEGF inhibitors had similar efficacy in improvement of VA, with approximately 8 letters gained. Bevacizumab was found to be less effective at decreasing the central subfield thickness on OCT. This study has helped clinicians in guiding which of the three currently available anti-VEGF agents should be used to initiate therapy. However, care must be taken when extrapolating the results to treatment regimens that differ from the one used in protocol T [24]. Also, in some parts of the world, not all three anti-VEGF agents are available.

Anti-VEGF therapy has revolutionized the treatment of DME by allowing a mean improvement in VA outcome. In fact, it is now the standard first-line therapy for most patients with center involved DME with vision loss. Nevertheless, DME does not resolve completely on OCT in a significant percentage of patients, and some patients continue to have decreased VA despite monthly anti-VEGF therapy. In these refractory cases, switching from one anti-VEGF agent to another is one option. Aflibercept has theoretical advantages over bevacizumab and ranibizumab by having stronger binding affinity to VEGF and by binding placental growth factor. There is also indirect evidence that aflibercept may have a longer duration of action. A retrospective chart review of 21 eyes showed a significant visual improvement upon conversion from bevacizumab or ranibizumab to aflibercept [25]. Pharmacogenetics could partially explain why some patients respond better to one agent *versus* another, but more studies are needed to address this topic. In current clinical practice, patients are often switched to aflibercept, despite limited evidence supporting this strategy. Further clinical trials may help answer the role of switching therapies.

Anti-VEGF Treatment Regimens for DME

In addition to the financial burden related to drug costs, the multitude of clinic visits and intravitreal injections required with anti-VEGF therapy can be onerous to patients. Therefore, individualized treatment strategies, such and PRN and treat-and-extend (T&E) have been developed to limit the treatment burden. While PRN treatment does decrease the number of treatments, it may not affect the number of clinic visits if patients still need to be monitored monthly, as was the case for the neovascular age-related macular degeneration (AMD) trials. The T&E strategy, which is the most commonly used regimen for neovascular AMD among retina specialists in the United States, decreases both the number of clinic visits and the number of intravitreal injections for the patient. The RETAIN trial compared T&E plus laser, T&E alone, and PRN ranibizumab regimens for DME and showed that both T&E arms were non-inferior to PRN arm with a 46% reduction in clinic visits [26]. There are no multicenter randomized controlled trials comparing T&E strategy to monthly treatment for DME. In the DRCR.net trials, "defer and extend" strategy was used such that if the eye was stable in two consecutive visits based on VA and OCT thickness after the first year, the treatment was deferred, and the follow-up was extended from monthly visits to every two months. If the eye continued to be stable, then the injections were deferred again and the follow-up interval was extended to every four months. The five-year data from DRCR.net protocol I study showed that the number of intravitreal injections decrease substantially with each year of follow up, such that an average of nine injections were needed in the first year, but no injections were needed on average in years four and five [27]. Thus, while there is a large treatment burden initially, the patients can be reassured that the injections may not have to be continued indefinitely for DME therapy.

Safety and Potential Side Effects of Anti-VEGF Therapy

While the introduction of anti-VEGF therapy has revolutionized the care of center-involved DME, some are concerned that long-lasting VEGF antagonism may be detrimental to the health of cells that rely on its trophic activity such as neurons and endothelial cells both in the retina and systemically. Studies have shown that all three anti-VEGF agents are detectable in serum after intravitreal injection and levels of plasma free VEGF decrease. There is a notable difference in the amount of reduction of VEGF levels and rate of drug clearance with ranibizumab being cleared fastest and having the lowest reduction in systemic VEGF levels and aflibercept being cleared slowest and having the highest reduction in systemic VEGF levels [28]. Systemically delivered anti-VEGF agents are known to promote the development of elevated blood pressure, and arterial thromboembolic events such as stroke, myocardial infarction, and death; however, their doses are more than 100 times higher than what is used in intravitreal injections [29, 30]. Thus far, there has been no statistically significant signals derived from Level 1 evidence that directly point to a greater risk of developing arterial thromboembolic events in the anti-VEGF cohorts compared with control groups. However, none of these trials were powered to statistically answer this question. Such trials are unlikely to be carried out, as each arm of the study would need more than 10,000 patients to detect a meaningful difference for these rare events.

Other ocular side effects of intravitreal anti-VEGF are well established. Infectious endophthalmitis remains one of the most devastating complications of any intravitreal injection with a reported incidence rate of 0.02% to 0.05%. A recent analysis of over 1 million injections found a rate of 0.035% or one endophthalmitis in 2857 injections [31]. Other risks include retinal tears, detachments, vitreous hemorrhage, and traumatic iatrogenic cataract. However, these are quite uncommon and much less visually debilitating than endophthalmitis [32]. Intravitreal injection of anti-VEGF causes a transient, volume-dependent elevation of intraocular pressure (IOP) that typically resolves within 30 to 60 minutes [33]. However, the post hoc analysis of various studies demonstrated that a subset of patients (1.7% - 11%) developed persistent ocular hypertension. While there is no evidence yet that this ocular hypertension has lead to retinal nerve fiber layer thinning, it seems prudent to monitor patients for the development of ocular hypertension and glaucomatous changes [34].

Future Developments in Anti-VEGF Therapy for DME

The multi-center, phase III trials that established the use of anti-VEGF therapy for DME excluded patients with VA better than 20/32 or 20/40. In practice, many physicians will still treat patients with center-involving or center-threatening DME with very good VA, particularly if the patient is symptomatic. DRCR.net protocol V, a randomized multicenter clinical trial, found that, among eyes with center-involved DME and VA 20/25 or better, there was no significant difference in vision loss at 2 years whether eyes were initially managed with laser photocoagulation, aflibercept, or observation and given aflibercept only if visual acuity worsened. It demonstrated that observation without treatment unless visual acuity worsened was a reasonable strategy for DME with good VA [35].

Given the proven benefit of targeting VEGF as a therapy for DME, recent efforts have been made to develop treatments that suppress VEGF for longer duration. Designed ankyrin repeat proteins (DARPins) are a novel class of proteins selected for high-affinity binding to a target protein. For instance, a DARPin compound abicar pegol (Abicipar, Allergan. Dublin, Ireland) selectively binds all VEGF-A isoforms and has been studied in a phase I/II study to determine the safety and biologic activity in patients with DME [36]. At 3 months, drug levels were still detectable in the aqueous humor at a concentration several orders of magnitude higher than the half-maximal inhibitory concentration. Clinical trials using DARPins, other longer-acting anti-VEGF agents, and other drug delivery systems including port delivery system and gene therapy are underway for neovascular AMD, central retinal vein occlusion, and DME.

Laser Photocoagulation for DME

Anti-VEGF therapy has firmly replaced focal/grid laser photocoagulation for the treatment of ci-DME. Thus, the role of laser in treating this disease has become less clear. Combining ranibizumab with prompt macular laser photocoagulation has not been shown to offer a significant benefit to ranibizumab treatment alone in terms of VA improvement or decreasing the number of intravitreal injections. The RESTOR study even showed greater VA improvement in patients treated with ranibizumab alone compared to ranibizumab plus laser at the 36-month endpoint, though this difference was not statistically significant [16, 17]. DRCR.net protocol I showed greater VA improvement with ranibizumab plus deferred laser compared to ranibizumab plus prompt laser at two years, although there was no statistically significant difference [19].

There are some advantages to laser photocoagulation over anti-VEGF therapy, including no risk of endophthalmitis, lower cost and treatment burden. Currently most clinicians will consider focal/grid laser treatment in eyes with DME that is not center-involving but is juxta-foveal and has one or more clearly identifiable microaneurysms that are a source of leakage on fluorescein angiography. These microaneurysms should be located far enough away from the fovea such that they can be easily and safely laser photocoagulated. These eyes respond well to laser photocoagulation with decrease in macular edema often with just one or two sessions of treatment. However, the time course to decreasing edema may take longer than following injections with intravitreal anti-VEGF agents or intravitreal corticosteroids. It is unclear whether addition of laser is better for the eyes that are refractory to anti-VEGF therapy or whether it is better to consider one of the other treatment strategies such as switching to another anti-VEGF agent, or switching to another class of medication such as corticosteroids, which will be discussed below.

Micropulse Laser Treatment for DME

Conventional laser photocoagulation treats with heat and causes visible retinal scars, which can enlarge over time. This can lead to adverse effects, such as encroachment of chorioretinal scars into the fovea, development of subretinal fibrosis, rupture of Bruch's membrane with development of choroidal neovascularization, loss of visual field sensitivity, and development of paracentral scotomas. Advances in laser technology have led to the development of micropulse laser systems, which are designed to selectively target the retinal pigment epithelium (RPE), while having a minimal effect on the neurosensory retina [37]. The repetitive pulsed delivery of laser in microseconds rather than in milliseconds aims to treat the RPE with sub-lethal thermal energy to initiate a therapeutic cellular cascade, while avoiding many of the detrimental effects of conventional suprathreshold retinal photocoagulation [38, 39]. Small retrospective studies on yellow micropulse laser have shown improved visual acuity and decreased central retinal thickness in previously treatment-naïve eyes with no signs of retinal damage [40, 41]. Larger prospective studies are needed to determine the potential role of micropulse laser for DME.

Targeted Peripheral Laser Photocoagulation for DME

The use of ultrawide-field fluorescein angiography (UWFA) has drawn attention to large areas of peripheral retinal nonperfusion that are often seen in patients with DME. Since retinal ischemia may be associated with increased production of VEGF, scatter laser photocoagulation of these nonperfused areas has been discussed as a potential treatment for refractory DME. RaScaL is a pilot study that compared the efficacy of a single treatment of ranibizumab plus peripheral laser scatter *versus* triamcinolone plus macular laser. At six months, the scatter treatment group had fewer recurrences requiring treatment, although VA and central foveal thickness were similar between the two groups [42]. However, this was a small study with short follow-up. Also the DAVE trial, a 3-year randomized trial of 40 eyes with DME, did not find that combination therapy with ranibizumab and targeted peripheral laser improved visual outcomes or reduced treatment burden compared with ranibizumab alone [43]. Larger prospective studies using UWFA-guided scatter laser treatment may be needed to determine the role of this treatment modality for DME refractory *versus* anti-VEGF monotherapy, but given lack of clear benefit from these smaller studies, this may not be a favored treatment modality.

Corticosteroids for DME

Kenalog-40 (Bristol-Myers Squibb Company, Princeton, NJ, USA) is a form of triamcinolone acetonide suspension that is not FDA-approved for intraocular use, although it has been used for many years to treat various ocular conditions off-label, including for DME. Trivaris (Allergan, Inc, Irvine, CA, USA) was the form of triamcinolone that was used in DRCR.net protocol I. Triesence (Alcon, Fort Worth, TX, USA) is a preservative-free form of triamcinolone that is FDA-approved for intraocular use. Several clinical trials have been performed to assess the efficacy of both sub-Tenon and intravitreal delivery of triamcinolone for the treatment of DME, since it was available prior to the use of anti-VEGF agents, and inflammation is implicated in development of DME. Intravitreal triamcinolone has not shown benefit over focal/grid laser photocoagulation and has been associated with higher adverse effects [44, 45], such as cataract formation and IOP elevation requiring medical or surgical intervention. However, smaller studies have shown a modest improvement in VA for diffuse DME [46]. In DRCR.net protocol I, intravitreal triamcinolone with prompt laser treatment was not superior to laser treatment, though when analysis was limited to pseudophakic eyes, the VA outcome was similar to the ranibizumab groups with less number of intravitreal injections [18]. This suggests that progression of cataract contributes significantly to the worse visual outcome in patients treated with intravitreal triamcinolone and should be a consideration when needing to treat patients who are phakic.

Sustained-release corticosteroid delivery systems have been developed to potentially reduce the treatment burden, as well as to decrease the incidence of cataract and glaucoma, while preserving the effects seen with corticosteroid delivered in a bolus manner, as in intravitreal triamcinolone injections. The dexamethasone delivery system (Ozurdex, Allergan, Irvine, CA, United States) and the fluocinolone acetonide insert (Iluvien, Alimera Sciences, Alpharetta, GA, United States) have both been FDA-approved for the treatment of DME in pseudophakic eyes or eyes that will undergo cataract surgery in the near future and are not steroid responders in terms of IOP elevation. The sustained-release fluocinolone acetonide insert can provide substantial benefit for up to three years with a single injection, though the VA gains are slightly less than those seen with anti-VEGF therapy [47, 48]. The FAME trial demonstrated that patients with chronic DME for greater than three years at the initiation of treatment responded better than those with DME for a shorter duration [49]. The reason for this discrepancy is not fully understood, but it is possible that chronic DME is more chemokine-driven, while non-chronic DME is more VEGF-driven. Currently, there are no multi-center randomized trials comparing sustained-release corticosteroids to anti-VEGF therapy for the treatment of DME. Most clinicians use intraocular steroid injection as a second line therapy in patients who are not steroid responders and who do not respond well to monthly anti-VEGF therapy or needing treatment during pregnancy.

Vitrectomy for DME

Vitrectomy has been used as treatment for DME, particularly when it is associated with vitreomacular traction (VMT) or visually significant epiretinal membrane (ERM). In DRCR.net protocol D, vitrectomy improved central retinal thickness but not VA for eyes with poorly-responsive DME or VMT-associated DME [50, 51]. A systematic review of 11 studies found little evidence to support vitrectomy as an intervention for DME unless ERM or VMT was present [52]. More recently, a retrospective study using spectral-domain optical coherence tomography (SD-OCT) found that external limiting membrane (ELM) integrity is a positive predictor for VA improvement in eyes undergoing vitrectomy for medically non-responsive DME [53]. The ELM status was a better predictor than the ellipsoid zone integrity or central retinal thickness. More studies are needed before SD-OCT findings can be used as a sensitive and specific prognostic indicator in the management of DME. There is a possibility that VMT may be released by injection of intraocular gas alone in the office without the need for surgical intervention. This treatment modality is currently being investigated for various ocular conditions including VMT, stage 2 macular holes, and DME with VMT.

Treatment of Proliferative Diabetic Retinopathy

The Diabetic Retinopathy Study (DRS) in the 1970's showed that prompt pan-retinal photocoagulation (PRP) for high-risk PDR decreases the risk of severe vision loss by over 50% [54]. Loss of VA and constriction of the peripheral visual field were noted in some eyes following treatment. The two-year risk of severe vision loss without treatment was felt to outweigh these adverse effects for eyes with neovascularization and preretinal or vitreous hemorrhage and eyes with neovascularization on or within a disc diameter of the optic disc equaling or exceeding ¼ to ⅓ disc area in extent.

More recently, intravitreal anti-VEGF therapy has been shown to cause regression of neovascularization in PDR with recurrences occurring by 12 weeks after an initial injection [55]. Anti-VEGF has been used in PDR to hasten the resolution of vitreous hemorrhage, diminish intraoperative complications, and prevent post-operative vitreous hemorrhage [56, 57].

The use of anti-VEGF therapy is now being considered as an alternative to PRP, given the potential for preserving visual function by avoiding retinal damage. DRCR.net protocol S compared ranibizumab *versus* PRP for the treatment of PDR with or without DME [58]. Monthly injections of ranibizumab were given through 12 weeks, followed by a structured re-treatment protocol in the ranibizumab arm. Even in the PRP arm, if DME was present at baseline, intravitreal ranibizumab injections were administered to treat DME. The result showed that ranibizumab is non-inferior to PRP in terms of visual acuity change and may be better in terms of VA improvement throughout the two years of the study when the area under the curve was analyzed. Ranibizumab had the added benefits over PRP of less peripheral vision loss, less frequency of vitrectomy, and decreased incidence of DME. The ranibizumab group also demonstrated regression of neovascularization at two years and was noted to have two-step diabetic retinopathy severity score improvement. Anti-VEGF therapy may be a favorable alternative to PRP for the treatment of PDR, especially in patients who are deemed to be compliant with follow-up or in eyes with PDR with coexisting DME. 5 year follow-up of patients in protocol S provided additional information regarding the long-term benefit and the durability of anti-VEGF treatment for PDR. Although the loss to follow up was relatively high in both groups, VA in most patients who completed follow up was very good with a mean VA of 20/25 (approximate Snellen equivalent) in both groups. Serious vision loss or serious PDR complications were uncommon in both groups. The ranibizumab group had lower rates of developing diabetic macular edema (22% *vs* 38%) and had less visual field loss (-330 dB *vs* -527 dB) supporting that both anti-VEGF therapy and PRP are viable treatment options for patients with PDR [59]. If the patient is deemed not reliable for follow-up, the clinicians may still choose to treat with PRP rather than with anti-VEGF in eyes with PDR without DME. In parts of the world where the cost of medical care or physician supply is an issue, PRP may be preferred over anti-VEGF therapy. Even in compliant patients with PDR without DME, the clinician may recommend a combination of anti-VEGF injections followed by PRP to decrease the incidence of PRP-induced macular edema while reducing the treatment burden. In summary, we now have anti-VEGF agents in addition to PRP as therapeutic modalities for eyes with PDR, which is a significant benefit to our patients.

Vitrectomy for PDR

If an eye has progressed to advanced PDR with traction retinal detachment threatening the fovea or nonclearing vitreous hemorrhage, pars plana vitrectomy (PPV) could be considered. In recent years, various instruments for PPV have evolved and improved greatly such that the surgery can be carried out with greater safety and success. Therefore, most retina surgeons do not wait as long as in the past before recommending surgery, in hopes of preventing vision loss or more rapid restoration of vision, allowing the patients to return to their daily activities. However, as with any intraocular surgery, careful discussion should be performed prior to surgery that includes potential side effects of surgery, including progression of cataract in phakic patients, possible need for post-operative positioning if intraocular gas injection were needed, and possible need for returning to the operating room for recurrent or new retinal detachment. However, with removal of vitreous with posterior hyaloid, PPV allows removal of a scaffold for growth of neovascularization and may reduce progression of PDR.

CONCLUSION

Diabetic retinopathy is a major cause of vision loss in both the developed and developing world. The treatment of DME, and more recently of PDR, has been revolutionized in the last decade by the development and improvement of intravitreal anti-VEGF therapy. This therapy is capable of not only preventing vision loss but also significantly improving visual outcome in most treated patients. The current treatment strategies of diabetic retinopathy also pose challenges, as the optimal treatments are often expensive and require more office visits than have historically been needed with laser photocoagulation alone. Nevertheless, the future of diabetic retinopathy treatment continues to look promising with multiple new drugs and trials in development that could offer patients better visual outcomes with increased safety, reduced costs, and decreased treatment burdens.

CONSENT FOR PUBLICATION

Not applicable.

CONFLICT OF INTEREST

The author declares no conflict of interest, financial or otherwise.

ACKNOWLEDGEMENTS

Declared none.

REFERENCES

[1]   Fong DS, Aiello LP, Ferris FL III, Klein R. Diabetic retinopathy. Diabetes Care 2004; 27(10): 2540-53.
[http://dx.doi.org/10.2337/diacare.27.10.2540] [PMID: 15451934]

[2]   Peach CJ, Mignone VW, Arruda MA, *et al.* Molecular Pharmacology of VEGF-A Isoforms: Binding

and Signalling at VEGFR2. Int J Mol Sci 2018; 19(4): E1264.
[http://dx.doi.org/10.3390/ijms19041264] [PMID: 29690653]

[3]   Harper SJ, Bates DO. VEGF-A splicing: the key to anti-angiogenic therapeutics? Nat Rev Cancer 2008; 8(11): 880-7.
[http://dx.doi.org/10.1038/nrc2505] [PMID: 18923433]

[4]   Ferrara N. Vascular endothelial growth factor: basic science and clinical progress. Endocr Rev 2004; 25(4): 581-611.
[http://dx.doi.org/10.1210/er.2003-0027] [PMID: 15294883]

[5]   Witmer AN, Vrensen GF, Van Noorden CJ, Schlingemann RO. Vascular endothelial growth factors and angiogenesis in eye disease. Prog Retin Eye Res 2003; 22(1): 1-29.
[http://dx.doi.org/10.1016/S1350-9462(02)00043-5] [PMID: 12597922]

[6]   Fong DS, Aiello L, Gardner TW, *et al.* American Diabetes Association. Diabetic retinopathy. Diabetes Care 2003; 26 (Suppl. 1): S99-S102.
[http://dx.doi.org/10.2337/diacare.26.2007.S99] [PMID: 12502630]

[7]   Lueder GT, Silverstein J. American academy of pediatrics section on ophthalmology and section on endocrinology. Screening for retinopathy in the pediatric patient with type 1 diabetes mellitus. Pediatrics 2005; 116(1): 270-3.
[http://dx.doi.org/10.1542/peds.2005-0875] [PMID: 15995070]

[8]   American academy of ophthalmology retina/vitreous panel. Preferred Practice Pattern Guidelines 2016. www.aao.org/ppp

[9]   Hipwell AE, Sturt J, Lindenmeyer A, *et al.* Attitudes, access and anguish: a qualitative interview study of staff and patients' experiences of diabetic retinopathy screening. BMJ Open 2014; 4(12): e005498.
[http://dx.doi.org/10.1136/bmjopen-2014-005498] [PMID: 25510885]

[10]   Mukamel DB, Bresnick GH, Wang Q, Dickey CF. Barriers to compliance with screening guidelines for diabetic retinopathy. Ophthalmic Epidemiol 1999; 6(1): 61-72.
[http://dx.doi.org/10.1076/opep.6.1.61.1563] [PMID: 10384685]

[11]   Thompson AC, Thompson MO, Young DL, *et al.* Barriers to follow-up and strategies to improve adherence to appointments for care of chronic eye diseases. Invest Ophthalmol Vis Sci 2015; 56(8): 4324-31.
[http://dx.doi.org/10.1167/iovs.15-16444] [PMID: 26176869]

[12]   Palmer JJ, Chinanayi F, Gilbert A, *et al.* Trends and implications for achieving VISION 2020 human resources for eye health targets in 16 countries of sub-Saharan Africa by the year 2020. Hum Resour Health 2014; 12: 45.
[http://dx.doi.org/10.1186/1478-4491-12-45] [PMID: 25128287]

[13]   Rajalakshmi R, Arulmalar S, Usha M, *et al.* Validation of smartphone based retinal photography for diabetic retinopathy screening. PLoS One 2015; 10(9): e0138285.
[http://dx.doi.org/10.1371/journal.pone.0138285] [PMID: 26401839]

[14]   Walton OB IV, Garoon RB, Weng CY, *et al.* Evaluation of automated teleretinal screening program for diabetic retinopathy. JAMA Ophthalmol 2016; 134(2): 204-9.
[http://dx.doi.org/10.1001/jamaophthalmol.2015.5083] [PMID: 26720694]

[15]   Early treatment diabetic retinopathy study research group. Photocoagulation for diabetic macular edema. Early Treatment Diabetic Retinopathy Study report number 1. Early Treatment Diabetic Retinopathy Study research group. Arch Ophthalmol 1985; 103(12): 1796-806.
[http://dx.doi.org/10.1001/archopht.1985.01050120030015] [PMID: 2866759]

[16]   Mitchell P, Bandello F, Schmidt-Erfurth U, *et al.* RESTORE study group. The RESTORE study: ranibizumab monotherapy or combined with laser *versus* laser monotherapy for diabetic macular edema. Ophthalmology 2011; 118(4): 615-25.
[http://dx.doi.org/10.1016/j.ophtha.2011.01.031] [PMID: 21459215]

[17]   Schmidt-Erfurth U, Lang GE, Holz FG, *et al.* RESTORE Extension Study Group. Three-year outcomes of individualized ranibizumab treatment in patients with diabetic macular edema: the RESTORE extension study. Ophthalmology 2014; 121(5): 1045-53.
[http://dx.doi.org/10.1016/j.ophtha.2013.11.041] [PMID: 24491642]

[18]   Elman MJ, Aiello LP, Beck RW, *et al.* Diabetic Retinopathy Clinical Research Network. Randomized trial evaluating ranibizumab plus prompt or deferred laser or triamcinolone plus prompt laser for diabetic macular edema. Ophthalmology 2010; 117(6): 1064-1077.e35.
[http://dx.doi.org/10.1016/j.ophtha.2010.02.031] [PMID: 20427088]

[19]   Elman MJ, Bressler NM, Qin H, *et al.* Diabetic Retinopathy Clinical Research Network. Expanded 2-year follow-up of ranibizumab plus prompt or deferred laser or triamcinolone plus prompt laser for diabetic macular edema. Ophthalmology 2011; 118(4): 609-14.
[http://dx.doi.org/10.1016/j.ophtha.2010.12.033] [PMID: 21459214]

[20]   Nguyen QD, Brown DM, Marcus DM, *et al.* RISE and RIDE Research Group. Ranibizumab for diabetic macular edema: results from 2 phase III randomized trials: RISE and RIDE. Ophthalmology 2012; 119(4): 789-801.
[http://dx.doi.org/10.1016/j.ophtha.2011.12.039] [PMID: 22330964]

[21]   Boyer DS, Nguyen QD, Brown DM, Basu K, Ehrlich JS. RIDE and RISE Research Group. Outcomes with as-needed ranibizumab after initial monthly therapy: Long-term outcomes of the phase III RIDE and RISE trials. Ophthalmology 2015; 122(12): 2504-13.e1.
[http://dx.doi.org/10.1016/j.ophtha.2015.08.006] [PMID: 26452713]

[22]   Korobelnik J-F, Do DV, Schmidt-Erfurth U, *et al.* Intravitreal aflibercept for diabetic macular edema. Ophthalmology 2014; 121(11): 2247-54.
[http://dx.doi.org/10.1016/j.ophtha.2014.05.006] [PMID: 25012934]

[23]   Wells JA, Glassman AR, Ayala AR, *et al.* Diabetic Retinopathy Clinical Research Network. Aflibercept, bevacizumab, or ranibizumab for diabetic macular edema. N Engl J Med 2015; 372(13): 1193-203.
[http://dx.doi.org/10.1056/NEJMoa1414264] [PMID: 25692915]

[24]   Heier JS, Bressler NM, Avery RL, *et al.* American society of retina specialists anti-vegf for diabetic macular edema comparative effectiveness panel. Comparison of aflibercept, bevacizumab, and ranibizumab for treatment of diabetic macular edema: extrapolation of data to clinical practice. JAMA Ophthalmol 2016; 134(1): 95-9.
[http://dx.doi.org/10.1001/jamaophthalmol.2015.4110] [PMID: 26512939]

[25]   Lim LS, Ng WY, Mathur R, *et al.* Conversion to aflibercept for diabetic macular edema unresponsive to ranibizumab or bevacizumab. Clin Ophthalmol 2015; 9: 1715-8.
[http://dx.doi.org/10.2147/OPTH.S81523] [PMID: 26396494]

[26]   Prünte C, Fajnkuchen F, Mahmood S, *et al.* RETAIN Study Group. Ranibizumab 0.5 mg treat-an-extend regimen for diabetic macular oedema: the RETAIN study. Br J Ophthalmol 2016; 100(6): 787-95.
[http://dx.doi.org/10.1136/bjophthalmol-2015-307249] [PMID: 26453639]

[27]   Elman MJ, Ayala A, Bressler NM, *et al.* Diabetic retinopathy clinical research network. Intravitreal ranibizumab for diabetic macular edema with prompt *versus* deferred laser treatment: 5-year randomized trial results. Ophthalmology 2015; 122(2): 375-81.
[http://dx.doi.org/10.1016/j.ophtha.2014.08.047] [PMID: 25439614]

[28]   Avery RL, Castellarin AA, Steinle NC, *et al.* Systemic pharmacokinetics and pharmacodynamics of intravitreal aflibercept, bevacizumab, and ranibizumab. Retina 2017; 37(10): 1847-58.
[http://dx.doi.org/10.1097/IAE.0000000000001493] [PMID: 28106709]

[29]   Bevacizumab full prescribing information. http://www.gene.com/download/pdf/avastin_prescribing.pdf

[30]   Z-aflibercept full prescribing information. https://www.regeneron.com/zaltrap/zaltrap-fpi.pdf

[31]   Bavinger JC, Yu Y, VanderBeek BL. Comparative risk of endophthalmitis after intravitreal injection with bevacizumab, aflibercept, and ranibizumab. Retina 2019; 39(10): 2004-11.
[http://dx.doi.org/10.1097/IAE.0000000000002351] [PMID: 30312260]

[32]   Jager RD, Aiello LP, Patel SC, Cunningham ET Jr. Risks of intravitreous injection: a comprehensive review. Retina 2004; 24(5): 676-98.
[http://dx.doi.org/10.1097/00006982-200410000-00002] [PMID: 15492621]

[33]   Kim JE, Mantravadi AV, Hur EY, Covert DJ. Immediate intraocular pressure changes following intravitreal injections with anti-VEGF agents. Am J Ophthalmol 2008; 146: 930-4.
[http://dx.doi.org/10.1016/j.ajo.2008.07.007] [PMID: 18775528]

[34]   Bracha P, Moore NA, Ciulla TA, WuDunn D, Cantor LB. The acute and chronic effects of intravitreal anti-vascular endothelial growth factor injections on intraocular pressure: A review. Surv Ophthalmol 2018; 63(3): 281-95.
[http://dx.doi.org/10.1016/j.survophthal.2017.08.008] [PMID: 28882597]

[35]   Baker CW, Glassman AR, Beaulieu WT, *et al.* DRCR retina network. Effect of initial management with aflibercept *vs* laser photocoagulation *vs* observation on vision loss among patients with diabetic macular edema involving the center of the macula and good visual acuity: a randomized clinical trial. JAMA 2019; 321(19): 1880-94.
[http://dx.doi.org/10.1001/jama.2019.5790] [PMID: 31037289]

[36]   Campochiaro PA, Channa R, Berger BB, *et al.* Treatment of diabetic macular edema with a designed ankyrin repeat protein that binds vascular endothelial growth factor: a phase I/II study. Am J Ophthalmol 2013; 155(4): 697-704, 704.e1-704.e2.
[http://dx.doi.org/10.1016/j.ajo.2012.09.032] [PMID: 23218689]

[37]   Pollack JS, Kim JE, Pulido JS, Burke JM. Tissue effects of subclinical diode laser treatment of the retina. Arch Ophthalmol 1998; 116(12): 1633-9.
[http://dx.doi.org/10.1001/archopht.116.12.1633] [PMID: 9869794]

[38]   Friberg TR, Karatza EC. The treatment of macular disease using a micropulsed and continuous wave 810-nm diode laser. Ophthalmology 1997; 104(12): 2030-8.
[http://dx.doi.org/10.1016/S0161-6420(97)30061-X] [PMID: 9400762]

[39]   Mainster MA. Decreasing retinal photocoagulation damage: principles and techniques. Semin Ophthalmol 1999; 14(4): 200-9.
[http://dx.doi.org/10.3109/08820539909069538] [PMID: 10758220]

[40]   Nicolò M, Musetti D, Traverso CE. Yellow micropulse laser in diabetic macular edema: a short-term pilot study. Eur J Ophthalmol 2014; 24(6): 885-9.
[http://dx.doi.org/10.5301/ejo.5000495] [PMID: 24905254]

[41]   Kwon YH, Lee DK, Kwon OW. The short-term efficacy of subthreshold Micropulse yellow (577-nm) laser photocoagulation for diabetic macular edema. Korean J Ophthalmol 2014; 28(5): 379-85.
[http://dx.doi.org/10.3341/kjo.2014.28.5.379] [PMID: 25276079]

[42]   Suñer IJ, Peden MC, Hammer ME, Grizzard WS, Traynom J, Cousins SW. RaScaL: a pilot study to assess the efficacy, durability, and safety of a single intervention with ranibizumab plus peripheral laser for diabetic macular edema associated with peripheral nonperfusion on ultrawide-field fluorescein angiography. Ophthalmologica 2014.
[PMID: 25427532]

[43]   Brown DM, Ou WC, Wong TP, Kim RY, Croft DE, Wykoff CC. DAVE study group. Targeted retinal photocoagulation for diabetic macular edema with peripheral retinal nonperfusion: three-year randomized DAVE trial. Ophthalmology 2018; 125(5): 683-90.
[http://dx.doi.org/10.1016/j.ophtha.2017.11.026] [PMID: 29336896]

[44]   Diabetic Retinopathy Clinical Research Network. A randomized trial comparing intravitreal

triamcinolone acetonide and focal/grid photocoagulation for diabetic macular edema. Ophthalmology 2008; 115(9): 1447-1449, 1449.e1-1449.e10.
[http://dx.doi.org/10.1016/j.ophtha.2008.06.015] [PMID: 18662829]

[45]   Chew E, Strauber S, Beck R, *et al.* Diabetic Retinopathy Clinical Research Network. Randomized trial of peribulbar triamcinolone acetonide with and without focal photocoagulation for mild diabetic macular edema: a pilot study. Ophthalmology 2007; 114(6): 1190-6.
[http://dx.doi.org/10.1016/j.ophtha.2007.02.010] [PMID: 17544778]

[46]   Jonas JB, Spandau UH, Kamppeter BA, Vossmerbaeumer U, Harder B, Sauder G. Repeated intravitreal high-dosage injections of triamcinolone acetonide for diffuse diabetic macular edema. Ophthalmology 2006; 113(5): 800-4.
[http://dx.doi.org/10.1016/j.ophtha.2006.01.002] [PMID: 16530840]

[47]   Boyer DS, Yoon YH, Belfort R Jr, *et al.* Ozurdex MEAD Study Group. Three-year, randomized, sham-controlled trial of dexamethasone intravitreal implant in patients with diabetic macular edema. Ophthalmology 2014; 121(10): 1904-14.
[http://dx.doi.org/10.1016/j.ophtha.2014.04.024] [PMID: 24907062]

[48]   Campochiaro PA, Brown DM, Pearson A, *et al.* FAME Study Group. Sustained delivery fluocinolone acetonide vitreous inserts provide benefit for at least 3 years in patients with diabetic macular edema. Ophthalmology 2012; 119(10): 2125-32.
[http://dx.doi.org/10.1016/j.ophtha.2012.04.030] [PMID: 22727177]

[49]   Cunha-Vaz J, Ashton P, Iezzi R, *et al.* FAME Study Group. Sustained delivery fluocinolone acetonide vitreous implants: long-term benefit in patients with chronic diabetic macular edema. Ophthalmology 2014; 121(10): 1892-903.
[http://dx.doi.org/10.1016/j.ophtha.2014.04.019] [PMID: 24935282]

[50]   Flaxel CJ, Edwards AR, Aiello LP, *et al.* Factors associated with visual acuity outcomes after vitrectomy for diabetic macular edema: diabetic retinopathy clinical research network. Retina 2010; 30(9): 1488-95.
[http://dx.doi.org/10.1097/IAE.0b013e3181e7974f] [PMID: 20924264]

[51]   Haller JA, Qin H, Apte RS, *et al.* Diabetic Retinopathy Clinical Research Network Writing Committee. Vitrectomy outcomes in eyes with diabetic macular edema and vitreomacular traction. Ophthalmology 2010; 117(6): 1087-1093.e3.
[http://dx.doi.org/10.1016/j.ophtha.2009.10.040] [PMID: 20299105]

[52]   Simunovic MP, Hunyor AP, Ho I-V. Vitrectomy for diabetic macular edema: a systematic review and meta-analysis. Can J Ophthalmol 2014; 49(2): 188-95.
[http://dx.doi.org/10.1016/j.jcjo.2013.11.012] [PMID: 24767227]

[53]   Chhablani JK, Kim JS, Cheng L, Kozak I, Freeman W. External limiting membrane as a predictor of visual improvement in diabetic macular edema after pars plana vitrectomy. Graefes Arch Clin Exp Ophthalmol 2012; 250(10): 1415-20.
[http://dx.doi.org/10.1007/s00417-012-1968-x] [PMID: 22354371]

[54]   Rndings DRS, Number DRSR. The Diabetic Retinopathy Study Research Group. Photocoagulation treatment of proliferative diabetic retinopathy. Clinical application of Diabetic Retinopathy Study (DRS) findings, DRS Report Number 8. Ophthalmology 1981; 88(7): 583-600.
[PMID: 7196564]

[55]   Jorge R, Costa RA, Calucci D, Cintra LP, Scott IU. Intravitreal bevacizumab (Avastin) for persistent new vessels in diabetic retinopathy (IBEPE study). Retina 2006; 26(9): 1006-13.
[http://dx.doi.org/10.1097/01.iae.0000246884.76018.63] [PMID: 17151487]

[56]   Zhang Z-H, Liu H-Y, Hernandez-Da Mota SE, *et al.* Vitrectomy with or without preoperative intravitreal bevacizumab for proliferative diabetic retinopathy: a meta-analysis of randomized controlled trials. Am J Ophthalmol 2013; 156(1): 106-115.e2.
[http://dx.doi.org/10.1016/j.ajo.2013.02.008] [PMID: 23791371]

[57] Spaide RF, Fisher YL. Intravitreal bevacizumab (Avastin) treatment of proliferative diabetic retinopathy complicated by vitreous hemorrhage. Retina 2006; 26(3): 275-8.
[http://dx.doi.org/10.1097/00006982-200603000-00004] [PMID: 16508426]

[58] Gross JG, Glassman AR, Jampol LM, *et al.* Writing committee for the diabetic retinopathy clinical research network. Panretinal photocoagulation *vs* intravitreous ranibizumab for proliferative diabetic retinopathy: a randomized clinical trial. JAMA 2015; 314(20): 2137-46.
[http://dx.doi.org/10.1001/jama.2015.15217] [PMID: 26565927]

[59] Gross JG, Glassman AR, Liu D, *et al.* Diabetic retinopathy clinical research network. Five-year outcomes of panretinal photocoagulation *vs* intravitreous ranibizumab for proliferative diabetic retinopathy: a randomized clinical trial. JAMA Ophthalmol 2018; 136(10): 1138-48.
[http://dx.doi.org/10.1001/jamaophthalmol.2018.3255] [PMID: 30043039]

CHAPTER 12

Future Direction in Diabetic Eye Disease

Gautam Vangipuram[*] and **Gaurav K. Shah**

The Retina Institute, Saint Louis, Missouri, USA

Abstract: Diabetic retinopathy is one of the leading causes of vision loss worldwide and its incidence is only projected to increase. Much effort has been dedicated to investigating new therapies and drug delivery approach in treating its complications, diabetic macular edema (DME) and proliferative diabetic retinopathy (PDR). Although anti-vascular endothelial growth factor (VEGF) has gained popularity in treatment for DR, patients who respond poorly to intravitreal injections have prompted the search for additional pathogenic pathways and thus therapeutic targets that may better control disease activity. These novel therapies, including various anti-angiogenic agents, growth factor inhibitors, integrin inhibitors, sustained delivery platforms, gene therapy, chemokine and other inflammatory inhibitors, and neuroprotective agents, are currently being evaluated for the management of DR. Optimal treatment paradigms in the management of PDR are also under investigation.

Keywords: Anti-VEGF, Angiogenic, Cytokine, Complications, DME, Diabetes, Integrin, Implant, Laser, Neovascularization, Proliferative, Retinopathy, Steroid, Target, Therapeutic.

INTRODUCTION

Diabetic retinopathy (DR) remains the leading cause of blindness among working-age individuals in developed countries. Unfortunately, given current demographic trends in population and obesity, the disease shows no sign of remission . As of 2013, the estimated incidence of diabetic macular edema (DME) disease worldwide has affected 26 million individuals and is expected to increase to 40 million by 2035 [1]. With DR being the most common complication of diabetes, vision-threatening conditions such as DME and proliferative diabetic retinopathy (PDR) have become a large portion of retinal subspecialty care [2]. The underlying pathogenesis of DR is still under investigation with vascular basement membrane thickening and pericyte loss leading to vascular permeability and capillary loss often cited as casual. However, multiple mechanisms to this disease have been postulated and are currently the target of novel treatment agents

[*] **Corresponding author Gautam Vangipuram:** The Retina Institute, Saint Louis, Missouri, USA; Tel: (314) 367-1181; Fax: (314) 968-5117; E-mail: gautam.vangipuram@gmail.com

(Fig. **1**). Therapies targeting alternative pathways responsible for promoting inflammation, including Ang2 and integrin, have shown early promise. Eventually with progressive non-perfusion, proliferative disease develops as a result of the release of Vascular Endothelial Growth Factor (VEGF) which leads to the development of neovascularization.

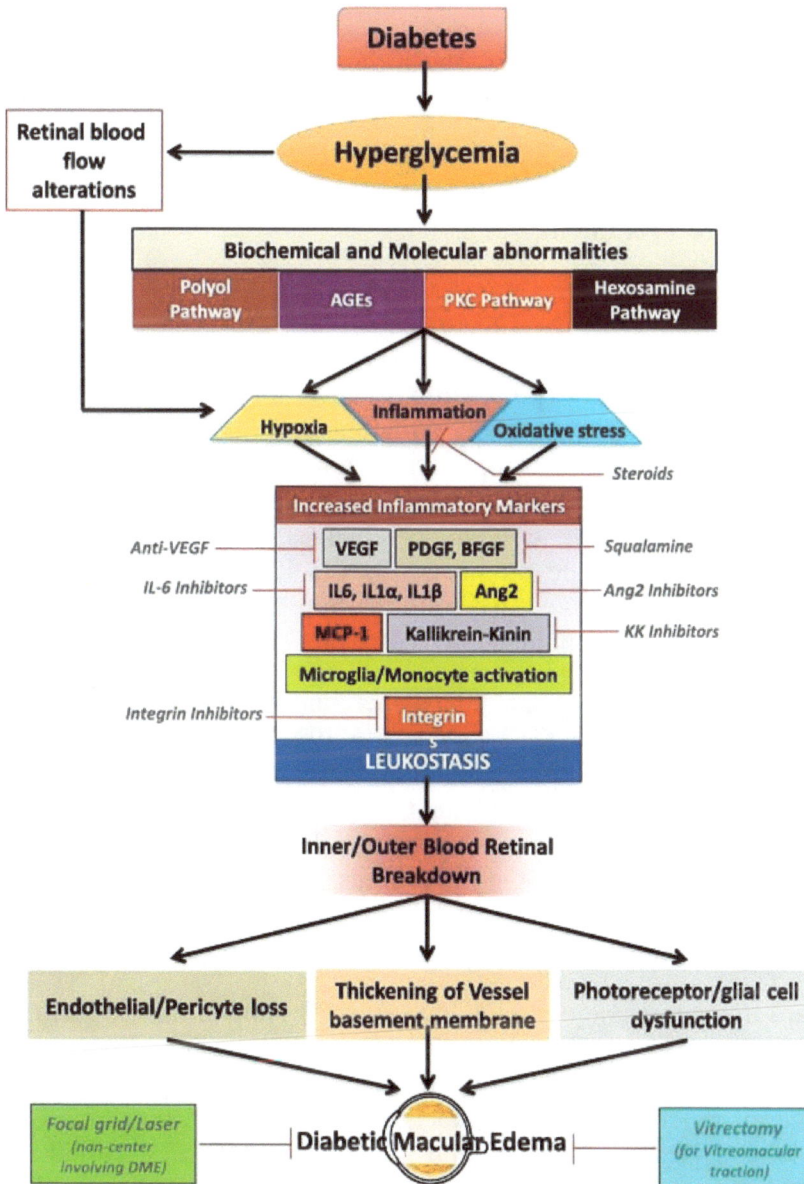

Fig. (1). Schematic pathway of pro-inflammatory cytokines and neovascular factors involved in the development of DME.[44] (Adapted from Urias EA *et al.*).

Current treatment for DR involves risk factor modification and working with a patient's primary care physician or endocrinologist to help manage blood sugar control and concomitant hypertension if present. In the treatment of DR, laser photocoagulation had been the mainstay of treatment for decades in managing both proliferative diabetic disease and diabetic macular edema (DME). With the advent of anti-VEGF agents, however, several randomized controlled studies have proven these medications as efficacious in some regards to the standard of care laser. Furthermore, exploration of the inflammatory mechanisms, combination therapy, and drug delivery platforms remains ongoing. The goal of this chapter is to briefly review current therapies and treatment modalities in diabetic retinopathy and discuss future directions in management.

Standard of Care Treatment

Addressing Risk Factors

Duration of diabetic disease is the main risk factor for developing DR along with poor glycemic control and hypertension, as several studies have investigated the effects of tight control over these parameters. Recently, there is increasing evidence to suggest diabetic complications may be linked by a series of faulty metabolic regulatory systems including oxidative stress, non-enzymatic glycosylation of proteins, epigenetic changes, and chronic inflammation producing a new "metabolic memory" [3, 47, 48]. Proponents of this theory, therefore, suggest aggressive early intervention once diabetes is diagnosed to restore the body's natural homeostasis.

In the United Kingdom Prospective Diabetes Study (UKPDS), intensive glycemic management in type 2 diabetes resulted in a 39% reduction in the risk for laser photocoagulation when compared with conventional glycemic control standards [3]. Similarly, the Diabetes Control and Complications Trial (DCCT) showed that tight glycemic control with insulin in type 1 diabetics reduced the risk of new retinopathy by 76% and decreased the progression of the existing disease by 54% [4]. It was recently reported that HbA1c maintenance below 7.6% may prevent PDR in type 1 diabetes for up to 20 years [5].

With regard to hypertension, the UKPDS study demonstrated a benefit in slowing DR progression by controlling blood pressure (systolic blood pressure <150 *vs.* <180 mmHg *vs.* standard control) using angiotensin-converting enzyme inhibitors or β-adrenergic blockers in type 2 diabetics [6]. In contrast, the Action in Diabetes and Vascular Disease: Preterax and Diamicron MR Controlled Evaluation (ADVANCE) and Action to Control Cardiovascular Risk in Diabetes (ACCORD) trials showed equivocal results for retinopathy with intensive management of blood pressure [7, 8]. Importantly, the UKPDS study required a baseline hypertension diagnosis to be enrolled in the blood pressure control group and the duration of follow-up was twice as long as the ADVANCE or ACCORD trials.

In the Early Treatment Diabetic Retinopathy Study (ETDRS), diabetic patients with diffuse edema, hard exudates, and poor response to laser had higher blood lipid levels [8]. The Fenofibrate Intervention and Event Lowering in Diabetes (FIELD) and ACCORD studies have shown that fenofibrate reduces DR progression in type II diabetes [9, 10]. In the FIELD study, 9795 patients aged 50–75 years with type 2 diabetes mellitus were randomly assigned to receive fenofibrate 200 mg/day (n=4895) or matching placebo (n=4900). The requirement for first laser treatment for all retinopathy was significantly lower in the fenofibrate group than in the placebo group (164 [3.4%] patients on fenofibrate *vs* 238 [4.9%] on placebo; hazard ratio [HR] 0.69, 95% CI 0·56–0·84; p=0·0002]). The mechanism-of-action driving this effect is thought to be due to the anti-inflammatory, anti-oxidant, anti-angiogenic, and anti-apoptotic capabilities of fenofibrate [10].

Anti-Vascular Endothelial Growth Factor (VEGF) Therapy

Laser photocoagulation remains the mainstay treatment for PDR and focal/grid laser remained a popular option for DME after the results of the ETDRS study. However, after the results of DRCR Protocol I showed superiority in visual acuity outcomes of Ranibizumab plus prompt or deferred laser *vs.* focal laser or triamcinolone, the popularity of anti-VEGF agents in managing DME has dramatically increased. DRCR Protocol T compared three anti-VEGF agents: ranibizumab (Lucentis, Genentech, San Francisco, CA), bevacizumab (Avastin, Genentech, San Francisco, CA), and aflibercept (Eylea, Regeneron, Tarrytown, NY), and showed no difference in visual acuity at 2 years among these three agents in eyes with visual acuity 20/40 or better. However, aflibercept was statistically more effective in improving vision compared to ranibizumab when baseline vision was 20/50 or worse at the 2 year mark [11]. Despite the promising results of anti-VEGF therapy for DME, treatment non-responders make up a minority of patients and alternative therapies are, at times, beneficial. Consideration of additional pathways besides those involving VEGF suppression may be essential for effective treatment in these eyes. In particular, the use of intravitreal anti-inflammatory therapy including triamcinolone, dexamethasone, and fluocinolone acetonide has shown promising results [11, 20]. The role of anti-VEGF in PDR has also expanded dramatically and will be discussed later in this chapter.

Anti-Inflammatory Therapy

Inflammation is known to play a key role in the pathogenesis of DR and studies have shown elevated cytokine and chemokine levels in eyes with DME [12]. The efficacy of intravitreal corticosteroids has been evaluated in studies such as DRCR Protocol I, a randomized controlled trial comparing focal/grid photocoagulation alone or with combined intravitreal injection of ranibizumab or intravitreal triamcinolone (IVTA) in patients with center-involving DME. Combined IVTA and laser significantly reduced central subfield thickness on optical coherence tomography at 12 months, but there was no significant improvement in visual acuity compared with laser alone, a phenomenon attributed to cataract formation [11]. Sub-analysis of pseudophakic patients showed the triamcinolone plus laser group was equivalent to the ranibizumab treatment group and superior to laser alone.

The benefit of steroids for DME has been further explored in several randomized clinical trials involving the dexamethasone and fluocinolone acetonide (FCa) intravitreal implants. In a large multicenter study of 1048 patients, dexamethasone intravitreal implants at two doses (0.7mg, 0.35 mg) were compared to sham injection over a 3 year study period. The percentage of patients with ≥15-letter improvement in BCVA from baseline at the study endpoint was greater with 0.7 mg (22.2%) and 0.35 mg (18.4%) than sham (12.0%; $P \leq 0.018$.). Although visual improvement was reported with both implants at low and high doses, cataract formation (64.1-69.7%) and increases in intraocular pressure (IOP) were common complications [13]. FCa is also an FDA approved intravitreal implant for DME with a theoretical advantage of longer duration of effect. However, given the higher incidence of IOP rise resulting in glaucoma surgery with fluocinolone, the FDA has approved a 0.19mg fluocinolone acetonide intravitreal implant for DME patients who have undergone a trial of corticosteroids without a steroid response. In an open-label, single-center, Phase IV study investigating the efficacy and safety of fluocinolone intravitreal implantation in chronic DME patients with insufficient response to laser and anti-VEGF, clinically significant reduction of central subfield thickness was noted compared with laser alone at 12 months. Furthermore, pseudophakic patients saw a clinically significant gain of visual activity 1 year after treatment and only 1 of 17 eyes had an elevated IOP >30mmHg that was treated medically [14].

Due to the side effects, including cataract formation and IOP rise, intravitreal steroids are often reserved as second-line treatment after a series of anti-VEGF injections fail or inadequately improve DME. In current practice, however, a combination of both steroids and anti-VEGF agents may be required to attain proper control of disease activity.

Because of the proven effect using steroids, non-steroidal anti-inflammatory (NSAID) agents have been investigated as potential drugs for the treatment of DME. Studies have suggested that high doses of aspirin may slow the progression of DR [15]; however, the ETDRS results did not find any benefit of aspirin in preventing vision loss in DME or severe non-PDR [16]. Additionally, DRCR Protocol R did not show a significant difference in visual outcomes at 1 year for patients with non-center involving DME treated with nepafenac 0.1% eye drops [17]. A summary of these various agents is shown in Table **1**.

Table 1. Anti-inflammatory medications currently approved for the use in diabetic retinopathy.

Drug	Target/Mechanism	Route of Administration	Clinical Development
Anti-Inflammatory			
Steroids	**Inhibits Action of Inflammatory Mediators, Induces Anti-Inflammatory Mediators**		
Triamcinolone	(above as steroid)	Intravitreal injection	Phase III; FDA approved
Dexamethasone	(above as steroid)	Intravitreal implant	Phase III; FDA approved
Fluocinolone acetonide	(above as steroid)	Intravitreal implant	Phase III; FDA approved
NSAIDS	**Inhibit Cyclooxygenase (COX) Activity, Decreases Prostaglandins & Thromboxanes**		
Aspirin	COX-1 & 2	Oral	ETDRS, DAMAD
Nepafenac	COX-1 & 2	Topical	Phase III; FDA approved

New Therapeutic Strategies for DME

Over the past decade, much focus has been on developing more potent agents targeting the VEGF pathway in treating DME. However, recent evidence in non-VEGF responders has led to a multimodal approach in treating DME that may require inhibition of multiple signaling pathways. Here we briefly discuss the novel agents and delivery platforms on the horizon in treating DME (Table **2**).

Table 2. Novel pharmaceutical therapies and drug delivery mechanisms in the treatment of DME.

Drug	Target/Mechanism	Route of Administration	Clinical Development	Outcomes
Anti-Vascular Endothelial Growth Factor				
Brolucizumab	VEGF	Intravitreal	Phase III	FDA approved for AMD
Faricimab	VEGF, Ang2	Intravitreal	Phase III	Phase II trial BOULEVARD: DME patients treated with 6mg of faricimab had a mean improvement of 13.9 letters at 24 weeks compared to 10.3 for ranibizumab control eyes (p=0.03) [19].
Conbercept	VEGF	Intravitreal	Approved in China, currently preclinical in US	Retrospective study of 107 patients with DME, mean improvement in best corrected visual acuity and central macular thickness improved compared to untreated controls at 12 months [20].
OPT 302	VEGF (C&D)	Intravitreal	Phase Ib/IIa	Early results from 35 eyes show an improvement in the combination therapy group *vs.* monotherapy group (+6.6 letters and +3.4 letters, respectively) with a favorable safety profile [21].
Port Delivery System	VEGF	Intravitreal	Phase III	Awaiting q24 week PAGODA results evaluating ranibizumab through PDS *vs.* monthly intravitreal 0.5 mg ranibizumab for patients with center involving DME.
AAV Gene Therapy	VEGF	Intravitreal, suprachoroidal, subretinal	Phase II	Awaiting phase I/IIa study results RGX-314) on gene therapy vector for neovascular AMD.
Inhibition of Other Growth Factors				
Src kinase inhibitor (TG 100081)	VEGF, PDGF, bFGF	Topical	Preclinical	

(Table 2) cont.....

Drug	Target/Mechanism	Route of Administration	Clinical Development	Outcomes
PF-655	RTP801 gene (small interfering RNA)	Intravitreal	Phase II (DEGAS & MATISSE). Did not meet phase III endpoint critieria	PF-04523655 3-mg group showed a trend for greater improvement in BCVA from baseline than laser (respectively 5.77 *vs.* 2.39 letters; P = 0.08 [45]
iCo-007	cRAF kinase mRNA blocks VEGF, IGF-1, HGF	Intravitreal	Phase II	Phase II trial terminated due to lack of efficacy in meeting clinical endpoint.
Teprotumumab	IGF-1 receptor	Intravenous	FDA approved for TED	Phase I open label study completed for DME. Awaiting initiation to phase II.
Inhibition of Inflammatory Response				
THR-149-001	pKAL	Intravitreal	Phase I	In 12 subjects, an average improvement of 6.4 ETDRS letters was noted after one injection of THR-149-001 with no reported dose limiting toxicity [26].
THR-687	Integrin pathway	Intravitreal	Phase I	Twelve patients with rescue ranibizumab and aflibercept as needed, mean BCVA improvement was 8.3 letters following a single injection of THR-687 [27].
OCS-01	Steroid	Topical	Phase II	In a study of 133 patients randomize to OCS-01 *vs.* control, a decrease in average CMT at 12 weeks compared to vehicle control (-53.6 μm *vs* -16.8 μm, P=.0115) was observed.
Risuteganib	Integrin pathway	Intravitreal	Phase II	Ina a sub-analysis of patients with prior-VEGF treatment, risuteganib performed much better control therapy with an improvement of 8.4 letters to 5.8 letters respectively [29].

(Table 2) cont.....

Drug	Target/Mechanism	Route of Administration	Clinical Development	Outcomes
AKB-9778	Ang2	Sub-cutaneous, topical	Phase II	In a randomized phase II study, 35.4% and 20.8% of study eyes gained ≥ 10 or ≥ 15 letters, respectively in the combination group compared to 29.8% and 17.0% respectively in the ranibizumab monotherapy group [1].
Xipere™	Steroid	Suprachoroidal	Phase II	Fewer treatment visits (2.8 visits *vs.* 4.7 visits) and similar BCVA improvement (12.3 letters *vs.* 13.5 letters) was noted in the combination treatment *vs.* monotherapy group at 24 weeks [30].
Photobiomodulation	Near-infrared light, multiple targets	Patch	Pilot	Pending
Doxycycline	Microglia, MMP	Oral	Phase II	mean BCVA improved continuously from baseline at 1, 2, 4, and 6 months by +1.0, +4.0, +4.0, and +5.8 letters, respectively, while mean retinal thickness (CST) on OCT decreased by −2.9%, −5.7%, −13.9, and −8.1% for the same time points.
Neurodegeneration and Other Potential Targets				
Somatostatin	Neuroprotection *via* survival signaling	Topical	Phase II/III	Topical treatment with somatostatin and brimonidine seems not useful for preventing the development of neurodegeneration, at least in a period of 2 years of follow-up. However, these neuroprotective treatments are effective in arresting the progression in those patients in whom some degree of neurodegeneration is already present [37].

FUTURE DIRECTIONS IN ANTI-VEGF

Brolucizumab

Brolucizumab (Novartis, RTH 258) is a humanized single-chain antibody fragment designed to inhibit VEGF-A. Due to its relatively small size (molecular weight: 26KD) compared to other anti-VEGF agents such as bevacizumab (molecular weight: 149 KD), it has a much higher dosing per volume of drug injected. The drug has shown promise in the treatment of neovascular AMD after two large phase III trials (HAWK, HARRIER) showed non-inferiority of visual endpoints at 48 weeks with q12 week dosing compared to q8 week aflibercept in roughly 50% of patients [18]. After FDA approval, the drug has failed to gain traction in the AMD marketplace however, due to its higher rates of intraocular inflammation. In an analysis of the 1088 patients enrolled in the HAWK/HARRIER studies, the overall rate of intraocular inflammation was 4.6% (50/1088) and an overall rate of 3.3% (36/1088) of retinal vasculitis. The role of brolucizumab in DME is currently being investigated in phase III KESTREL and KINGFISHER studies, assessing the efficacy and safety of brolucizumab *vs.* aflibercept in patients with diabetic macular edema.

Faricimab

The combination anti-VEGF-A and Ang-2 inhibitor drug, Abicipar, has shown promising results in early clinical trials. Ang-2 works through Tie2 receptor mediated tyrosine kinase to promote vessel destabilization and vascular leakage. In its phase II trial, BOULEVARD, patients treated with 6mg of faricimab had a mean improvement of 13.9 letters at 24 weeks compared to 10.3 for ranibizumab control eyes (p=0.03) [19]. Recently, enrollment has been completed on the phase III portion (YOSEMITE and RHINE) of this drug, which aims to be the largest prospective randomized control trial for DME.

Conbercept

Conbercept (KH902, Chengdu Kanghong Biotech Co, Ltd, Sichuan, China) is an engineered fusion protein of the extracellular domain 2 of VEGFr1 and extracellular domains 3 and 4 of VEGFr2 fused to the Fc portion of human IgG1. Its multitude of extracellular domains improve its binding affinity comparted to that of its anti-VEGF counterparts. The drug was approved in China for use in neovascular AMD in 2013 and DME in 2019. Studies on this medication for DME are limited to retrospective trials but have shown early promising results. In a 2018 study of 107 patients with DME, mean improvement in best corrected visual acuity and central macular thickness improved compared to untreated controls at 12 months in those with poor baseline initial acuity (8.0±15.0 letters *vs*

−4.0±6.0 letters, P<0.001, −212.8±11.9 *vs* −44.3±35.3 μm, P<0.001, respectively) [20]. Randomized clinical trials are underway in the United States for conbercept in the treatment of neovascular AMD, with plans to initiate similar trials for DME.

OPT-302

OPT-302 blocks the binding of VEGF-C and VEGF-D to its receptor VEGFR-3. Downstream activation of VEGFR-3 has been observed in response to upregulation of VEGF-A in diabetic retinopathy. It has been postulated that combination therapy of OPT-302 with aflibercept in a single intravitreal injection may produce broad downstream inactivation of the entire VEGF/PGF pathway. Currently, a phase Ib/IIa randomized clinical control trial is underway looking at combination OPT-302/aflibercept therapy compared to aflibercept/sham in previous treatment non-responders. Early results from 35 eyes show an improvement in the combination therapy group *vs.* monotherapy group (+6.6 letters and +3.4 letters, respectively) with a favorable safety profile [21].

Port Delivery System (PDS)

In addition to molecules targeting the VEGF pathway, novel systems are being investigated as to how most efficiently and safely deliver medications. The Port Delivery System (PDS, Genentech, Inc., South San Francisco, California) (Fig. **2**) is a permanent refillable silicone-coated implant designed to elute specific doses of anti-VEGF medication into the vitreous cavity. The hope is that through an implantable device, a large reservoir of medication can be stored in the implant as a depot, reducing patient treatment burden. A phase II dose escalation study (LADDER) of 220 patients with neovascular AMD showed comparable visual acuity results in a 100mg/ml PDS dosage of ranibizumab compared to monthly 0.5 ml injections with a median time to first refill of 15 (11.9-16.9 months, 80% CI) months [22]. Currently, a phase 3 randomized clinical trial (PAGODA) is actively recruiting in comparing q24 week ranibizumab through a PDS *vs.* monthly intravitreal 0.5 mg ranibizumab for patients with center involving DME.

Gene Therapy

Several gene therapy candidates have emerged as viable candidates in the treatment of DME. The concept involves intravitreal or subretinal delivery of an attenuated viral particle designed to deliver a gene therapy vector to retinal tissue, which in turn produces the encoded protein. Regenxbio (Rockville, MD) has begun phase I/IIa studies (RGX-314) on its gene therapy vector for neovascular AMD which is delivered either subretinal or suprachoroidal, and in turn produces a monocloncal antibody fragment mimicking ranibizumab in structure and function [23]. Plans are underway for phase II trials in patients with DME. ADVM-022 (Adverum Biotechnologies, Redwood City, CA) is a similar attenuated adenovirus vector encoding the cDNA of aflibercept protein. Its advantage is it can be delivered intravitreally, avoiding a potential operating room visit. A phase II study (INFINITY) is currently underway comparing visual and anatomical outcomes after one-time intravitreal injection of ADVM-022 *vs.* aflibercept.

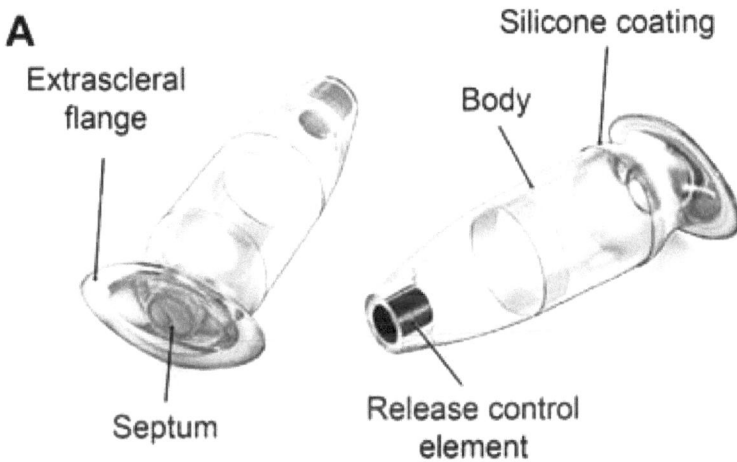

Fig. (2). Refillable Port Delivery System (PDS, Genentech, Inc., South San Francisco, California) used in LADDER and PAGODA clinical trials studies for treatment of neovascular AMD and DME, respectively.

Growth Factor Inhibition

The protein inhibitor targeting Src kinase (TG 100081), small interrupting RNA targeting RTP801 (PF-655; Quark Pharmeceuticals, Fremont, CA), and anti-sense inhibitor of C-raf kinase mRNA (iCo-007, iCo Therapeutics, Vancouver BC, Canada) have all shown success in reducing VEGF-associated vascular permeability in animal models. Of these, PF-655 has had several phase II studies (DEGAS and MATISSE) currently showing that the drug is safe, well tolerated, and may have a dose-related effect on improving visual acuity [24]. Likewise, intraocular insulin-like growth factor-1 (IGF-1) has been linked to blood-retina--barrier breakdown and vascular permeability [25, 26]. The IFG-1 receptor blocker teprotumumab (Genmab, Princeton, NJ) has been developed as an intravenous infusion and recently FDA approved for thyroid eye disease associated inflammation. It is currently in an open-label phase I trial being examined for its safety and efficacy in DME patients [27]. Overall, the results of these studies have not been as promising as their anti-VEGF or steroidal counterparts and further investigation is needed.

Inflammatory Response Inhibition

Though molecules targeting VEGFa have without doubt improved visual and functional outcomes in the treatment of DME, up to 40% of patients with this disease treated with anti-VEGF agents demonstrate a sub-optimal improvement in BCVA [11]. Thus evaluation of independent mechanisms outside of VEGF suppression are needed to adequately manage DME. Steroid-mediated inhibition of inflammation has been extensively investigated with several FDA approved medications for the treatment of DME. However, several other medications in the pipeline have shown promising results and are discussed here.

THR-149-001

THR-149 (Oxurion, NV) is a plasma Kallikrein (pKal) inhibitor with phase I data published on safety and efficacy in DME. The pKal/Kinin system has been found to be upregulated in patients with DR and preclinical models show this pathway to mediate vascular hyperpermeability, leukostasis, inflammation, and micro-hemorrhages. Importantly, vitreous levels of pKal have been shown to be independently elevated of VEGF, providing a potential pharmacological target in treatment non-responders. In a phase I dose escalation study of 12 subjects, an average improvement of 6.4 ETDRS letters was noted after one injection of THR-149-001 with no reported dose limiting toxicity. Plans are underway to advance to phase II clinic trial (KALAHARI) in the near future [26].

THR-687

THR-687 (Oxurion, NV) is a novel intravitreal pan-RGD integrin antagonist designed for the treatment of DME. Integrin receptors have been postulated to be involved in angiogenesis, inflammation, and vascular permeability both upstream and downstream of VEGF. In a phase I dose escalation study of 12 patients with rescue ranibizumab and aflibercept as needed, mean BCVA improvement was 8.3 letters following a single injection of THR-687 [27]. No significant adverse events or dose-related toxicity was noted in this initial study. Plans for a phase II clinical trial is currently underway.

OCS-01

The topical medicine OCS-01 (Oculis, Switzerland) incorporates a novel solubilizing nanoparticle technology to increase tear film solubility of its medication, dexamethasone, to decrease rapid tear film removal and promote delivery to the posterior segment. Though the utility of dexamethasone implant has been previously reported on in DME, the advantage of OCS-01 is its topical delivery and rapid on-off effect in terms of visual acuity and intraocular pressure fluctuations. In a prospective, multi-center, randomized, double-masked, parallel group, vehicle-controlled study phase II clinic study, a total of 133 patients with DME were randomized to OCS-01 topical therapy *vs.* control three times daily for 12 weeks followed by a 4 week washout period. Patients in the OCS-01 arm showed a decrease in average CMT at 12 weeks compared to vehicle control (-53.6 μm *vs* -16.8 μm, P=.0115). Furthermore, mean CMT worsened in the 4 week washout period in the OCS-01 arm with no significant change in control eyes. As expected, a mean IOP rise of 4.53 mmHg was seen in the OCS-01 arm at 12 weeks, however, this effect was almost totally mitigated in the washout period (0.35 mmHg) [28]. Further comparative studies are needed with this novel topical vehicle to standard of care steroid monotherapy including dexamethasone and fluocinolone.

Risuteganib

Risuteganib (Allegro Ophthalmics, San Juan Capistrano, CA) is a novel integrin inhibitor responsible for blocking a multitude of downstream pathways involved in vascular permeability and oxidative stress seen in DME. Animal models have shown risuteganib to have a complimentary role in VEGF suppression as well. A Phase II study was conducted (DELMAR) comparing 80 patients with DME randomized to either sequential therapy with 3 monthly injections of risuteganib (following one anti-VEGF injection), combination therapy, or monotherapy with bevacizumab (control arm). The study arm was not given any injections after the initial three study doses for the following 12 weeks. At 20 weeks, the mean improvement in BCVA was 7.1 letters for the study arm and 6.7 letters for the control arm. Interestingly, in a sub-analysis of patients with prior-VEGF treatment, risuteganib performed much better to the control with an improvement of 8.4 letters to 5.8 letters respectively [29]. The data may indicate that some patients have more profound VEGF mediated disease while others with DME may benefit with therapy through another mechanism.

AKB-9778 Tie2 Mediators

As previously mentioned, the modulation of vascular permeability in DME is regulated by a host of cytokines other than VEGF. Phosphorylation of the Tie2 receptor has been shown to suppress vascular leakage in mouse models with DME and neovascular AMD. (6). A recent phase IIa clinical study looked at subcutaneous AKB-9778 monotherapy or in combination with ranibizumab *vs.* ranibizumab therapy alone in 144 patients with DME. The main outcome measure was a change in central subfield thickness, with visual acuity and adverse events also investigated. At 12 weeks, mean change from baseline CST was significantly greater in the combination group (164.4 ± 24.2 mm) compared with the ranibizumab monotherapy group (110.4 ± 17.2 mm; P = 0.008). Furthermore, 35.4% and 20.8% of study eyes gained ≥ 10 or ≥ 15 letters, respectively in the combination group compared to 29.8% and 17.0% respectively in the ranibizumab monotherapy group [1]. Unfortunately, the endpoint for this drug formulation was not met in the Phase IIb trial and topical formulations are currently being developed in conjunction with anti-VEGF agents.

Xipere™

Xipere™ (Clearside Biomedical, Alpharetta, GA) is a patented suspension of corticosteroid triamcinolone acetonide designed to be delivered to the suprachoroidal space by an in-office procedure. The benefit to this delivery platform is its sustained release thereby decreasing the injection or medication administration burden of the patient. A phase II clinical trial (TYBEE) comparing suprachoroidal triamcinolone injection plus aflibercept to aflibercept monotherapy has been completed. Fewer treatment visits (2.8 visits *vs.* 4.7 visits) and similar BCVA improvement (12.3 letters *vs.* 13.5 letters) was noted in the combination treatment *vs.* monotherapy group at 24 weeks [30]. The delivery platform is in the stages of pursuing phase III clinical trials, which have already shown promising results in the treatment of non-infectious uveitis.

Photobiomodulation (PBM)

The DRCR.net is conducting an ongoing pilot study on photobiomodulation in the treatment of DME (Protocol AE). Far-red/near-infrared light (630-900 nm) has been shown in multiple in vitro and animal models to restore the function of damaged mitochondria and upregulate the production of cytoprotective factors. In diabetic mouse models, daily 4-minute treatment with PBM has been shown to reduce retinal ganglion cell apoptosis and improve photopic b-wave function on ERG. Study subjects will be asked to wear a PBM patch device twice daily for 90 seconds while still receiving standard of care therapy for DME. Results detailing changes *vs.* control in CST and BCVA are expected in 2021.

Targeting Neurodegeneration and Other Potential Targets

In addition to inflammation, a neurodegenerative mechanism has also been implicated as a contributing factor in early DR retinopathy [31]. Growing evidence highlighting lower intravitreal levels of somatostatin (SST) in both PDR and DME [32 - 34] suggests that replacing this down-regulated neuroprotective factor may be helpful. Previously, two pilot studies reported that patients with severe NPDR or early PDR receiving intramuscular administration of somatostatin analogs were less likely to require pan-retinal photocoagulation and had fewer vitreous hemorrhages, thus preserving visual acuity [35, 36]. A

European phase II/III study has looked at the effects of topical somatostatin and brimonidine, another known neuroprotective substance, in patients with NPDR with modest results [37].

Future Treatment Strategies for Proliferative Diabetic Retinopathy (PDR)

Since the seminal Diabetic Retinopathy Study (DRS) published in 1981 showing eyes treated with pan-retinal photocoagulation had a 50% reduction in severe vision loss (>5/200) at 5 years, laser therapy has become the mainstay for the proliferative disease [38]. Its advantages include its durability, cost, and relatively low treatment burden. The downsides include loss of peripheral vision, decreased dark adaption, need for patient cooperation and more rarely risk of pupillary dilation and cystoid macular edema. With the advent of anti-VEGF medications and the effect seen not only on improving DME but in dramatically regressing neovascularization, a growing amount of practitioners have incorporated anti-VEGF medications into their practice patterns for managing PDR. Finally, pars plana vitrectomy for non-clearing vitreous hemorrhage also has a place in the management of non-clearing vitreous hemorrhage associated with PDR; the optimal timing of surgery remains under investigation. Though these three modalities, laser photocoagulation, anti-VEGF therapy, and vitrectomy are likely to remain in the forefront of PDR management for the foreseeable future, the optimal effectively of each or combination therapy is widely debated. Here we touch briefly on updates to treatment strategies in PDR.

Protocol S

The DRCR.net conducted both two and five-year investigational analyses on treatment regimens of initial monthly ranibizumab *vs.* PRP in patients with PDR (Protocol S). The primary outcome measure was mean change in visual acuity with secondary outcome measures, including peripheral visual field, development of macular edema and vitreous hemorrhage and need for vitrectomy. Initial 2-year results showed surprising durability of anti-VEGF therapy, as these eyes had on average a 0.5 line BCVA improvement compared to those receiving PRP. In addition, the peripheral vision was largely persevered in these patients compared to PRP treated eyes. The 5-year analysis however showed similar visual improvement in both the ranibizumab and PRP treated groups. Interestingly, though still statistically significant, the change in cumulative visual field total point score in the ranibizumab treated group approached that of PRP eyes (−330 (645) dB *vs* −527 (635) dB, respectively, P = 0.04) [39]. This decrease in visual field signal in the anti-VEGF group may indicate the growing peripheral ischemic burden throughout the disease course. A major caveat to the 5-year investigation is the percent of study completers—only 60% of participants (66% excluding deaths) were able to complete the 5-year study visit. Though this study gives credence to anti-VEGF agents' ability to manage PDR, its success largely hinges on patient compliance and follow-up. Nonetheless, in the appropriate patient population, anti-VEGF agents should be considered in the treatment of PDR.

Adjuvant Anti-VEGF Usage

Visualization of tractional membranes and fibrovascular proliferation during diabetic vitrectomy is crucial to ensuring anatomical success. Intraoperative hemorrhage during manipulation of membranes often occurs and can be managed to a certain degree with control of infusion pressure, systemic blood pressure control or endo-cautery. The use of adjuvant anti-VEGF prior to surgery has been advocated by some to induce regression of fibrovascular proliferation and decrease the incidence of intraoperative bleeding. Its use should be cautioned as several retrospective studies have demonstrated increased rates of tractional retinal detachment or so-called "crunch" phenomenon due to rapid membrane contraction. In a retrospective study of 211 intravitreal injections in PDR refractory to PRP, 11 eyes (5.2%) developed or had progression of TRD in an average of 13 days (range 3-31 days) [40]. Somewhat contradictory to this, a retrospective pooled analysis of PDR eyes in DRCR protocols I, J, N, S, and T found a 1-year cumulative probability of TRD 4.8% (95% confidence interval: 3.2%–7.3%, 22 events) *vs.* 6.8% (95% confidence interval:4.6%–9.9%, 25 events) in control-group eyes (hazard ratio = 0.95 [95% confidence interval:0.54–1.66, P = 0.86]) [41]. In general, if patient compliance is not a concern, anti-VEGF injection up to 1 week prior to planned vitrectomy is a reasonable course of action. More randomized prospective data is needed to determine the risk and incidence of fibrovascular contraction following anti-VEGF in this patient population.

Hybrid-Gauge Surgery

Small gauge (25 and 27) surgery has now come into vogue as the instrumentation package of choice for some vitreoretinal surgeons. In addition to smaller incisions and less chance of post-operative wound leak, small gauge instruments are extremely adept and dissecting delicate fibrovascular membranes and delaminating attachments from the retina. The use of a hybrid model (23 or 25 gauge trocars with 25 or 27 gauge instrumentation) is also of benefit. As reported by Walter *et al.*, this hybrid model allows for more surgical surface area accessible, as bending of the instruments with traditional small gauge trocars in minimized [42]. As with all novel surgical methods, the cost of this hybrid methodology must be taken into account during preoperative planning.

CONCLUSION

Diabetic retinopathy remains a challenging disease spectrum to manage for even the most seasoned retina specialist. However, the progress the field has made in the last few decades has been monumental in terms of preventing the severe visual consequences of the unmitigated disease. Medical management of this disease in the future will require a multi-modal approach in not only treating established pathways of VEGF and inflammatory mediated disease but a nuanced understanding of the broader pathology. Fortunately, several promising pharmaceutical and drug delivery options exist in the current DR pipeline. Input and observation from retina specialists will be crucial in the upcoming years to determine the proper use effectiveness of these agents. Surgical management in PDR has also evolved from the era of the Diabetic Retinopathy Vitrectomy Study (DRVS), which showed early vitrectomy (<6 months duration) was particularly advantageous for patients with type 1 diabetes [43]. With the advent of small gauge vitrectomy and adjunctive anti-VEGF, retina specialists have an armamentarium to tackle even the most complex pathology. We look forward to what the next iteration of advancements will bring in DR management.

CONSENT FOR PUBLICATION

Not applicable.

CONFLICT OF INTEREST

The author declares no conflict of interest, financial or otherwise.

ACKNOWLEDGEMENTS

The authors would like to thank photographer Elaine Gonzales of MidAtlantic Retina for the photographs in this chapter.

REFERENCES

[1] Campochiaro PA, Khanani A, Singer M, *et al.* Enhanced benefit in diabetic macular edema from AKB-9778 tie2 activation combined with vascular endothelial growth factor suppression. Ophthalmology 2016; 123(8): 1722-30.

[2] UK Prospective Diabetes Study (UKPDS) Group. Intensive blood-glucose control with sulphonylureas or insulin compared with conventional treatment and risk of complications in patients with type 2 diabetes (UKPDS 33). Lancet 1998; 352(9131): 837-53.
[http://dx.doi.org/10.1016/S0140-6736(98)07019-6] [PMID: 9742976]

[3] Nathan DM, Genuth S, Lachin J, *et al.* Diabetes Control and Complications Trial Research Group. The effect of intensive treatment of diabetes on the development and progression of long-term complications in insulin-dependent diabetes mellitus. N Engl J Med 1993; 329(14): 977-86.
[http://dx.doi.org/10.1056/NEJM199309303291401] [PMID: 8366922]

[4] Nordwall M, Abrahamsson M, Dhir M, Fredrikson M, Ludvigsson J, Arnqvist HJ. Impact of HbA1c,

followed from onset of type 1 diabetes, on the development of severe retinopathy and nephropathy: the VISS Study (Vascular Diabetic Complications in Southeast Sweden). Diabetes Care 2015; 38(2): 308-15.
[http://dx.doi.org/10.2337/dc14-1203] [PMID: 25510400]

[5] King P, Peacock I, Donnelly R. The UK prospective diabetes study (UKPDS): clinical and therapeutic implications for type 2 diabetes. Br J Clin Pharmacol 1999; 48(5): 643-8.
[http://dx.doi.org/10.1046/j.1365-2125.1999.00092.x] [PMID: 10594464]

[6] Beulens JWJ, Patel A, Vingerling JR, *et al.* AdRem project team; ADVANCE management committee. Effects of blood pressure lowering and intensive glucose control on the incidence and progression of retinopathy in patients with type 2 diabetes mellitus: a randomised controlled trial. Diabetologia 2009; 52(10): 2027-36.
[http://dx.doi.org/10.1007/s00125-009-1457-x] [PMID: 19633827]

[7] Chew EY, Ambrosius WT, Davis MD, *et al.* ACCORD Study Group; ACCORD Eye Study Group. Effects of medical therapies on retinopathy progression in type 2 diabetes. N Engl J Med 2010; 363(3): 233-44.
[http://dx.doi.org/10.1056/NEJMoa1001288] [PMID: 20587587]

[8] Chew EY, Klein ML, Ferris FL, Remaley NA, Murphy RP, Chantry K, *et al.* Association of elevated serum lipid levels with retinal hard exudate in diabetic retinopathy. Early Treatment Diabetic Retinopathy Study (ETDRS) Report 22 Arch Ophthalmol Chic Ill 1960 1996; 114(9): 84-1079.

[9] Keech AC, Mitchell P, Summanen PA, *et al.* FIELD study investigators. Effect of fenofibrate on the need for laser treatment for diabetic retinopathy (FIELD study): a randomised controlled trial. Lancet 2007; 370(9600): 1687-97.
[http://dx.doi.org/10.1016/S0140-6736(07)61607-9] [PMID: 17988728]

[10] Simó R, Roy S, Behar-Cohen F, Keech A, Mitchell P, Wong TY. Fenofibrate: a new treatment for diabetic retinopathy. Molecular mechanisms and future perspectives. Curr Med Chem 2013; 20(26): 3258-66.
[http://dx.doi.org/10.2174/0929867311320260009] [PMID: 23745548]

[11] Elman MJ, Aiello LP, Beck RW, *et al.* Diabetic Retinopathy Clinical Research Network. Randomized trial evaluating ranibizumab plus prompt or deferred laser or triamcinolone plus prompt laser for diabetic macular edema. Ophthalmology 2010; 117(6): 1064-1077.e35.
[http://dx.doi.org/10.1016/j.ophtha.2010.02.031] [PMID: 20427088]

[12] Campochiaro PA, Brown DM, Pearson A, *et al.* FAME Study Group. Sustained delivery fluocinolone acetonide vitreous inserts provide benefit for at least 3 years in patients with diabetic macular edema. Ophthalmology 2012; 119(10): 2125-32.
[http://dx.doi.org/10.1016/j.ophtha.2012.04.030] [PMID: 22727177]

[13] Boyer DS, Yoon YH, Belfort R Jr, *et al.* Ozurdex MEAD Study Group. Three-year, randomized, sham-controlled trial of dexamethasone intravitreal implant in patients with diabetic macular edema. Ophthalmology 2014; 121(10): 1904-14.
[http://dx.doi.org/10.1016/j.ophtha.2014.04.024] [PMID: 24907062]

[14] Massin P, Erginay A, Dupas B, Couturier A, Tadayoni R. Efficacy and safety of sustained-delivery fluocinolone acetonide intravitreal implant in patients with chronic diabetic macular edema insufficiently responsive to available therapies: a real-life study. Clin Ophthalmol 2016; 10: 1257-64.
[http://dx.doi.org/10.2147/OPTH.S105385] [PMID: 27468222]

[15] The DAMAD Study Group. Effect of aspirin alone and aspirin plus dipyridamole in early diabetic retinopathy. A multicenter randomized controlled clinical trial. Diabetes 1989; 38(4): 491-8.
[http://dx.doi.org/10.2337/diab.38.4.491] [PMID: 2647556]

[16] Early Treatment Diabetic Retinopathy Study Research Group. Effects of aspirin treatment on diabetic retinopathy. ETDRS report number 8. Ophthalmology 1991; 98(5) (Suppl.): 757-65.
[http://dx.doi.org/10.1016/S0161-6420(13)38010-5] [PMID: 2062511]

[17]   Friedman SM, Almukhtar TH, Baker CW, *et al.* Diabetic Retinopathy Clinical Research Network. Topical nepafenec in eyes with noncentral diabetic macular edema. Retina 2015; 35(5): 944-56.
        [http://dx.doi.org/10.1097/IAE.0000000000000403] [PMID: 25602634]

[18]   Dugel PU, Koh A, Ogura Y, *et al.* HAWK and HARRIER Study Investigators. HAWK and HARRIER: phase 3, multicenter, randomized, double-masked trials of brolucizumab for neovascular age-related macular degeneration. Ophthalmology 2020; 127(1): 72-84.
        [http://dx.doi.org/10.1016/j.ophtha.2019.04.017] [PMID: 30986442]

[19]   Regillo C. Anti-VEGF/anti-angiopoietin-2 bispecific antibody faricimab in diabetic macular edema. Retina Society 51st annual Scientific Meeting. San Francisco, CA. 2018.

[20]   Li F, Zhang L, Wang Y, *et al.* One-year outcome of conbercept therapy for diabetic macular edema. Curr Eye Res 2018; 43(2): 218-23.
        [http://dx.doi.org/10.1080/02713683.2017.1379542] [PMID: 29265939]

[21]   Boyer D. Switching to combination OPT-302 with aflibercept from prior anti-VEGF-A monotherpay in eyes with persistent diabetic macular edema. Paper resented at American Society of Retina Specialists Meeting; Seattle, WA July 24th, 2020.

[22]   Campochiaro PA, Marcus DM, Awh CC, *et al.* The port delivery system with ranibizumab for neovascular age-related macular degeneration: results from the randomized phase 2 ladder clinical trial. Ophthalmology 2019; 126(8): 1141-54.
        [http://dx.doi.org/10.1016/j.ophtha.2019.03.036] [PMID: 30946888]

[23]   Heier J, Campochiaro P, Ho A, *et al.* Results of cohorts 1-5 for the RGX-314 phase I/IIa study of gene therapy for neovascular wAMD Presented at: Retina Subspecialty Day, American Academy of Ophthalmology; October 11, 2019; San Francisco, California

[24]   Das A, McGuire PG, Rangasamy S. Diabetic macular edema: pathophysiology and novel therapeutic targets. Ophthalmology 2015; 122(7): 1375-94.
        [http://dx.doi.org/10.1016/j.ophtha.2015.03.024] [PMID: 25935789]

[25]   Haurigot V, Villacampa P, Ribera A, *et al.* Increased intraocular insulin-like growth factor-I triggers blood-retinal barrier breakdown. J Biol Chem 2009; 284(34): 22961-9.
        [http://dx.doi.org/10.1074/jbc.M109.014787] [PMID: 19473988]

[26]   Dugel P. THR-149 for the treatment of DME: results of a phase 1, open-label, dose-escalation study. Talk Presented: September 8th 2019.

[27]   Khanani AM. A Phase 1 Study of the THR-687: An Integrin Antagonist for the Treatment of Diabetic Macular Edema (DME).

[28]   Dugel P. A Phase 2 Study of OCS-01: A Potential Topical Treatment for DME. Exudation and Degeneration Conference.

[29]   Risuteganib (LUMINATE®): Potential Paradigm Shift In the Treatment of Oxidative Stress-Induced DME https://ois.net/wp content/uploads/2018/10/CompanyShowcase_Allegro.pdf

[30]   Suprachoroidal CLS-TA with Intravitreal Aflibercept vsvs Aflibercept Alone in Subject with Diabetic Macular Edema (TYBEE) https://clinicaltrials.gov/ct2/show/NCT03126786

[31]   Barber AJ. A new view of diabetic retinopathy: a neurodegenerative disease of the eye. Prog Neuropsychopharmacol Biol Psychiatry 2003; 27(2): 283-90.
        [http://dx.doi.org/10.1016/S0278-5846(03)00023-X] [PMID: 12657367]

[32]   Hernández C, Carrasco E, Casamitjana R, Deulofeu R, García-Arumí J, Simó R. Somatostatin molecular variants in the vitreous fluid: a comparative study between diabetic patients with proliferative diabetic retinopathy and nondiabetic control subjects. Diabetes Care 2005; 28(8): 1941-7.
        [http://dx.doi.org/10.2337/diacare.28.8.1941] [PMID: 16043736]

[33]   Simó R, Lecube A, Sararols L, *et al.* Deficit of somatostatin-like immunoreactivity in the vitreous fluid of diabetic patients: possible role in the development of proliferative diabetic retinopathy.

Diabetes Care 2002; 25(12): 2282-6.
[http://dx.doi.org/10.2337/diacare.25.12.2282] [PMID: 12453974]

[34]   Simó R, Carrasco E, Fonollosa A, García-Arumí J, Casamitjana R, Hernández C. Deficit of somatostatin in the vitreous fluid of patients with diabetic macular edema. Diabetes Care 2007; 30(3): 725-7.
[http://dx.doi.org/10.2337/dc06-1345] [PMID: 17327350]

[35]   Grant MB, Mames RN, Fitzgerald C, *et al.* The efficacy of octreotide in the therapy of severe nonproliferative and early proliferative diabetic retinopathy: a randomized controlled study. Diabetes Care 2000; 23(4): 504-9.
[http://dx.doi.org/10.2337/diacare.23.4.504] [PMID: 10857943]

[36]   Boehm BO, Lang GK, Jehle PM, Feldman B, Lang GE. Octreotide reduces vitreous hemorrhage and loss of visual acuity risk in patients with high-risk proliferative diabetic retinopathy. Horm Metab Res 2001; 33(5): 300-6.
[http://dx.doi.org/10.1055/s-2001-15282] [PMID: 11440277]

[37]   Trial to assess the efficacy of neuroprotective drugs administered topically to prevent or arrest diabetic retinopathy. Available from: https://clinicaltrials.gov/ct2/show/NCT01726075

[38]   The Diabetic Retinopathy Study Research Group. Photocoagulation treatment of proliferative diabetic retinopathy. Clinical application of Diabetic Retinopathy Study (DRS) findings, DRS Report Number 8. Ophthalmology 1981; 88(7): 583-600.
[PMID: 7196564]

[39]   Gross JG, Glassman AR, Liu D, *et al.* Diabetic Retinopathy Clinical Research Network. Five-year outcomes of panretinal photocoagulation *vs* intravitreous ranibizumab for proliferative diabetic retinopathy: a randomized clinical trial. JAMA Ophthalmol 2018; 136(10): 1138-48. [published correction appears in JAMA Ophthalmol. 2019 Apr 1;137(4):467].
[http://dx.doi.org/10.1001/jamaophthalmol.2018.3255] [PMID: 30043039]

[40]   Arevalo JF, Maia M, Flynn HW Jr, *et al.* Tractional retinal detachment following intravitreal bevacizumab (Avastin) in patients with severe proliferative diabetic retinopathy. Br J Ophthalmol 2008; 92(2): 213-6.
[http://dx.doi.org/10.1136/bjo.2007.127142] [PMID: 17965108]

[41]   Bressler NM, Beaulieu WT, Bressler SB, *et al.* DRCR Retina Network. Anti-vascular endothelial growth factor therapy and risk of traction retinal detachment in eyes with proliferative diabetic retinopathy: pooled analysis of five DRCR retina network randomized clinical trials. Retina 2020; 40(6): 1021-8.
[http://dx.doi.org/10.1097/IAE.0000000000002633] [PMID: 31567817]

[42]   Walter SD, Mahmoud TH. Hybrid-gauge and Mixed-gauge Microincisional Vitrectomy Surgery. Int Ophthalmol Clin 2016; 56(4): 85-95.
[http://dx.doi.org/10.1097/IIO.0000000000000141] [PMID: 27575760]

[43]   The Diabetic Retinopathy Vitrectomy Study Research Group. Early vitrectomy for severe vitreous hemorrhage in diabetic retinopathy. Two-year results of a randomized trial. Diabetic Retinopathy Vitrectomy Study report 2. Arch Ophthalmol 1985; 103(11): 1644-52.
[http://dx.doi.org/10.1001/archopht.1985.01050110038020] [PMID: 2865943]

[44]   Urias EA, Urias GA, Monickaraj F, McGuire P, Das A. Novel therapeutic targets in diabetic macular edema: Beyond VEGF. Vision Res 2017; 139: 221-7.
[http://dx.doi.org/10.1016/j.visres.2017.06.015] [PMID: 28993218]

[45]   Nguyen QD, Schachar RA, Nduaka CI, *et al.* DEGAS Clinical Study Group. Dose-ranging evaluation of intravitreal siRNA PF-04523655 for diabetic macular edema (the DEGAS study). Invest Ophthalmol Vis Sci 2012; 53(12): 7666-74.
[http://dx.doi.org/10.1167/iovs.12-9961] [PMID: 23074206]

[46]   Randomized A. A Randomized, Multi-center, Phase II Study of the Safety, Tolerability and

Bioactivity of Repeated Intravitreal Injections of iCo-007 as Monotherapy or in Combination With Ranibizumab or Laser Photocoagulation in the Treatment of Diabetic Macular Edema (the iDEAL Study) (iDEAL) https://clinicaltrials.gov/ct2/show/results/NCT01565148

[47] Berezin A. Metabolic memory phenomenon in diabetes mellitus: Achieving and perspectives. Diabetes Metab Syndr 2016; 10(2) (Suppl. 1): S176-83.
[http://dx.doi.org/10.1016/j.dsx.2016.03.016] [PMID: 27025794]

[48] Reddy MA, Zhang E, Natarajan R. Epigenetic mechanisms in diabetic complications and metabolic memory. Diabetologia 2015; 58(3): 443-55.
[http://dx.doi.org/10.1007/s00125-014-3462-y] [PMID: 25481708]

SUBJECT INDEX

A

Abducens nerve palsies 81, 84
  acquired unilateral 84
  isolated 84
Accumulation 19, 27, 109, 130, 131, 148, 150
  subretinal fluid 150
  visceral fat 27
Activity 112, 131, 186, 208
  antioxidant enzyme 131
Acute leukemia 35
Adenomas 19
  advanced 19
Adenomatous polyps 19
Adiponectin 6
Advances in laser technology 193
Aflibercept monotherapy 217
Aflibercept protein 214
Agents 22, 23, 38, 89, 137, 138, 139, 186,
    189, 190, 203, 206, 208, 220
  alkylating 138
  anti-angiogenic 203
  anticholinergic 138
  anti-inflammatory 89
  chronic immunosuppressive 38
  cycloplegic 139
  neuroprotective 203
  therapeutic 186
Aldose reductase 6, 90, 116
  inhibitors 116
  pathway 6
Altered collagen synthesis 111
American diabetes association (ADA) 22, 34,
    39, 40
AMP-activated protein kinase 22
Amphotericin 72, 73, 74
  intravenous 72, 73
Analysis, retrospective pooled 219
Ang-2 inhibitor drug 212
Angiogenesis 179, 185, 215
Angiogenic 134, 179
  growth factors 134

stimulus 179
Angiography 161
Angle 52, 133, 134, 135, 137
  aqueous fluid drainage 52
  neovascularization 52, 134, 135, 137
  iridocorneal 133, 134, 135
Anti-inflammatory treatment 27
Antioxidant therapy 27
Anti-VEGF 182, 185, 191, 193, 195, 196, 203,
    206, 207, 212, 214, 219, 220
  adjunctive 220
  adjuvant 219
Anti-VEGF agents 137, 138, 186, 188, 189,
    191, 193, 194, 196, 205, 206, 207, 215,
    217, 219
Anti-VEGF injections 183, 196, 207, 216,
    218, 219
  serial intravitreal 183
Anti-VEGF intravitreal 93, 98
  injections 93
  treatment 98
Anti-VEGF therapy 139, 182, 185, 189, 190,
    191, 192, 193, 194, 195, 196, 218
  adjunctive 139
  monthly 189, 195
Anti-VEGF treatment 91, 196
  post-operative 91
Apoptosis 19, 36, 130, 134
  cardiomyocyte 19
Aseptic technique 188
Atheroembolic disease 21
Atherosclerosis, accelerated 19, 20
ATPase 111, 112
  activity 112
  enzyme 112
Autoreactive, inhibiting 36
Autosomal recessive syndrome 85

B

Bi-hormonal 32
  systems 32

www.ingramcontent.com/pod-product-compliance
Lightning Source LLC
Chambersburg PA
CBHW050827220326
41598CB00006B/327